Diastolic Heart Failure

Otto A. Smiseth and Michał Tendera (Eds.)

Diastolic Heart Failure

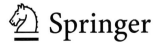

Otto A. Smiseth, MD, PhD
Professor of Medicine
Head, Heart-Lung Clinic
Department of Cardiology
Rikshospitalet
University of Oslo
Oslo, Norway

Michał Tendera, MD, PhD
Professor of Medicine
Head, 3rd Division of Cardiology
Medical University of Silesia
Katowice, Poland

British Library Cataloguing in Publication Data
Diastolic heart failure
1. Heart failure
I. Smiseth, Otto A. II. Tendera, Michał
616.1′29

Library of Congress Control Number: 2007925712

ISBN: 978-1-84628-890-6   e-ISBN: 978-1-84628-891-3

© Springer-Verlag London Limited 2008

Apart from any fair dealing for the purposes of research or private study, or criticism or review, as permitted under the Copyright, Designs and Patents Act 1988, this publication may only be reproduced, stored or transmitted, in any form or by any means, with the prior permission in writing of the publishers, or in the case of reprographic reproduction in accordance with the terms of licences issued by the Copyright Licensing Agency. Enquiries concerning reproduction outside those terms should be sent to the publishers.

The use of registered names, trademarks, etc. in this publication does not imply, even in the absence of a specific statement, that such names are exempt from the relevant laws and regulations and therefore free for general use.

Product liability: The publisher can give no guarantee for information about drug dosage and application thereof contained in this book. In every individual case the respective user must check its accuracy by consulting other pharmaceutical literature.

9 8 7 6 5 4 3 2 1

Springer Science+Business Media
springer.com

To our wives Kaja and Ewa

Preface

It is estimated that approximately 20 million people suffer from heart failure worldwide. Moreover, the prevalence of heart failure still tends to increase. A significant proportion of patients with this condition have normal left ventricular systolic function, as measured by the ejection fraction. It is believed that in these patients, heart failure is the result of diastolic dysfunction. This condition is, therefore, frequently referred to as diastolic heart failure.

While heart failure with impaired left ventricular systolic function has been extensively studied, patients with preserved systolic function have been grossly underinvestigated, and underlying mechanisms, diagnostic criteria, and definition have been controversial. More recently, however, we gained important new insights into pathophysiology and natural history of diastolic heart failure and we have a better understanding of how patients with this condition should be evaluated and managed.

This book is written to bring together in a clear and concise manner, the current knowledge about diastolic heart failure. It is written primarily for clinicians, and the aim has been to provide insights which will be useful in the daily care of heart failure patients. We also hope the book will be of interest to scientists involved in heart failure research.

The first chapters describe the essential physiology of left ventricular filling and the pathophysiology of diastolic heart failure. This includes the role of disturbances in myocardial relaxation, changes in myocardial compliance, chamber stiffness, and interactions with extraventricular structures, as well as the neurohormones. The diagnostic criteria are reviewed and we present an algorithm for a practical diagnostic work-up in patients with suspected diastolic heart failure. We explain how Doppler flow velocities in combination with tissue Doppler can be utilized to diagnose diastolic heart failure and to provide a noninvasive estimate of left ventricular filling pressure. Furthermore, we suggest how atrial natriuretic peptides may be utilized as a supplementary diagnostic tool.

Recent important data on epidemiology are presented, and challenges related to specific diseases are addressed, including hypertension, diabetes mellitus, cardiomyopathies, and pericardial disease. Finally, we review the therapeutic options and discuss different treatment strategies.

We are fortunate to have several leading experts in the field of diastolic function and diastolic heart failure as authors, and they are thanked for their valuable contributions. This book is the first to give a comprehensive overview not only of the diastolic heart failure, but also of different aspects of left ventricular diastolic function in general. The aim of the authors was to summarize the existing knowledge on the role of diastolic dysfunction in heart failure, and also to identify the gaps in our understanding of the problem. We hope that the book will prove useful for both scientists and clinicians involved in research and clinical care of patients with heart failure.

Otto A. Smiseth
Michał Tendera

Contents

Preface vii
Contributors xi

Section 1   Pathophysiology

1 Molecular Mechanisms of Diastolic Dysfunction.............. 3
   Gilles W. De Keulenaer and Dirk L. Brutsaert

2 Pathophysiologic Aspects of Myocardial Relaxation and
   End-Diastolic Stiffness of Cardiac Ventricles 21
   Thierry C. Gillebert and Adelino F. Leite-Moreira

3 Ventricular Interaction via the Septum and Pericardium....... 41
   Israel Belenkie, Eldon R. Smith, and John V. Tyberg

4 Role of the Left Atrium 53
   Sergio Macciò and Paolo Marino

5 Role of Neurohormones and Peripheral Vasculature 71
   Gretchen L. Wells and William C. Little

6 Filling Velocities as Markers of Diastolic Function 81
   Otto A. Smiseth

7 Myocardial Velocities as Markers of Diastolic Function........ 99
   Jarosław D. Kasprzak and Karina A. Wierzbowska-Drabik

8 Diastolic Versus Systolic Heart Failure 119
   Hidekatsu Fukuta and William C. Little

Section 2   Diagnosis of Diastolic Heart Failure

9 Invasive Evaluation of Diastolic Left
   Ventricular Dysfunction 137
   Loek van Heerebeek and Walter J. Paulus

10 Echocardiographic Assessment of Diastolic Function and
    Diagnosis of Diastolic Heart Failure 149
    Grace Lin and Jae K. Oh

11 Magnetic Resonance Imaging. 163
    Frank E. Rademakers and Jan Bogaert

12 Natriuretic Peptides in the Diagnosis of Diastolic
    Heart Failure 175
    Michał Tendera and Wojciech Wojakowski

13 Noninvasive Estimation of Left Ventricular
    Filling Pressures 187
    Sherif F. Nagueh

Section 3 Epidemiology, Prognosis, and Treatment

14 Epidemiology of Diastolic Heart Failure 205
    Michał Tendera and Wojciech Wojakowski

15 Prognosis in Diastolic Heart Failure 213
    Piotr Ponikowski, Ewa A. Jankowska, and Waldemar Banasiak

16 Treatment of Diastolic Heart Failure 223
    Michał Tendera and Ewa Gaszewska-Żurek

Section 4 Specific Disease-Related Problems in Diastolic Heart Failure

17 Coronary Artery Disease and Diastolic Left
    Ventricular Dysfunction 243
    Jean G.F. Bronzwaer and Walter J. Paulus

18 Hypertension and Diastolic Function. 263
    Raymond Gaillet and Otto M. Hess

19 Diastolic Disturbances in Diabetes Mellitus 271
    Thomas H. Marwick

20 Hypertrophic Cardiomyopathy 285
    Saidi A. Mohiddin and William J. McKenna

21 Constrictive Pericarditis and Restrictive Cardiomyopathy 311
    Farouk Mookadam and Jae K. Oh

22 Summary 329
    Otto A. Smiseth and Michał Tendera

Index 339

Contributors

Waldemar Banasiak, MD, PhD
Cardiology Department
Centre for Heart Disease
Military Hospital
Wroclaw, Poland

Israel Belenkie, MD, PhD
Department of Cardiac Sciences
University of Calgary
Calgary, AB, Canada

Jan Bogaert, MD, PhD
Department of Radiology
Gasthuisberg University Hospital
Leuven, Belgium

Jean G.F. Bronzwaer, MD, PhD
Department of Cardiology
VU University Medical Center
Amsterdam, The Netherlands

Dirk L. Brutsaert, MD, PhD
Cardiology Department
AZ Middelheim — University of
   Antwerp
Antwerp, Belgium

Gilles W. De Keulenaer, MD, PhD
Cardiology Department
AZ Middelheim — University of
   Antwerp
Antwerp, Belgium

Hidekatsu Fukuta, MD, PhD
Department of Internal Medicine
Cardiology Section
Wake Forest University School of Medicine
Winston-Salem, NC, USA

Raymond Gaillet, MD
Department of Cardiology
Swiss Cardiovascular Center
University Hospital
Bern, Switzerland

Ewa Gaszewska-Żurek, MD
3rd Division of Cardiology
Silesian School of Medicine
Katowice, Poland

Thierry C. Gillebert, MD, PhD
Department of Cardiovascular Diseases
University Hospital
Ghent, Belgium

Otto M. Hess, MD
Department of Cardiology
Swiss Cardiovascular Center
University Hospital
Bern, Switzerland

Ewa A. Jankowska, MD, PhD
Cardiology Department
Centre for Heart Disease
Military Hospital
Wroclaw, Poland

Section 1
Pathophysiology

1
Molecular Mechanisms of Diastolic Dysfunction

Gilles W. De Keulenaer and Dirk L. Brutsaert

Introduction

Heart failure is a clinical syndrome characterized by symptoms and signs of decreased tissue perfusion and increased tissue water. Defining the cause of this syndrome requires measurements of both systolic and diastolic functions. When abnormalities in diastolic function are predominant and abnormalities in hemodynamic pump function are absent or mild (e.g., preserved ejection fraction [EF]), this syndrome is called "diastolic heart failure" (DHF) or "heart failure with preserved ejection fraction."

Therefore, DHF can be defined as *a clinical syndrome characterized by the symptoms and signs of heart failure, a preserved EF, and diastolic dysfunction.* Importantly, as we discuss later, a preserved EF indicates that the ventricular hemodynamic pump performance is preserved, whereas systolic function of the ventricular muscular pump may already be compromised significantly. From a conceptual perspective, DHF occurs when the ventricular chamber is unable to accept an adequate volume of blood during diastole at normal diastolic pressures and at volumes sufficient to maintain an appropriate stroke volume. These abnormalities are caused by an impaired ventricular relaxation and/or an increase in ventricular stiffness and may result in higher filling pressures at rest; it more frequently produces elevated filling pressures during exercise, which results in exercise dyspnea.

In this chapter, we discuss the pathophysiologic mechanisms underlying diastolic dysfunction and failure. After describing the pathophysiology at the level of the ventricular muscular pump, we outline the molecular mechanisms underlying disturbances of ventricular relaxation and compliance. Subsequently, we address the question to what extent abnormalities of the ventricular muscular pump and molecular machinery observed in DHF are typical for DHF or whether these abnormalities are part of a more general pathophysiologic trajectory common to different forms of chronic heart failure that progresses toward end-stage hemodynamic pump failure.

Pathophysiology of Diastolic Dysfunction and Failure at the Level of the Ventricular Muscular Pump

Discussion about normal and abnormal diastolic functions of the ventricle is inevitably linked to the fact that the heart is as much a muscle as it is a pump. When evaluating the function of this muscular pump, one thus should always take into account the mechanical properties of the cardiac muscle as well as those of the cardiac pump. As further illustrated in Figure 1.1, the most important consequence of these aspects of the ventricular muscular pump, at least with respect to the analysis of cardiac diastole, is that pressure fall during isovolumic relaxation in the pump (which fully completes at end-systolic volumes) and the increase in pump volume during early rapid filling are part of the contraction–relaxation cycle of the ventricular muscular "systole."[1-3] "True" diastole of the ventricular muscular pump thus starts after early rapid ventricular filling and hence encompasses diastasis and the atrial contraction phase. At normal rest heart rates, diastole usually lasts for approximately 50% of the total duration of the cardiac cycle. By contrast, on a pressure–volume

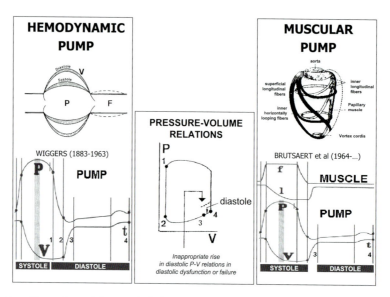

FIGURE 1.1. Subdivision of the cardiac cycle in a ventricular hemodynamic pump versus a ventricular muscular pump. (**Left**) Wiggers' traditional subdivision, with systole ending slightly prior to aortic valve closure. (**Middle**) Ventricular pressure-volume relations, illustrating upward shift at (end-) diastole in patients with diastolic dysfunction and/or diastolic failure. (**Right**) Novel insights, since the early 1960s, into the intracellular physiological and pathophysiological mechanisms of the heart as a muscular pump, which were obviously unknown in the Wiggers' era, have logically led to reconsidering the traditional Wiggers' subdivision of the cardiac cycle. The figure compares the time traces (t) of an afterloaded twitch in cardiac muscle (f, force; l, length) with the synchronized time traces of pressure (P) and volume (V) of a ventricular hemodynamic pump. The similarity between the corresponding time traces has led to the inclusion of isovolumic relaxation into systole of a ventricular muscular pump. Although the rapid filling phase should, on the same conceptual grounds, also be seen as part of systole, we prefer — because of a number of (non-muscular) hemodynamic, i.e. mostly flow-related variables — to consider this phase rather as a transition between systole and diastole. This subtle modification to our previous reappraisal of the cardiac cycle emphasizes that during early rapid filling, the properties of a pump may indeed diverge somewhat from those of a muscle.

(PV) diagram, diastole represents only the last 5%–15% ventricular filling (points 3 to 4 in Figure 1.1).[1,2]

Consistent with the above definition, DHF then refers to a disease process that shifts the *end portion* of the PV diagram inappropriately upward so that left ventricular (LV) filling pressures are increased disproportionately to the magnitude of LV dilatation. The causes of such a shift can be subdivided into the following:

1. Inappropriate tachycardia (e.g., transient atrial fibrillation, supraventricular tachyarrhythmias) resulting in inappropriate abbreviation of diastolic duration
2. A decrease in ventricular diastolic compliance
3. Impairment in ventricular systolic relaxation, that is, impaired isovolumic pressure fall (and/or impaired early rapid filling)
4. A combination of 1, 2, and 3, as is usually the case

By extension, it follows that impaired ventricular relaxation — as it is the last part of the systole of the muscular pump — should not be called "diastolic dysfunction." Instead, it should be retained as an early and isolated manifestation of systolic dysfunction. Nevertheless, impaired ventricular relaxation can in many conditions itself be the cause of an upward shift of the end portion of the PV diagram and therefore lead to DHF.

Obviously, in daily clinical practice, it is not trivial to diagnose at the patient's bedside whether impaired ventricular relaxation (e.g., recorded during an echo Doppler study by virtue of a prolonged isovolumic relaxation time and/or reversed early-diastolic velocity [E]/atrial-induced [A] velocity relationship) does or does not cause such an upward shift of the end portion of the PV diagram, even not when simplifying the problem by only considering the patient at rest. Fortunately, there is emerging evidence that additional diagnostic efforts, for example, by applying tissue

1. Diastolic Dysfunction

Doppler or by assessing serum brain natriuretic peptide (BNP) or the N-terminal prohormone BNP (NT-pro-BNP), may help to distinguish between the different clinical conditions.

Molecular Mechanisms of Impaired Ventricular Relaxation and Decreased Ventricular Compliance

Diastolic dysfunction of the heart can be secondary to impaired ventricular systolic relaxation (in fact a process of systole but at the same time a possible cause of DHF when disturbed; see earlier discussion) and by decreased diastolic compliance (defined by the PV relationship), resulting in exaggerated ventricular tension during filling of the ventricular cavity. Causes of impaired relaxation and/or compliance (Table 1.1) can be divided into the following:

1. Factors intrinsic to the cardiomyocyte
2. Factors within the extracellular matrix (ECM) that surrounds the cardiomyocytes
3. Factors that activate the production of neurohormones and paracrine substances

To varying extents, these factors play a role in DHF, but much remains to be learned about how these factors interplay and to what extent therapeutic targeting would result in prognostic or symptomatic improvements. For diastolic dysfunction of the left ventricle caused by extraventricular constraint (by pericardium or right ventricle) the interested reader is referred to Chapter 3.

Cardiomyocyte

Elements and processes intrinsic to the cardiomyocyte contributing to diastolic (dys)function are summarized in Table 1.1 and Figure 1.2. In general, they relate to processes responsible for calcium removal from the myocyte cytosol (calcium homeostasis), to processes involved in cross-bridge detachment, and to cytoskeletal functional elements. Changes in any of the processes and elements can lead to abnormalities in both active relaxation and passive stiffness.

Calcium Homeostasis

Calcium released from the sarcoplasmic reticulum (SR) through the SR calcium release channel (RyR) is removed from the cardiomyocyte cytosol as an important component of active relaxation. This removal depends on the reuptake of calcium into the SR by a calcium pump known as SERCA2, a process that is highly regulated in the normal heart, and on the extrusion of calcium in the extracellular fluid by the combined activity of the sarcolemmal sodium–calcium exchanger and the

TABLE 1.1. Causes leading to diastolic heart failure.

Inappropriate tachycardia	Impaired systolic relaxation	Decreased compliance
Intermittent atrial fibrillation or atrial tachyarrhythmias	➢ **Load-induced** ■ Pressure-volume overload ➢ **Impaired inactivation processes** ■ Calcium homeostasis ∨ calcium overload ∨ calcium transport (sarcolemma, SR) ∨ modifying proteins (phospholamban, calmodulin, . . .) ■ Myofilaments ∨ Tn-C calcium binding ∨ Tn-I phosphorylation ∨ myofilament calcium sensitivity ■ Energetics ∨ ADP/ATP ratio ∨ ADP and Pi concentration ➢ **Non-uniformity of load or inactivation processes in space or time** ■ E.g., "asynchrony" by conduction disturbances ➢ **Abnormal activity of RAAS, OS, ANP/BNP, cardiac endothelial system**	➢ **Extracellular matrix** ■ Fibrillar collagen ■ Basement membrane proteins ■ Proteoglycans ■ MMP/TIMP ➢ **Abnormal activity of cardiac endothelial system (especially NO)** ➢ **Cytoskeletal abnormalities** ■ Microtubules ■ Intermediates filaments (desmin) ■ Titin ■ Nebulin

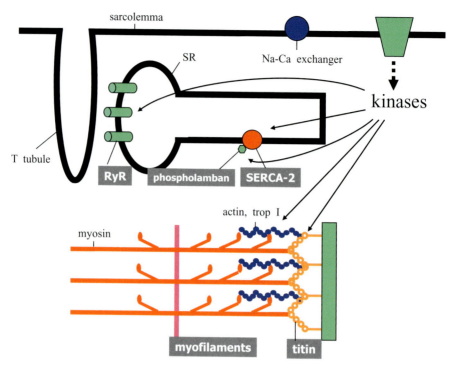

FIGURE 1.2. Diastolic dysfunction is induced by molecular changes at different molecular levels of contraction and relaxation. Abnormal relaxation and stiffness can be caused by modifications of contractile filaments (thick and thin filaments), the linkage protein titin, and disturbed calcium homeostasis. Discovered modifications include gene mutations, changes in gene expression, isoform switching, and changed phosphorylation ratios by kinases that are activated by receptor-ligand binding. At the level of calcium homeostasis, abnormalities of sarcoplasmic reticulum (SR) calcium release through the hyperphosphorylated ryanodine-sensitive calcium release channel (RyR) and abnormalities of calcium reuptake proteins (SERCA2, phospholamban, and sodium–calcium [Na-Ca] exchanger) have been described. Modulatory effects of diastolic function by receptor-induced kinases are indicated.

sarcolemmal calcium pump, with the latter pump playing a minor role.

Abnormal activity of SERCA2 has been implicated in the impaired relaxation in heart failure. The SERCA2 activity declines in LV hypertrophy and heart failure by reduced gene and protein expression and by reduced phosphorylation of its inhibitory modulatory protein phospholamban.[4–7] Conversely, experimental gene transfer with SERCA2a or a negative phospholamban mutant improves relaxation.[8,9] Despite these observations, however, it is as yet unclear at which stages of chronic heart failure SERCA2 activity becomes affected, as variable observations have been made depending on the type of heart failure and on the applied experimental methodology.[10,11] By all means, impaired SERCA2 activity is certainly not specific for DHF, as it will become more pronounced when global pump performance is reduced.[4]

Apart from an insufficient removal of calcium from the cytosol, leakage of calcium from the SR through RyR during the inactivation phase of the cardiac cycle ("diastolic calcium sparks") may cause impaired relaxation and increased stiffness, but to what extent this really occurs in heart failure and may be linked to the reported protein kinase A–induced hyperphosphorylation of RyR are still controversial.[12,13]

Cross-Bridge Detachments

Impaired relaxation and increased stiffness may also result from slow or incomplete cross-bridge detachment. In heart failure, abnormal cross-bridge detachment may result from reduced phosphorylation of troponin I, which increases calcium sensitivity of the myofibrils to calcium. Importantly, reduced phosphorylation of troponin I has been observed in end-stage human heart failure[14] at a stage of severely impaired pump performance but not yet at stages of preserved global pump performance.[15] Nevertheless, deficient cyclic guanosine monophosphate–mediated phosphorylation of troponin I due to reduced availability of nitric oxide is a potential mechanism of impaired relaxation and increased stiffness at earlier stages of heart failure and ventricular hypertrophy.[16]

Relaxation may also be impaired by alterations in the thick myofilaments. Severe relaxation abnormalities have indeed been observed in experimental mutations of the myosin heavy chain that affect its binding to actin[17] even at stages prior to ventricular hypertrophy and myofibrillar disarray. Whether such changes in the thick myofilaments also contribute to the development of relaxation disturbances during the progression of heart failure is, however, still unknown.

Obviously, cross-bridge detachment can be disturbed, in addition to impaired inactivation, by perturbations in loading. In heart failure, both at preserved and reduced EF, ventricular load is usually enhanced both before contraction (preload) and during relaxation. Enhanced preload delays onset and rate of relaxation, an effect that may become particularly relevant during β-adrenergic stimulation as the lusitropic effects of adrenergic stimulation in tachycardia may be blocked.[18,19] Also during relaxation, ventricular load is enhanced in heart failure because of enhanced afterload. Effects of loading on the timing and rate of relaxation are complex and dependent on the timing of load.[3,20] The importance of inappropriate loading has, however, been reemphasized in recent studies demonstrating abnormal ventricular–arterial interaction due to a disproportionate cardiovascular stiffening in patients with DHF. Stiffening-induced imbalances of the ventricular–arterial load may exacerbate systemic afterload, that is, arterial impedance and reflected waves, and hence affect onset and rate of LV relaxation.[1,21]

Cytoskeletal Abnormalities

Proteins within the sarcomere, other than the myofibrils that generate active force, contribute substantially to the stiffness of the cardiac muscle over the normal range of the sarcomere length (<2.2 μm). These molecules include titin, tubulin,

and desmin, but most of the elastic force of the sarcomere is now thought to reside in titin.[22] Interestingly, titin is the subject of intense regulation, including isoform switching, calcium binding, and phosphorylation, indicating that myocardial resting tension can be dynamically regulated.

The two titin isoforms (N2B and N2BA) differ substantially in length and stiffness, with the N2B isoform being small and stiff. The distribution of these isoforms differs among species, heart chambers, and disease states and seems to track the corresponding variations in diastolic muscle stiffness.[23] With respect to the development of heart failure, increased expression of the stiffer N2B isoform has been demonstrated in tachycardia-induced cardiomyopathy in dogs[24] and in spontaneously hypertensive rats along with increased diastolic muscle stiffness,[25] whereas N2BA was more apparent in end-stage human ischemic cardiomyopathy.[26]

Despite the rapid accumulation of these convincing observations, many questions about the relation between titin and diastolic function remain unanswered. These questions relate to the mechanisms of isoform switching, the relevance for human disease, and the importance of other modifications of titin besides isoform switching. For example, recent observations indicate that phosphorylation of titin may reverse the increased stiffness of cardiomyocytes in DHF.[15,27] Importantly, titin isoform switching seems to be coordinated somehow with the development of interstitial myocardial fibrosis, but the temporal relation between both processes may differ among species and types of disease and may be affected by therapeutic interventions.[23] This observation should caution against premature conclusions about the specific role for either titin or the ECM in any measured change in diastolic distensibility if data on both components are not available together.

Extracellular Matrix

Changes in the structures within the ECM can also affect diastolic function (see Figure 1.2). The myocardial ECM is composed of three important constituents: (1) fibrillar protein, such as collagen types I and III and elastin; (2) proteoglycans; and (3) basement membrane proteins such as collagen

The CARDIAC ENDOTHELIUM modulates onset and rate of LV relaxation, and LV distensibility

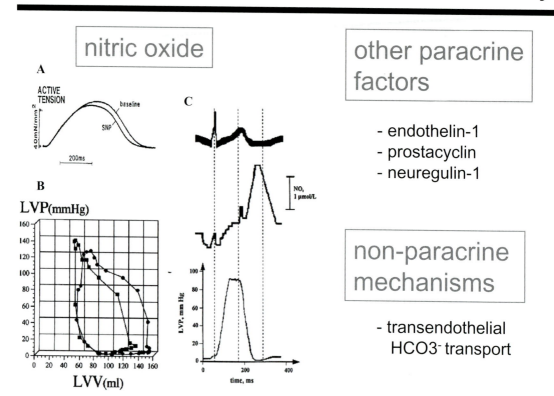

FIGURE 1.3. The cardiac endothelium modulates onset and rate of left ventricular relaxation and left ventricular distensibility.[53] (A) Acute effect of the nitric oxide synthase activating effects of sodium nitroprusside on isometric twitch performance of isolated cat papillary muscle. Relaxation hastening effects are mediated by nitric oxide released from the cardiac endothelium. (Modified with permission from Mohan et al.[83]) (B) Intracoronary, but not intraatrial, infusion of substance P increases diastolic distensibility of the ventricle in the human heart as manifested by the rightward shift of the diastolic pressure–volume relation. LVP, left ventricular pressure; LVV, left ventricular volume. (Modified with permission from Paulus et al.[34]) (C) The beating heart, in the absence of endothelial dysfunction, exhibits cyclic changes of nitric oxide concentration that peak during relaxation and diastasis. Changes in preload are tracked by parallel changes of nitric oxide release, demonstrating an autoregulatory mechanism of load-dependent control of relaxation. The illustrated nitric oxide–mediated autoregulatory control of the cardiac endothelium on relaxation and ventricular distensibility of the heart may explain diastolic dysfunction in the aging, diabetic, or hypertensive heart. Apart from nitric oxide, endothelin-1, prostacyclin, and neuregulin-1, released from the cardiac endothelium, affect myocardial performance, usually by affecting onset and rate of relaxation and distensibility.[53,84–87] In addition, transendothelial ion fluxes, at least in the endocardium, regulate intracellular pH and mechanical performance of adjacent cardiomyocytes.[53,88]

type IV, laminin, and fibronectin. It has been hypothesized that the most important components within the ECM that contribute to the development of diastolic dysfunction are fibrillar collagen (amount, geometry, distribution, especially as perimysial fibers), degree of cross-linking, and ratio of collagen type I to III.[28–30] Collagen synthesis is altered by load, both preload and afterload, by neurohormonal activation (e.g., the renin-angiotensin-aldosterone system and the sympathetic nervous systems), and by growth factors. Collagen degradation is under the control of proteolytic enzymes, including matrix metalloproteinases. Any change in the regulatory processes affecting collagen degradation and synthesis can thus alter diastolic function.

1. Diastolic Dysfunction

Several studies have made correlations between modifications of the collagen network and diastolic muscle stiffness but usually with rather extreme collagen modifications only.[30–32] A direct linkage between fibrosis and stiffness is thus still controversial, especially because in some other studies correlations between the amount of fibrosis and muscle stiffness were lacking. Hence, whether these inconsistencies point toward a role for the posttranslational structure of collagen rather than the amount of collagen or instead indicate that titin plays a more important role than ECM in general is still the subject of debate.[33]

Neurohormonal and Cardiac Endothelial Activation

Both acutely and chronically, neurohormonal and cardiac endothelial activation and/or inhibition have been shown to alter diastolic function. Chronic activation of the renin-angiotensin-aldosterone system has been shown to increase ECM fibrillar collagen. Inhibition of the renin-angiotensin-aldosterone system prevents or reverses this increase. Generally, but not consistently, these changes have been shown to affect myocardial stiffness. Acute activation of the cardiac endothelial system has been shown to alter relaxation and stiffness (Figure 1.3).[34] These acute changes in endothelial function induce rapid responses too fast to involve the ECM; therefore, the cardiac endothelium seems to act on the cardiomyocyte directly and to affect one or more cellular determinants of diastolic function within a very short time frame.[1,53] For example, in the heart there is cyclical release of nitric oxide that is mostly subendocardial and that peaks at the time of relaxation and filling. These brief bursts of nitric oxide release provide a beat-to-beat modulation of relaxation and stiffness.[35,36]

Is Diastolic Heart Failure a Distinct Disease Entity?

From the other chapters in this book it will be seen that in a muscular pump approach to cardiac performance, systole and diastole are strongly related and that relaxation disturbances, although part of the muscular systolic contraction–relaxation cycle, can be responsible for diastolic failure. In addition, when looking at the (sub)cellular and the molecular mechanisms, there is no indication that the disturbances of cardiomyocytes or ECM observed in heart failure are typical for either DHF or hemodynamic pump heart failure, suggesting that both disease presentations may be more closely related than previously anticipated.

Consistent with these observations, recent studies on the mechanical ventricular properties in patients diagnosed with DHF have revealed abnormalities of LV systolic function. For example, performance of longitudinal myocardial fibers has been measured by long axis M-mode echo or tissue Doppler imaging in patients with heart failure and preserved EF. These measurements revealed depressed contractile performance in patients with DHF and in patients with asymptomatic diastolic dysfunction despite a preserved EF (Figure 1.4).[3,37] Hence, the conjecture that DHF is a distinct disease in which systolic myocardial function is preserved seems at least inaccurate. Diastolic heart failure should, instead, be regarded as a variant form of systolic heart failure (SHF) but one in which symptoms and signs develop prematurely.[38–46]

Perhaps this novel view may, at first glance, appear contradictory with previous studies on ventricular performance in DHF. In these studies[47] parameters of global systolic performance of the LV (stroke work, preload recruitable stroke work, EF, systolic stress-shortening relationship, end-systolic PV relationship, and peak +dP/dt) in patients with DHF were not different from control patients. Importantly, however, it should be kept in mind that these parameters of ventricular performance merely reflect the function of the heart as a *hemodynamic pump* as historically proposed by Wiggers,[48] Rushmer,[49] and Sarnoff.[50] From the observations by Abbott and Mommaerts[51] and Sonnenblick,[52] it became clear, however, that any evaluation of cardiac performance ought to include,[1] in addition, some properties of cardiac muscle.

From the perception of a traditional hemodynamic pump, preservation of peripheral perfusion pressure, stroke volume, and cardiac output (blood flow) — as well as all related or derived

IN DIASTOLIC HEART FAILURE
longitudinal myocardial systolic function is impaired despite normal LVEF

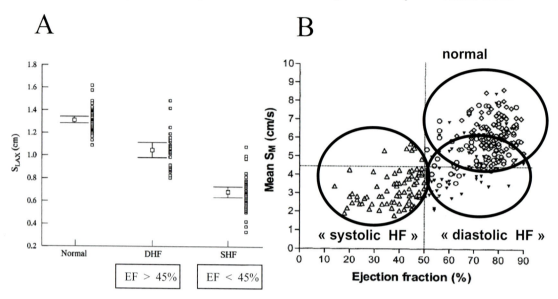

FIGURE 1.4. Heart failure (HF) with preserved ejection fraction (EF) is commonly accompanied by various degrees of systolic dysfunction. (A) Systolic/mitral annular amplitude by long axis M-mode echocardiography (S_{LAX}) reveals a significant decrease in systolic function in diastolic heart failure despite preserved ejection fraction (EF >45%). (Modified with permission from Yip et al.[39]) (B) Mean regional myocardial sustained systolic velocity (mean S_M) from a six-basal segmental model by tissue Doppler image has been plotted as a function of ejection fraction in four groups of patients: controls (open circles), diastolic dysfunction (open diamonds), diastolic heart failure (closed triangles), and systolic heart failure (open triangles). Importantly, in the lower right quadrant of this scatter plot, mean S_M has already significantly decreased in about 50% and 15% of patients with diastolic heart failure and diastolic dysfunction, respectively, despite a preserved ejection fraction >50%. (Reprinted with permission from Bruch et al.[40])

parameters such as stroke work, PV and stress-shortening relations, and +dP/dt — is of key importance. In normal conditions, the higher the end-diastolic volume, the higher the stroke volume, the ratio of stroke volume to end-diastolic volume being calculated as the *EF*, which remains constant. Under stress (e.g., after an acute myocardial infarction), the heart is able to maintain stroke volume, as well as peripheral flow and perfusion pressure, hence *hemodynamic pump* performance, constant for some time, but only at the expense of an inappropriately increased end-diastolic volume with concomitant ventricular remodeling. The ensuing progressive decline in calculated EF must, therefore, be seen as an early sensitive sign of this inappropriately increased end-diastolic volume and remodeling, hence of hemodynamic pump failure.

Regional and temporal contractile properties of ventricular cardiac muscle are, however, most often impaired at a much earlier stage. Hence, consistent with recent echo-Doppler analysis,[38-46] particularly in hearts with concentric hypertrophy that are hampered somehow to increase their end-diastolic volume, substantial *systolic dysfunction* of the *ventricular muscular pump* may be present already when mean overall hemodynamic pump performance, including its most sensitive mechanical index EF, is still well *preserved*. In addition to myocardial temporal and regional nonuniformities, this early stage of systolic dysfunction of the ventricular muscular pump is also characterized by significant LV relaxation abnormalities in time of onset and rate of ventricular relaxation. Importantly, in a muscular, unlike a hemodynamic, pump, ventricular relaxation should be regarded as an intrinsic part of systole.[1,2] Moreover, as the hemodynamic pump index EF is *blind* for such early changes in cardiac muscular pump performance,[1] it is too insensitive, hence inappropriate, to characterize a group of patients with symptoms of heart failure resulting from such abnormalities, that is, DHF, as being distinct from other patients with chronic heart failure.

Accordingly, from reviewing (1) the definitions of diastolic dysfunction and failure, (2) the molecular mechanisms of diastolic dysfunction, (3) the significant systolic abnormalities of the muscular properties of the left ventricle in DHF during both contraction and relaxation, and (4) that a preserved left ventricular ejection fraction (LVEF) merely indicates that overall cardiac performance as a hemodynamic pump is adequately compensated despite substantial systolic dysfunction of the muscular pump, we conclude that chronic heart failure must progress along a single pathophysiologic trajectory common to both DHF and SHF. How then does this conjecture fit within the current pathophysiologic paradigms of chronic heart failure?

Diastolic Heart Failure and Alternative Paradigms of Chronic Heart Failure

In a traditional conceptual view of the pathophysiology of chronic heart failure, cardiac function is regarded as evolving within a vicious circle of (de)compensatory mechanisms, gradually and irreversibly spiraling down until end-stage pump failure or until death ensues prematurely. This pathophysiologic model is most suitable to illustrate the complementary contribution of the underlying systemic (mal)adaptive reactions, that is, hemodynamic overload, neurohormonal activation, enhanced proinflammatory cytokine activity, and endothelial dysfunction.[53] A disadvantage of this model is, however, that it lacks a time dimension, thereby neglecting the time-dependent evolution of symptom severity. In clinical practice, the symptoms in many patients, especially those with DHF, evolve clearly out of phase with the pathophysiologic progression of overall pump dysfunction. As this important

paradox of chronic heart failure remains unappreciated, DHF does not seem to fit within the above traditional paradigm of chronic heart failure. In the following paragraphs we will, therefore, review two alternative paradigms of chronic heart failure and investigate how their pathophysiologies relate to DHF.

A Time-Dependent Progression Model of Chronic Heart Failure

In a time-dependent model of chronic heart failure, depicted in Figure 1.5 as a time trajectory of cardiac pump performance, the progression of chronic heart failure can be subdivided in three consecutive pathophysiologic stages. Under stress, the heart recruits various compensatory autoregulatory mechanisms. A fundamental feature of this first and very early "systolic activation" or reversible prediseae stage is the capacity of the heart to delay the onset of ventricular relaxation. This often ignored or underestimated feature allows the ventricle to modulate systolic time duration during which a given amount of stroke work is delivered.[1–3] In a second stage ("systolic dysfunction"), as commonly observed during the initial phases of myocardial hypertrophy and ischemia, the above autoregulatory mechanisms become maladaptive. Typically, ventricular relaxation either regionally or globally becomes abnormally slow and impaired with a progressive loss of the ventricle to modulate the timing of onset of relaxation. It can be commonly detected as an abnormal mitral inflow signal during Doppler echocardiography (E/A inversion). Impaired relaxation is caused by three major processes, including (1) dysfunction of intracellular myocardial inactivation processes; (2) inappropriate loading, including those induced by arterial elastance abnormalities inducing an abnormal ventricular–arterial interaction that may exacerbate effects of enhanced systemic afterload[21]; and (3) excessive nonuniformity.[2,3] During this second "systolic dysfunction" stage, hemodynamic pump performance, as reflected by the EF (>50%) is well preserved.

Finally, during a third stage ("hemodynamic pump failure"), deteriorating hemodynamic pump performance may reach a critical threshold

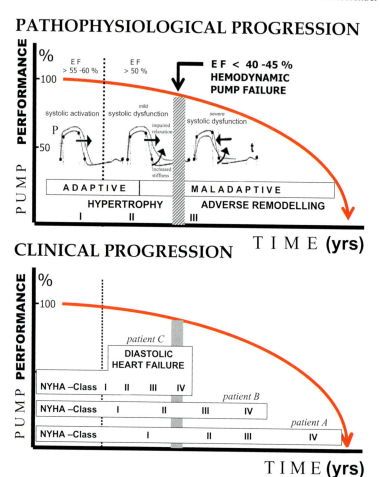

FIGURE 1.5. Time progression paradigm of chronic heart failure. The pathophysiologic as well as the clinical progression of chronic heart failure can be understood only by studying overall pump performance of the heart as a trajectory in the "time" domain. **(Top)** Pathophysiologic progression. Deterioration of pump performance during the progression of chronic heart failure typically evolves in successive stages, the contribution and duration of which may vary from patient to patient. A first stage is a reversible, compensatory stage during which systolic function is activated. Subsequently, the adaptive compensatory mechanisms become maladaptive leading to some degree of maladaptation, that is, impaired left ventricular relaxation as well as systolic dysfunction of the longitudinal myocardial components. On transition from the systolic activation to the systolic dysfunction stage, ejection fraction (EF) as a measure of overall pump performance will hardly decline and remain above 50% (i.e., preserved ejection fraction). Below an ejection fraction of 45%–50%, systolic function and pump performance are severely compromised and evolve toward full-blown — mostly a combination of systolic and diastolic — pump failure. P, pressure. **(Bottom)** Clinical progression. This diagram illustrates the paradox between the pathophysiologic progression as depicted by a single time trajectory and its divergence from the concomitant clinical time progression (New York Heart Association [NYHA] classification). The variable progression of clinical signs and symptoms in different patients (e.g., patients A, B, and C) has led to misinterpretations concerning "diastolic heart failure" or "heart failure with preserved ejection fraction" as a separate disease entity.

as evident from an EF below 40%–45% with severe systolic and diastolic abnormalities. Meanwhile, hypertrophy of the ventricle irreversibly evolves into so-called adverse remodeling. Adverse remodeling is still an ill-defined term indicating the presence of a number of structural and functional abnormalities that may result in myocardial fibrosis/necrosis and irreversible dilatation.

An advantage of this model is that the time progression of the clinical symptoms of chronic heart failure can be superimposed on the time trajectory of the above pathophysiologic progression. In chronic heart failure, it is silently assumed

1. Diastolic Dysfunction

that the severity of clinical symptoms develops uniformly in all patients and synchronously with the severity of pump failure, in which New York Heart Association (NYHA) class IV symptoms occur at EFs below 20% (e.g., patient A in Figure 1.5, bottom). The latter presentation does not, however, comply with daily clinical practice and with the observation that LVEF poorly correlates with exercise tolerance. Indeed, a large proportion of heart failure patients in NYHA classes III and IV may already be diagnosed clinically at an earlier pathophysiologic stage of pump failure, that is, with EFs clearly above 30%–40% (e.g., patient B in Figure 1.5, bottom) or even above 45%–50%, indicating that overall pump performance is preserved. Importantly, as indicated earlier, in the latter patients systolic abnormalities, including significant myocardial contraction–relaxation nonuniformities and impaired relaxation can be detected (e.g., patient C in Figure 1.5, bottom). The latter group corresponds to patients with so-called DHF and are sometimes denoted, erroneously, as having heart failure with preserved systolic function.

Accordingly, superimposing symptom progression and pathophysiologic progression in a time-progression model of chronic heart failure allows us to incorporate DHF and SHF within one and the same pathophysiologic time trajectory in which the two types of heart failure differ only in the onset of their clinical manifestation but not in the presence or absence of systolic abnormalities.

A Phenotype Model of Chronic Heart Failure

In the phenotype model shown in Figure 1.6 (top), chronic heart failure is, again, presented as one disease but with multiple patient-specific diverging *phenotypical trajectories*. Each patient follows his or her own distinct individual time trajectory of progressively deteriorating pump performance, the trajectory depending on a number of *disease modifiers*. In a large group of heart failure patients, a wide spectrum of different phenotypes can thus be identified, with two extreme presentations at each end of the spectrum. At the far left, patients suffer from primary diastolic dysfunction; at end stage these patients have nondilated ventricles, normal or high EF, high filling pressures, and

NYHA class IV symptoms but no signs of even mild global or regional systolic dysfunction, a disease that is probably nonexistent. At the far right, patients develop NYHA class IV symptoms at a stage when diastolic function is normal and only contractile dysfunction is apparent, a disease that is also nonexistent. In this regard, an important recent study by Yotti et al.[54] suggests that in patients with dilated cardiomyopathy, ventricular dilatation itself impairs diastolic filling by enhancing convective deceleration; along with slowed relaxation, reduced elastic recoil, and displacement onto the stiff portion of the LV end-diastolic pressure–LV end-diastolic volume relation, increased convective deceleration may thus also contribute to the substantial diastolic dysfunction observed in these patients.[55]

Accordingly, most if not all cases of heart failure (e.g., patients A, B, and C in Figure 1.5), are *hybrids within this spectrum* with combined systolic and diastolic abnormalities and with symptoms developing at normal, slightly reduced, moderately reduced, or severely reduced LVEF, the latter being an index of global hemodynamic pump performance rather than of systolic function. The direction of the patient's trajectory toward a heart failure phenotype with either preserved or reduced EF depends on a number of disease modifiers in which genetic, molecular, environmental, and phenotypic factors may interact.[56,57]

Comparing the *clinical characteristics* of heart failure patients with either preserved or reduced EF can easily identify a number of important modifier candidates. In Figure 1.6 (bottom), for example, gender and incidences of hypertension and of diabetes have been compared for three different groups of heart failure patients, those with normal (>50%), slightly reduced (>40%) or markedly impaired (<40%) EFs, respectively.[58–60] Strikingly, female gender, diabetes, and hypertension were much more common in the first group than in the last group and at intermediate incidence in the second group. Based on these observations, it is attractive to speculate that in each individual patient a *set of disease modifiers* (which probably also include age, myocardial hypertrophy, physical fitness, cholesterol levels, etc.) will influence the phenotypic trajectory of heart failure. In other words, after a cardiac insult, disease modifiers may, independent of whether they affect the on Ca^{2+} transport and mechanics in compensated pressure-overload hypertrophy and congestive heart failure. Circ Res 1995;77:759–764.

12. Ginsburg KS, Bers DM. Modulation of excitation-contraction coupling by isoproterenol in cardiomyocytes with controlled SR Ca load and ICa trigger. J Physiol 2004;556:463–480.

13. Li Y, Kranias EG, Mignery GA, Bers DM. Protein kinase A phosphorylation of the ryanodine receptor does not affect calcium sparks in mouse ventricular myocytes. Circ Res 2002;90:309–316.

14. Bodor S, Oakeley AE, Allen PD. Troponin I phosphorylation in the normal and failing adult human heart. Circulation 1997;96:1495–1500.

15. Borbely A, van der Velden J, Papp Z, Bronzwaer JG, Edes I, Stienen GJ, Paulus WJ. Cardiomyocyte stiffness in diastolic heart failure. Circulation 2005;111: 774–781.

16. Bronzwaer JG, Paulus WJ. Matrix, cytoskeleton, or myofilaments: which one to blame for diastolic left ventricular dysfunction? Prog Cardiovasc Dis 2005; 47:276–284.

17. Geisterfer-Lowrance AA, Christe M, Conner DA, Ingwall JS, Schoen FJ, Seidman CE, Seidman JG. A mouse model of familial hypertrophic cardiomyopathy. Science 1996;272:731–734.

18. Paulus WJ, Bronzwaer JG, Felice H, Kishan N, Wellens F. Deficient acceleration of left ventricular relaxation during exercise after heart transplantation [abstr]. Circulation 1992;86:1175–1185.

19. Vantrimpont PJ, Felice H, Paulus WJ. Does dobutamine prevent the rise in left ventricular filling pressures observed during exercise after heart transplantation? Eur Heart. 1995;16:1300–1306a.

20. Hori M, Inoue M, Kitakaze M, Tsujioka K, Ishida Y, Fukunami M, Nakajima S, Kitabatake A, Abe H. Loading sequence is a major determinant of afterload-dependent relaxation in intact canine heart. Am J Physiol 1985;249:H747–H754.

21. Kawaguchi M, Hay I, Fetics B, Kass DA. Combined ventricular systolic and arterial stiffening in patients with heart failure and preserved ejection fraction: implications for systolic and diastolic reserve limitations. Circulation 2003;107:714–720.

22. Granzier HL, Irving TC. Passive tension in cardiac muscle: contribution of collagen, titin, microtubules and intermediate filaments. Biophys J 1995; 68:1027–1044.

23. Wu Y, Cazorla O, Labeit D, et al. Changes in titin and collagen underlie diastolic stiffness diversity of cardiac muscle. J Mol Cell Cardiol 2000;32:2151–2162.

24. Wu Y, Bell SP, Trombitas K, et al. Changes in titin isoform expression in pacing-induced cardiac failure give rise to increased passive muscle stiffness. Circulation 2002;106:1384–1389.

25. Yamamoto K, Masuyama T, Sakata Y, et al. Myocardial stiffness is determined by ventricular fibrosis but not by compensatory or excessive hypertrophy in hypertensive heart. Cardiovasc Res 2002;55:76–82.

26. Neagoe C, Kulke M, del Monte F, et al. Titin isoform switch in ischemic human heart. Circulation 2002; 106:1333–1341.

27. Yamasaki R, Wu Y, McNabb M, et al. Protein kinase A phosphorylates titin's cardiac-specific N2B domain and reduces passive tension in rat cardiac myocytes. Circ Res 2002;90:1181–1188.

28. Jalil JE, Doering CW, Janicki JS, Pick R, Shroff SG, Weber KT. Fibrillar collagen and myocardial stiffness in the intact hypertrophied rat left ventricle. Circ Res 1989;64:1041–1050.

29. Weber KT, Janicki JS, Pick R, Capasso J, Anversa P. Myocardial fibrosis and pathologic hypertrophy in the rat with renovascular hypertension. Am J Cardiol 1990;65:1G–7G.

30. Kato S, Spinale FG, Tanaka R, Johnson W, Cooper G 4th, Zile MR. Inhibition of collagen cross-linking: effects on fibrillar collagen and ventricular diastolic function. Am J Physiol 1995;269:H863–H868.

31. Stroud JD, Baicu CF, Barnes MA, Spinale FG, Zile MR. Viscoelastic properties of pressure overload hypertrophied myocardium: effect of serine protease treatment. Am J Physiol Heart Circ Physiol 2002;282:H2324–H2335.

32. Brower GL, Janicki JS. Contribution of ventricular remodeling to pathogenesis of heart failure in rats. Am J Physiol Heart Circ Physiol 2001;280:H674–H683.

33. Kass DA, Bronzwaer JG, Paulus WJ. What mechanisms underlie diastolic dysfunction in heart failure? Circ Res 2004;94:1533–1542.

34. Paulus WJ, Vantrimpont PJ, Shah AM. Paracrine coronary endothelial control of left ventricular function in humans. Circulation. 1995;92:2119–2126.

35. Pinsky DJ, Patton S, Mesaros S, Brovkovych V, Kubaszewski E, Grunfeld S, Malinski T. Mechanical transduction of nitric oxide synthesis in the beating heart. Circ Res 1997;81:372–379.

36. Paulus WJ. Beneficial effects of nitric oxide on cardiac diastolic function: "the flip side of the coin." Heart Fail Rev 2000;5:337–344.

37. Zile MR, Brutsaert DL. New concepts in diastolic dysfunction and diastolic heart failure. Part II: causal mechanisms and treatment. Circulation 2002;105:1503–1508.

38. Yu CM, Lin H, Yang H, Kong SL, Zhang Q, Lee SW. Progression of systolic abnormalities in patients with "isolated" diastolic heart failure and diastolic dysfunction. Circulation 2002;105:1195–1201.

39. Yip G, Wang M, Zhang Y, Fung JW, Ho PY, Sanderson JE. Left ventricular long axis function in diastolic heart failure is reduced in both diastole and systole: time for a redefinition? Heart 2002;87:121–125.

40. Bruch C, Gradaus R, Gunia S, Breithardt G, Wichter T. Doppler tissue analysis of mitral annular velocities: evidence for systolic abnormalities in patients with diastolic heart failure. J Am Soc Echocardiogr 2003;16:1031–1036.

41. Sanderson JE. Diastolic heart failure: fact or fiction? Heart 2003;89:1281–1282.

42. Petrie MC, Caruana L, Berry C, McMurray JJ. "Diastolic heart failure" or heart failure caused by subtle left ventricular systolic dysfunction? Heart 2002;87:29–31.

43. Nikitin NP, Witte KK, Clark AL, Cleland JG. Color tissue Doppler-derived long-axis left ventricular function in heart failure with preserved global systolic function. Am J Cardiol 2002;90:1174–1177.

44. Vinereanu D, Nicolaides E, Tweddel AC, Fraser AG. "Pure" diastolic dysfunction is associated with long-axis systolic dysfunction. Implications for the diagnosis and classification of heart failure. Eur J Heart Fail 2005;7:820–828.

45. Vinereanu D, Lim PO, Frenneaux MP, Fraser AG. Reduced myocardial velocities of left ventricular long-axis contraction identify both systolic and diastolic heart failure-a comparison with brain natriuretic peptide. Eur J Heart Fail 2005;7:512–519.

46. Hasegawa H, Little WC, Ohno M, Brucks S, Morimoto A, Cheng HJ, Cheng CP. Diastolic mitral annular velocity during the development of heart failure. J Am Coll Cardiol. 2003;41:1590–1597.

47. Baicu CF, Zile MR, Aurigemma GP, Gaasch WH. Left ventricular systolic performance, function, and contractility in patients with diastolic heart failure. Circulation 2005;111:2306–2312.

48. Wiggers CJ. Determinants of cardiac performance. Circulation 1951;4:485–495.

49. Rushmer RF. Anatomy and physiology of ventricular function. Physiol Rev 1956;36:400–425.

50. Sarnoff SJ. Related myocardial contractility as described by ventricular function curves; observations on Starling's law of the heart. Physiol Rev 1955;35:107–122.

51. Abbott BC, Mommaerts WF. A study of inotropic mechanisms in the papillary muscle preparation. J Gen Physiol 1959;42:533–551.

52. Sonnenblick EH. Force–velocity relations in mammalian heart muscle. Am J Physiol 1962;202:931–939.

53. Brutsaert DL. Cardiac endothelial–myocardial signaling: its role in cardiac growth, contractile performance, and rhythmicity. Physiol Rev 2003;83:59–115.

54. Yotti R, Bermejo J, Antoranz JC, Desco MM, Cortina C, Rojo-Alvarez JL, Allue C, Martin L, Moreno M, Serrano JA, Munoz R, Garcia-Fernandez MA. A noninvasive method for assessing impaired diastolic suction in patients with dilated cardiomyopathy. Circulation 2005;112:2921.

55. Little WC. Related diastolic dysfunction beyond distensibility: adverse effects of ventricular dilatation. Circulation 2005;112:2888–2890.

56. De Keulenaer GW, Brutsaert DL. Systolic and diastolic heart failure: different phenotypes of the same disease? Eur J Heart Fail 2007;9:136–143.

57. Brutsaert DL, De Keulenaer GW. Diastolic heart failure: a myth. Curr Opin Cardiol 2006;21:240–248.

58. Klapholz M, Maurer M, Lowe AM, Messineo F, Meisner JS, Mitchell J, Kalman J, Phillips RA, Steingart R, Brown EJ Jr, Berkowitz R, Moskowitz R, Soni A, Mancini D, Bijou R, Sehhat K, Varshneya N, Kukin M, Katz SD, Sleeper LA, Le Jemtel TH. Hospitalization for heart failure in the presence of a normal left ventricular ejection fraction: results of the New York Heart Failure Registry. J Am Coll Cardiol 2004;43:1432–1438.

59. CHARM Investigators and Committees, Yusuf S, Pfeffer MA, Swedberg K, Granger CB, Held P, McMurray JJ, Michelson EL, Olofsson B, Ostergren J. Effects of candesartan in patients with chronic heart failure and preserved left-ventricular ejection fraction: the CHARM-Preserved Trial. Lancet 2003;362:777–781.

60. The Merit-HF study group. Effect of metoprolol CR/XL in chronic heart failure: Metoprolol CR/XL Randomised Intervention Trial in Congestive Heart Failure (MERIT-HF). Lancet 1999;353:2001–2007.

61. Vasan RS, Larson MG, Benjamin EJ, Evans JC, Reiss CK, Levy D. Congestive heart failure in subjects with normal versus reduced left ventricular ejection fraction: prevalence and mortality in a population-based cohort. J Am Coll Cardiol 1999;33:1948–1955.

62. Chen HH, Lainchbury JG, Senni M, Bailey KR, Redfield MM. Diastolic heart failure in the community: clinical profile, natural history, therapy, and impact of proposed diagnostic criteria. J Card Fail 2002;8:279–287.

63. Kalantar-Zadeh K, Block G, Horwich T, Fonarow GC. Reverse epidemiology of conventional cardiovascular risk factors in patients with chronic heart failure. J Am Coll Cardiol 2004;43:1439–1444.

64. Solomon SD, St John Sutton M, Lamas GA, Plappert T, Rouleau JL, Skali H, Moye L, Braunwald E, Pfeffer MA. Ventricular remodeling does not accompany the development of heart failure in diabetic patients after myocardial infarction. Circulation 2002;106:1251–1255.

65. Kenchaiah S, Evans JC, Levy D, Wilson PWF, Benjamin EJ, Larson MG, Kannel WB, Vasan RS. Obesity and the risk of heart failure. N Engl J Med 2002;347:305–313.

66. Horwich TB, Fonarow GC, Hamilton MA, MacLellan WR, Woo MA, Tillisch JH. The relationship between obesity and mortality in patients with heart failure. J Am Coll Cardiol 2001;38:789–795.

67. Horwich TB, Hamilton MA, Maclellan WR, Fonarow GC. Low serum total cholesterol is associated with marked increase in mortality in advanced heart failure. J Card Fail 2002;8:216–224.

68. Poole-Wilson PA, Uretsky BF, Thygesen K, Cleland JG, Massie BM, Ryden L; Atlas Study Group. Assessment of treatment with lisinopril and survival. Mode of death in heart failure: findings from the ATLAS trial. Heart 2003;89:42–48.

69. Weinberg EO, Mirotsou M, Gannon J, Dzau VJ, Lee RT, Pratt RE. Sex dependence and temporal dependence of the left ventricular genomic response to pressure overload. Physiol Genomics 2003;12:113–127.

70. Haghighi K, Schmidt AG, Hoit BD, Brittsan AG, Yatani A, Lester JW, Zhai J, Kimura Y, Dorn GW 2nd, MacLennan DH, Kranias EG. Superinhibition of sarcoplasmic reticulum function by phospholamban induces cardiac contractile failure. J Biol Chem 2001;276:24145–24152.

71. Dash R, Schmidt AG, Pathak A, Gerst MJ, Biniakiewicz D, Kadambi VJ, Hoit BD, Abraham WT, Kranias EG. Differential regulation of p38 mitogen-activated protein kinase mediates gender-dependent catecholamine-induced hypertrophy. Cardiovasc Res 2003;57:704–714.

72. Leinwand LA. Sex is a potent modifier of the cardiovascular system. J Clin Invest 2003;112:302–307.

73. Hay I, Rich J, Ferber P, Burkhoff D, Maurer MS. The role of impaired myocardial relaxation in the production of elevated left ventricular filling pressure. Am J Physiol Heart Circ Physiol 2005;288:H1203–H1208.

74. Skaluba SJ, Litwin SE. Mechanisms of exercise intolerance: insights from tissue Doppler imaging. Circulation 2004;109:972–977.

75. Fischer M, Baessler A, Hense HW, Hengstenberg C, Muscholl M, Holmer S, Doring A, Broeckel U, Riegger G, Schunkert H. Prevalence of left ventricular diastolic dysfunction in the community. Results from a Doppler echocardiographic-based survey of a population sample. Eur Heart J 2003;24:320–328.

76. Alpert MA, Terry BE, Mulekar M, Cohen MV, Massey CV, Fan TM, Panayiotou H, Mukerji V. Cardiac morphology and left ventricular function in normotensive morbidly obese patients with and without congestive heart failure, and effect of weight loss. Am J Cardiol 1997;80:736–740.

77. Perhonen MA, Zuckerman JH, Levine BD. Deterioration of left ventricular chamber performance after bed rest: "cardiovascular deconditioning" or hypovolemia? Circulation 2001;103:1851–1857.

78. Arbab-Zadeh A, Dijk E, Prasad A, Fu Q, Torres P, Zhang R, Thomas JD, Palmer D, Levine BD. Effect of aging and physical activity on left ventricular compliance. Circulation 2004;110:1799–1805.

79. Lakatta EG, Yin FC. Myocardial aging: functional alterations and related cellular mechanisms. Am J Physiol 1982;242:H927–H941.

80. Yelamarty RV, Moore RL, Yu FT, Elensky M, Semanchick AM, Cheung JY. Relaxation abnormalities in single cardiac myocytes from renovascular hypertensive rats. Am J Physiol 1992;262:C980–990.

81. Nishikawa N, Yamamoto K, Sakata Y, Mano T, Yoshida J, Miwa T, Takeda H, Hori M, Masuyama T. Differential activation of matrix metalloproteinases in heart failure with and without ventricular dilatation. Cardiovasc Res 2003;57:766–774.

82. Diamant M, Lamb HJ, Groeneveld Y, Endert EL, Smit JW, Bax JJ, Romijn JA, de Roos A, Radder JK. Diastolic dysfunction is associated with altered myocardial metabolism in asymptomatic normotensive patients with well-controlled type 2 diabetes mellitus. J Am Coll Cardiol 2003;42:328–335.

83. Mohan P, Brutsaert DL, Paulus WJ, Sys SU. Myocardial contractile response to nitric oxide and cGMP. Circulation 1996;93:1223–1229.

84. De Keulenaer GW, Andries LJ, Sys SU, Brutsaert DL. Endothelin-mediated positive inotropic effect induced by reactive oxygen species in isolated cardiac muscle. Circ Res 1995;76:878–884.

85. Leite-Moreira AF, Bras-Silva C, Pedrosa CA, Rocha-Sousa AA. ET-1 increases distensibility of acutely loaded myocardium: a novel ETA and Na+/H+ exchanger-mediated effect. Am J Physiol 2003;284:H1332–H1339.

86. Mohan P, Brutsaert DL, Sys SU. Myocardial performance is modulated by interaction of cardiac endothelium derived nitric oxide and prostaglandins. Cardiovasc Res 1995;29:637–640.

87. Cote GM, Miller TA, Lebrasseur NK, Kuramochi Y, Sawyer DB. Neuregulin-1alpha and beta isoform expression in cardiac microvascular endothelial cells and function in cardiac myocytes in vitro. Exp Cell Res 2005;311:135–146.

88. Fransen P, Lamberts RR, Hendrickx J, De Keulenaer GW. Endocardial endothelium modulates subendocardial pH(i) of rabbit papillary muscles: role of transendothelial HCO(3)(−) transport. Cardiovasc Res 2004;63:700–708.

2
Pathophysiologic Aspects of Myocardial Relaxation and End-Diastolic Stiffness of Cardiac Ventricles

Thierry C. Gillebert and Adelino F. Leite-Moreira

Introduction

- Cardiovascular congestion with preserved ejection fraction is not necessarily diastolic heart failure.
- Diastolic left ventricular dysfunction may be induced by overload, is present in systolic heart failure, and is the hallmark of diastolic heart failure.
- Distensibility, compliance, and left ventricular size are the main determinants of the diastolic pressure–volume relation.
- Myocardial relaxation may importantly affect end-diastolic left ventricular properties.
- Knowledge of intracellular calcium fluxes is essential to understand myocardial relaxation.
- Myocardial stiffness is regulated by extracellular matrix, by the cytoskeleton, and by myofilament interaction.
- Myocardial tone is regulated by phosphorylation of myofilaments, load, endothelin-1, β-adrenergic receptor stimulation, and angiotensin II.
- Diastolic heart failure is a combined disorder due to increased stiffness of heart and vessels.

Cardiovascular Congestion

When we observe symptoms and signs of cardiovascular congestion, we have to look for various conditions leading to these symptoms. These conditions may relate to overload (pressure or volume), to pump failure due to systolic dysfunc-

tion, or to pump failure due to diastolic dysfunction (Table 2.1).

Cardiovascular Congestion in Overload

Cardiovascular congestion may relate to volume and/or to pressure overload of the ventricle. Volume overload increases circulating volume, venous return, and filling pressures. What is true for volume overload is true as well for reduced compliance of the vascular bed, which consists for the major part of the venous vascular bed. Guyton[1] showed us that venous vasoconstriction has the same effect on venous return as a transfusion. It is the balance between circulating volume and total compliance of the vascular bed that determines venous return to the heart, hence filling pressures.

Pressure and volume overload may profoundly affect timing, rate, and completion of myocardial relaxation.[2–4] Practical relevance of the effects of cardiovascular pressure and volume on diastolic function are illustrated with two clinical examples from the literature.

Patients, presenting exertional hypertension (pressure overload) developed pressure-dependent diastolic dysfunction, a rise in filling pressures, and dyspnea. In these patients, angiotensin II receptor blockade with losartan blunted the hypertensive response to exercise and increased exercise tolerance and quality of life.[5]

Leg lifting in uncomplicated coronary artery bypass graft (CABG) patients with preserved systolic function (ejection fraction [EF] >0.45) increased venous return to the heart (volume

Table 2.1. Conditions resulting in cardiovascular congestion and elevated filling pressures.

1. Cardiovascular overload
   a. Pressure overload
      i. Elevated systemic pressures
      ii. Stress and exercise
      iii. Elevated pulmonary pressures, congenital heart diseases
      iv. Outflow tract obstruction or valvular stenosis
      v. Pharmacologic interactions (e.g., sympathomimetics)
   b. Volume overload
      i. Administration of fluid and electrolytes
      ii. Fluid retention due to hepatic or renal failure
      iii. Fluid retention due to neurohumoral and renal responses to forward failure of the heart
      iv. Regurgitant valvular heart diseases, right–left shunts
      v. High-output states (anemia, thyrotoxicosis, vitamin B_1 deficiency)
      vi. Pharmacologic interactions (e.g., nonsteroidal antiinflammatory drugs, corticoids)
2. Systolic heart failure
   a. Decreased contractile performance and use of the Frank-Starling mechanism
   b. Forward failure and secondary fluid retention (see 1.b.iii)
   c. Remodeling, dilatation, abnormalities of myocardial relaxation and compliance
3. Diastolic heart failure
   a. Abnormalities of myocardial relaxation and compliance
   b. Forward failure and secondary fluid retention (see 1.b.iii)

*Edema caused by, for example, venous insufficiency, hypoalbuminemia, and calcium antagonists are not mentioned as they are not a cause of elevated filling pressures.

overload).[6] Some CABG patients adapted according to the Frank-Starling mechanism, with enhanced contraction, enhanced relaxation, and almost unchanged filling pressures. Most patients displayed indifferent changes. Surprisingly, 15%–20% of these CABG patients responded with a marked elevation of filling pressures. Increased left ventricular (LV) filling pressures during leg lifting were explained by slowed and incomplete myocardial relaxation and by a position on the descending limb of the Frank-Starling curve.[2] This contraction–relaxation coupling deficit was due to increased venous return.

Cardiovascular Congestion in Systolic Heart Failure

In acute systolic heart failure (SHF), such as in acute myocardial infarction, the heart uses the Frank-Starling mechanism to compensate. This leads to elevated filling pressures by moving to the right on a still unaltered end-diastolic pressure–volume (PV) relation.

In SHF, neurohumoral and renal adjustments result in fluid and electrolyte retention, therefore in increased venous return. This retention contributes as well to the movement on the diastolic PV relation and elevation of filling pressures.

In chronic SHF, the process of myocardial relaxation is impaired to the same extent as the process of myocardial contraction. Both processes are coupled[6,7] and constitute a continuous process of contraction–relaxation. In chronic heart failure, end-diastolic stiffness of the ventricle is increased because the ventricle operates on the steep part of the curve and because the entire curve is altered because of remodelling and fibrosis.[8] Impaired myocardial relaxation and properties of the myocardium both contribute to elevating filling pressures in SHF. We discuss later in this chapter why the poorly contracting ventricle will necessarily have slow and incomplete myocardial relaxation. In these ventricles, myocardial relaxation is highly dependent on the level of operating pressures and volumes.

A study by Eichhorn et al.[9] illustrates this issue. Nitroprusside was administered to patients with SHF in order to assess the coupling between contraction and relaxation. The authors analyzed end-systolic elastance as a measure of contractility and load dependence of myocardial relaxation, evaluated with the slope R (ms/mm Hg) of the linear relation between the time constant tau and the end-systolic LV pressure. They found a hyperbolic relation between R and end-systolic elastance. With normal or subnormal systolic function, relaxation is normal and not load dependent. With systolic dysfunction, relaxation appeared to be very load dependent. Delayed and incomplete myocardial relaxation was present at baseline and could be reverted with nitroprusside.

Cardiovascular Congestion in Diastolic Heart Failure

In diastolic heart failure (DHF), the ventricle is not enlarged, the EF is preserved, and stroke volume is normal. Filling pressures are elevated to the same extent as in SHF, mainly because of a shift upward and leftward of the diastolic PV relation. The main pathophysiologic mechanisms of the alteration of the diastolic PV curve are delayed myocardial relaxation and altered properties of the LV wall. Similarly as in SHF, there are neurohumoral and renal adjustments leading to fluid and electrolyte retention.

The cardiovascular system, both heart and vessels, of aged patients with DHF is less compliant and therefore sensitive to even small changes in cardiovascular volume.[10] It will respond to small increases with frank elevation of systolic pressures and diastolic pressures. The opposite is also true, and removing some fluid from such a cardiovascular system with diuretics will rapidly decrease blood pressures and cardiac output, compromising blood supply to critical organs such as the kidney. As a whole, the cardiovascular system of such a patient with DHF can only operate in a narrow range of cardiovascular volumes, balancing between low output and congestion. An illustrative clinical example is hypertensive pulmonary edema in elderly patients.[11] In hypertensive pulmonary edema, elevated filling pressures are the consequence of pressure-dependent delayed myocardial relaxation and altered properties of the LV wall rather than the consequence of pressure-dependent impairment of contractility. The relative contribution of impaired relaxation and abnormal stiffness is still a debated issue in this clinical setting.[12]

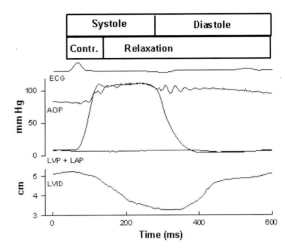

FIGURE 2.1. Hemodynamic aspects of the cardiac cycle. Data recorded in anaesthetized open-chest dog model. **(Top)** Limb electrocardiogram (ECG). **(Middle)** Pressures recorded with a fluid-filled manometer in the aortic root (AOP) and with a high fidelity microtip-manometer in left ventricle (LVP) and atrium (LAP). **(Bottom)** Left ventricular internal diameter (LVID) measured with implanted sonomicrometers. This measurement is comparable to an M-mode echocardiographic measurement of the left ventricular cavity at the tip of the mitral valve. The cardiac cycle is commonly subdivided into systole and diastole. The cyclic interaction of myofilaments is subdivided into contraction and relaxation. (From Gillebert et al.[15])

The Cardiac Cycle, Systole and Diastole

The Heart as a Pump

The pump performance of the LV depends on its ability to cycle between two states: (1) a compliant chamber in diastole that allows the LV to fill from a low left atrial pressure and (2) a stiff chamber in systole that ejects the stroke volume at arterial pressures.[13] The ventricle has two alternating functions: systolic ejection and diastolic filling. Furthermore, the stroke volume must be able to increase in response to stress, such as exercise, without much increase in left atrial pressures.[14] The theoretically optimal pressure domain curve of the LV is rectangular with instantaneous pressure rise, elevated systolic pressures, instantaneous fall, and low diastolic pressures.[15] This theoretically optimal situation is approached by cyclic interaction of myofilaments and supposes competent mitral and aortic valves. From a hemodynamic point of view, the classic Wiggers cycle[16] with systole until aortic valve closure and diastole thereafter remains valid and most useful (Figure 2.1).

The Heart as a Muscle

From a pathophysiologic point of view, the cyclic interaction of myofilaments includes muscular contraction and muscular relaxation. The transition from contraction to relaxation occurs simultaneously with the plateau phase of the cellular action potential and simultaneously with the descending limb of the cytoplasmic Ca^{2+} transient.[17] The transition from contraction to relaxation occurs during early ejection in healthy hearts and even prior to aortic valve opening in

(Figure 2.3, top). Typical examples are the heart in aortic stenosis, the hypertensive heart, and the remodeled heart of the aged subject.

The distinction between distensibility, compliance, and cavity size matters, however, when changes in the descriptors of the diastolic PV relation go in opposite directions. This is illustrated by SHF, for example, the ischemic cardiomyopathy (Figure 2.3, bottom). These hearts have an enlarged LV cavity but operate on a steep portion of their PV curve, with small increases in volume leading to sharp increases in diastolic LV pressures. There is an apparent increase in distensibility,[14] which could be explained solely by an increase in the constant A instead of an increase in the intercept P_0: this actually means an increase in LV size but no increase in LV distensibility.

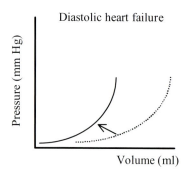

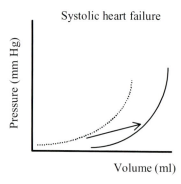

FIGURE 2.3. End-dastolic pressure–volume relations in diastolic and chronic systolic heart failure. **(Top)** The relation is shifted leftward and upward and is steeper. This is the manifestation of smaller cavity size and reduced compliance. **(Bottom)** In chronic systolic heart failure, the relation is shifted rightward and is steeper. Cavity size is increased and compliance is reduced. The hallmark of heart failure in both conditions is the reduced compliance and the steep curve accordingly.

The ventricle operates on a steep portion of the curve because of a combination of overfilling and decreased compliance of the ventricle. These severely diseased hearts are no more able to work at smaller volumes and respond to exercise, elevated cardiac output, and increased cardiovascular volumes by pulmonary congestion and symptoms. William Little recently referred to this situation as "diastolic dysfunction beyond distensibility," pointing out that, in addition to distensibility and compliance issues, these hearts developed less elastic recoil and disturbed diastolic acceleration of blood flow from the mitral inflow to the LV apex.[14]

For practical purposes, the concept of distensibility/compliance may be simplified to two or slightly more PV combinations allowing calculating a linear slope, $\Delta P/\Delta V$ (operational stiffness) or $\Delta V/\Delta P$ (operational compliance) without assumptions regarding the entire diastolic PV relation. This simplified representation focuses on the clinical relevance of the end-diastolic LV properties. According to Little, the only thing that really matters is the slope of the curve at operating conditions. When this slope is steep, the patients are in a labile balance. Slightly decreased LV volumes will result in decreased cardiac output and impaired tissue perfusion. Slightly increased LV volumes will restore cardiac output but at the expense of elevated filling pressures and pulmonary edema. This remains valid regardless of the mechanism of heart failure (systolic or diastolic) and regardless of the size of the ventricle. This discussion focuses on passive material properties of the ventricle of the cardiac chamber. In addition, it is relevant to derive passive tissue, myocardial properties by normalizing chamber stiffness according to chamber geometry. This latter aspect is covered in other chapters of this textbook.

In the normal heart, working under normal load and at a normal heart rate, relaxation is completed by end diastole and should not influence end-diastolic properties. When relaxation is delayed, when load is abnormal, when diastole is short, or when a combination of these factors concurs, relaxation may interfere to an important extent with filling pressures and with end-diastolic LV properties. Considering that relaxation is completed and neglecting extraventricular

2. Myocardial Relaxation and End-Diastolic Stiffness

constraint, compliance of the ventricle is determined by (1) ventricular geometry, (2) mechanical myocardial properties commonly alluded to as myocardial stiffness, and (3) myocardial tone. Myocardial tone is a recently expanded concept referring to dynamic aspects of distensibility and stiffness such as titin phosphorylation and neurohumoral modulation of myocardial distensibility.

Myocardial Relaxation and Its Time Course

Relaxation is the process whereby the myocardium returns to an unstressed length and force. In the normal heart, it comprises the major part of ventricular ejection, pressure fall, and the initial part of rapid filling.

Left Ventricular Pressure Fall

Left ventricular pressure fall is the hemodynamic manifestation of myocardial relaxation. Its analysis allows adequate description of the course of myocardial relaxation.[7] It has a nonuniform course that encompasses two consecutive phases, an initial acceleration and a subsequent deceleration, that are subjected to a distinct regulation by afterload.[3,4] The initial phase starts at peak LV pressure, before aortic valve closure, and ends close to peak rate of LV pressure fall (dP/dt_{min}). The subsequent phase begins at dP/dt_{min} and can be further subdivided into intermediate and terminal phases by mitral valve opening. The intermediate phase corresponds to the isovolumetric relaxation, whereas the terminal phase occurs during early LV diastolic filling. Analysis of LV pressure fall commonly includes indices that evaluate either time of onset or rate of the intermediate phase of pressure decline.[7] Time of onset is measured by ejection duration and by time from end diastole to aortic valve closure or to peak rate of LV pressure fall (dP/dt_{min}). Among the indices that evaluate rate of pressure decline, dP/dt_{min}, isovolumetric relaxation time and time constant tau are the most commonly used. Note that the later two indices mainly evaluate the rate of intermediate LV pressure fall and provide no informa-

tion on the rate of initial pressure fall. The time constant tau uses data from dP/dt_{min} until mitral valve opening and a logarithmic, exponential, or logistic formula.[21,26-28] Decreases in right ventricular (RV) and LV pressures follow distinct time courses, with the initial acceleration phase being relatively longer in the RV and the subsequent deceleration phase being relatively longer in the LV. As afterload increases, the course of RV pressure decrease becomes progressively more similar with that of LV pressure decrease. We must, therefore, be aware that with normal pulmonary systolic pressures, RV tau only evaluates a minor portion of RV pressure decrease.[29]

Determinants of Myocardial Relaxation

Myocardial relaxation is modulated by load, inactivation, and nonuniformity.[30]

Modulation of Relaxation by Load

Load changes influence calcium regulatory mechanisms and myofilament properties. Effects of load on relaxation depend on its type (preload vs. afterload), magnitude, duration, and time in the cardiac cycle at which it occurs.[7] Afterload elevations have a biphasic effect on relaxation rate and end-diastolic PV relation.[3,4] When they occur early in the cardiac cycle, a mild to moderate afterload elevation will, in the normal heart, delay the onset and accelerate the rate of pressure fall without affecting the end-diastolic PV relation (Figure 2.4). This reflects a compensatory response and the presence of diastolic tolerance to afterload. On the contrary, a severe afterload elevation or an afterload elevation that occurs later in ejection will induce a premature onset and a pronounced slowing of pressure fall, even in a healthy heart. Such slowing might lead to incomplete relaxation and therefore to elevation of filling pressures, a phenomenon that is exacerbated when preload is elevated (Figure 2.5).[20] This reflects a decompensatory response and the presence of diastolic intolerance to afterload. As marked hypertension represents a heavy afterload to the LV, this mechanism might contribute to exacerbation of diastolic dysfunction and pulmonary congestion in hypertensive crisis.[11,12]

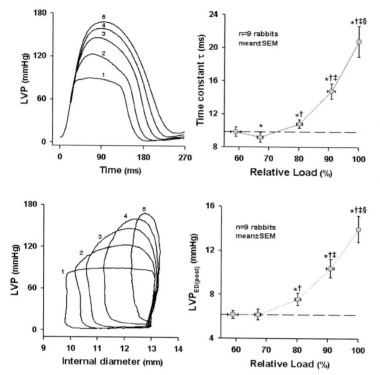

FIGURE 2.4. Systolic load and diastolic function. Five superimposed heartbeats in rabbits: one baseline and four variably afterloaded heartbeats. Each of the afterloaded beats was the first beat following an aortic clamp. With a moderate afterload (beat 2), tau does not increase (it actually decreases slightly) and end-diastolic left ventricular pressure remains unaltered. With elevated afterload (beats 3 to 5), tau and end-diastolic pressure increase as a function of the magnitude of the load. Elevated systolic load induces diastolic dysfunction. From Leite-Moreira et al.,[4] with permission of The European Society of Cardiology.)

The level of afterload above which a decompensatory response occurs may be shifted by pharmacologic agents,[31,32] varies among animal species,[4,33] is distinct in the two ventricles,[34] and is lower in the failing heart.[15] Potential underlying mechanisms for these differences in the diastolic tolerance to afterload include changes in the activity of the sarcoplasmic reticulum Ca^{2+} ATPase (SERCA2a) or the Na^+/Ca^{2+} exchanger, in troponin I phosphorylation or in myosin heavy chain isoforms.[32,34–36]

Modulation of Relaxation by Inactivation

Myocardial inactivation relates to the processes underlying calcium extrusion (Figure 2.6) from

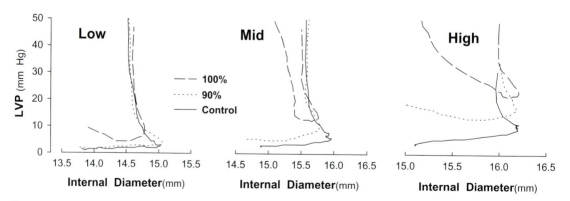

FIGURE 2.5. Diastolic portion of left ventricular pressure (LVP)– internal left ventricular diameter loops of a control and two afterloaded (90% and isovolumetric) heartbeats at low, mid, and high preload. The diastolic portion of the loops was shifted upward when afterload was elevated. This upward shift was exacerbated at higher preload. (From Leite-Moreira and Correira-Pinto,[20] with permission of The American Physiological Society.)

2. Myocardial Relaxation and End-Diastolic Stiffness

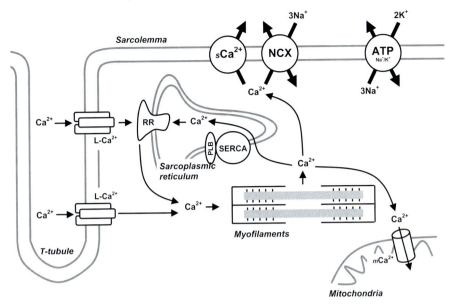

FIGURE 2.6. Excitation–contraction and inactivation–relaxation coupling in cardiomyocytes. Cardiomyocyte depolarization promotes Ca^{2+} entry through sarcolemmal L-type Ca^{2+} channels (L-Ca^{2+}), leading to Ca^{2+} release from the sarcoplasmic reticulum through ryanodine receptors (RR), thereby inducing contraction. During relaxation, the four pathways involved in calcium removal from the cytosol are phospholamban (PLB)–modulated uptake of Ca^{2+} into the sarcoplasmic reticulum by a Ca^{2+}-ATPase (SERCA), Ca^{2+} extrusion via the sodium–calcium exchanger (NCX), mitochondrial Ca^{2+} uniport, and sarcolemmal Ca^{2+}-ATPase, with the latter two being responsible for only about 1% of total. (Adapted from Roncon-Albuquerque R Jr, Leite-Moreira AF. A cinética do cálcio na progressão da insuficiência cardíaca. Rev Portuguesa Cardiol 2004;24(Suppl II):25–44.)

the cytosol in order to achieve its diastolic levels and cross-bridge detachment.[37] Determinants of myocardial inactivation, listed in Table 2.3, therefore include mechanisms related to calcium homeostasis and myofilament regulators of cross-bridge cycling.[38]

The four pathways involved in calcium extrusion from the cytosol are phospholamban-modulated uptake of Ca^{2+} by SERCA2a, Ca^{2+} extrusion via Na^+/Ca^{2+} exchange, mitochondrial Ca^{2+} uniport, and sarcolemmal Ca^{2+}-ATPase, with the two latter being responsible for about only 1% of total.[37] Recent evidence suggests that the main role of the sarcolemmal Ca^{2+} pump may be related to signal transduction in the cardiovascular system.[39] The quantitative importance of the two first major routes varies among species.[37]

Decreased levels or activity of SERCA2a can slow the removal of calcium from the cytosol. Increased levels or activity of phospholamban, a SERCA-inhibitory protein, can also impair relaxation. Increased cyclic adenosine monophosphate, resulting from ß-adrenergic stimulation or inhibition of cardiac phosphodiesterase, phosphorylates phospholamban to remove its inhibitory effect on SERCA. The net effect is an improvement in diastolic relaxation. Pathologic LV hypertrophy secondary to hypertension or aortic stenosis results in decreased SERCA and increased phospholamban, again leading to impaired relaxation. Similar changes are seen in the myocardium of patients with hypertrophic or dilated

TABLE 2.3. Determinants of myocardial inactivation.

Ca^{2+} homeostasis
  Ca^{2+} concentration
  Sarcolemmal and sarcoplasmic reticulum Ca^{2+} transport
  Modifying proteins (phospholamban, calmodulin, calsequestrin)
Myofilaments
  Troponin C Ca^{2+} binding
  Troponin I phosphorylation
  Ca^{2+} sensitivity
  α/β-Myosin heavy chain adenosine triphosphatase ratio
Energetics
  Adenosine diphosphate/adenosine triphosphate ratio
  Adenosine diphosphate and inorganic phosphate concentrations

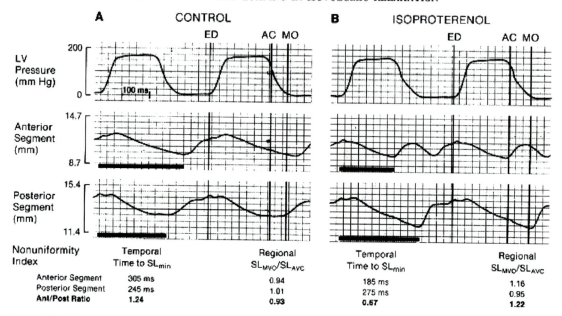

FIGURE 2.7. Effects of isoproterenol-induced asynchrony of segment reextension on the rate of left ventricular (LV) pressure fall (ED, end diastole). In the control situation (A), the segments shorten synchronously, wall movement during pressure fall (between aortic closure [AC] and mitral opening [MO]) is limited, and both segments lengthen after MO. The thick horizontal line represents time from end-diastole to minimum segment length. After isoproterenol (B), the stimulated anterior segment develops premature early segment reextension. This leads to abrupt and early onset of LV pressure fall. Pressure fall is slower. Between AC and MO early reextension of the anterior segement is accompanied by postsystolic shortening of the posterior segment. (From Gillebert and Lew,[46] with permission of The American Physiological Society.)

cardiomyopathy. Interestingly, levels of SERCA decrease with age, coincident with impaired diastolic function. As adenosine triphosphate hydrolysis is required for myosin detachment from actin, calcium dissociation from troponin C, and active sequestration of calcium by the sarcoplasmic reticulum, energetic factors must also be taken into consideration. Modification of any of these steps, the myofilament proteins involved in these steps, or the ATPase that catalyzes them can alter diastolic function.[36,40–42] It is therefore not surprising that ischemia leads to impaired relaxation.

Modulation of Relaxation by Nonuniformity

Pacing-induced asynchrony of contraction and relaxation leads to impaired systolic performance.[43] When myocardial relaxation starts at different times in various segments of the LV, one segment still contracts while the other relaxes. This leads to asynchronous early segment reextension[44] and premature closure of the aortic valve. During isovolumetric relaxation, reextension of one ventricular segment is accompanied by postsystolic shortening of another segment (Figure 2.7). The ventricle remains isovolumic but changes its shape and produces intraventricular volume displacement. Asynchronous early segment reextension and regional nonuniformity induce a slower rate of ventricular pressure fall and might contribute to the diastolic disturbances observed in myocardial ischemia and with intraventricular conduction disturbances.[45–47]

End-Diastolic Properties of Muscle and Heart

End-diastolic properties of the ventricular wall are influenced by myocardial stiffness, wall thickness, and chamber geometry. Determinants of myocardial stiffness include factors intrinsic to

2. Myocardial Relaxation and End-Diastolic Stiffness

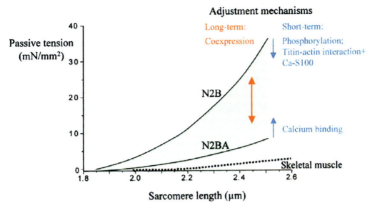

FIGURE 2.8. Sarcomere passive length–tension relation between cardiac myocytes that predominately express N2B titin and those that predominately express N2BA titin. Coexpression of titin isoforms at variable ratios allows intermediate passive tensions (double-headed arrow) as a long-term passive stiffness adjustment mechanism. It has been postulated that short-term adjustment mechanisms differentially impact the isoforms, decreasing stiffness of N2B titin and increasing stiffness of N2BA titin. (From Granzier and Labeit.[48] © 2004 American Heart Association, Inc. All rights reserved. Reprinted with permission.)

the cardiomyocytes themselves (cytoskeleton) and the extracellular matrix (ECM). The cardiomyocyte cytoskeleton is composed of microtubules, intermediate filaments (desmin), microfilaments (actin), and endosarcomeric proteins (titin, α-actinin, myomesin, and M protein). Changes in some of these cytoskeletal proteins have been shown to alter diastolic function.[36,40]

Most of the elastic force of the cardiomyocytes is now thought to reside in the macromolecule titin (Figure 2.8), whereas contributions of microtubules (tubulin) and intermediate filaments (desmin) appear <10% at operating sarcomere lengths.[48] Titin is expressed as varying isoforms that impart different mechanical properties, and this likely plays a role in altering passive stiffness in failing hearts. Titin can also be posttranslationally modified by Ca^{2+} (even in the diastolic range) and by phosphorylation, blurring notions of passive versus active tone.[15,36]

Phosphorylation of sarcomeric proteins by protein kinase A was recently shown to normalize increased stiffness of cardiomyocytes from patients with DHF.[49] Changes in the structures within the ECM can also affect diastolic function. Myocardial ECM is composed of (1) fibrillar protein (e.g., collagen types I and III and elastin); (2) proteoglycans; and (3) basement membrane proteins (e.g., collagen type IV, laminin, and fibronectin). Fibrillar collagen apparently is the most important component within the ECM contributing to the development of DHF.[36,40] The role played by other fibrillar proteins (basement membrane proteins and proteoglycans) remains largely unexplored.

Extracellular membrane fibrillar collagen, particularly in terms of its amount, geometry, distribution, degree of cross-linking, and ratio of collagen type I/type III are often altered in disease processes that alter diastolic function. The regulatory control of collagen biosynthesis and degradation includes (1) transcriptional regulation by physical (e.g., preload and afterload), neurohumoral (e.g., renin-angiotensin-aldosterone, endothelin-1, and sympathetic nervous systems), and growth factors; (2) posttranslational regulation, including collagen cross-linking; and (3) enzymatic degradation. Collagen degradation is under the control of matrix metalloproteinases.[36,40] Changes in either synthesis or degradation and their regulatory processes have been shown to alter diastolic function and lead to the development of DHF. In addition, it is now increasingly recognized that quality of collagen (specifically cross-linking and glycation) plays a key role in translating quantity into myocardial stiffness.[36] Recent demonstration that 16 weeks of treatment with a glucose cross-link breaker decreased LV mass and improved diastolic filling and quality of life in patients with DHF further reinforces this view.[15,36,50]

In addition to posttranslational modifications of titin, other evidence suggests that diastolic stiffness is actively modulated. Cross-bridge interaction occurs even at low diastolic calcium producing resting muscle tone. Modifications of myofilament calcium sensitivity by heart failure might also alter active tone.[50] This includes changes associated with protein kinase A (or guanosine monophosphate–dependent protein kinase) phosphorylation of myosin light chain 2 and troponin I (Figure 2.9). In this setting, nitric oxide and cyclic guanosine monophosphate increase resting diastolic cell length as a result of guanosine monophosphate–dependent protein kinase–mediated phosphorylation of myofilaments, and in patients with dilated cardiomyopathy administration of intracoronary substance P (a nitric oxide stimulator) decreases LV stiffness.[51] Furthermore, myocardial stiffness is acutely modulated by load, endothelin-1,[52] β-adrenoceptor stimulation,[53] and angiotensin II.[54]

With regard to load, as outlined above, a severe afterload elevation or an afterload elevation that occurs later in ejection will induce a pronounced slowing of pressure fall that might lead to incomplete relaxation and therefore to elevation of filling pressures.[4] This phenomenon is exacerbated when preload is elevated.[2,20] With regard to β-adrenergic receptor stimulation, it decreases myocardial stiffness through protein kinase A–induced phosphorylation of titin.[53] This posttranslational modification of titin was shown to acutely shift the diastolic length–tension relation downward (i.e., decrease stiffness) both in animal models[53] and in healthy and diseased human myocardium.[49]

It is widely accepted that when chronically elevated in pathologic conditions, endothelin-1 and angiotensin II might increase diastolic stiffness by inducing myocardial hypertrophy and altering ECM, leading to fibrosis.[55–58] However, recent studies convincingly demonstrated that both agents acutely decreased myocardial stiffness.[52,54] The acute direct myocardial effects of endothelin-1 and angiotensin II on myocardial stiffness were overlooked until recently, possibly because the few studies looking at this issue analyzed the effects of exogenously administered supraphysiologic doses. In these circumstances, coronary and/or systemic vasoconstriction could potentially have masked any effect on the intrinsic properties of the myocardium. In fact, both myocardial ischemia and severe afterload elevations potentially shift the end-diastolic PV relation upward, reflecting an decrease in myocardial distensibility.[4,20,23,59]

With regard to endothelin-1, the above-mentioned study[52] showed that this agent increases diastolic distensibility of acutely loaded cardiac muscles by binding to endothelin A receptors and activating the Na^+/H^+ exchanger (Figure 2.10). Although angiotensin II also acutely decreases myocardial stiffness,[54] its effect is observed even in the nonoverloaded myocardium (Figure 2.11). This effect is mediated by angiotensin II type 1 receptors and is dependent on the activation of

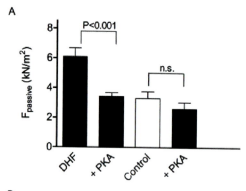

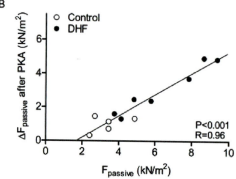

FIGURE 2.9. (A) Protein kinase A (PKA) treatment reduces passive force ($F_{passive}$) in cardiomyocytes from diastolic heart failure (DHF) patients to values observed in a control group at baseline and after PKA treatment. (B) Correlation between PKA-induced fall in $F_{passive}$ and baseline value of $F_{passive}$. (From Borbely et al.[49] © 2005 American Heart Association, Inc. All rights reserved. Reprinted with permission.)

2. Myocardial Relaxation and End-Diastolic Stiffness

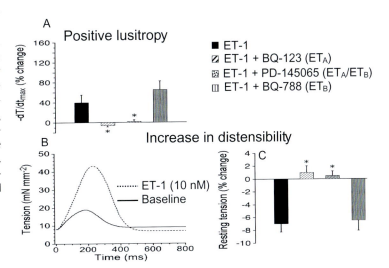

FIGURE 2.10. Effects of endothelin-1 (ET-1) on diastolic function in rabbits. Endothelin-1 increases the rate of myocardial relaxation (positive lusitropy, **(A)** and increases myocardial distensibility **(B,C)**. Increased distensibility is apparent as a decrease in resting tension after a heavily loaded (isometric) twitch **(lower left)**. The increases in both relaxation rate and distensibility were inhibited by selective ET_A (BQ-123) and nonselective ET_A/ET_B (PD-145065) receptor blockers, but not by the selective ET_B receptor blocker BQ-788. (From Leite-Moreira et al.,[52] with permission of The American Physiological Society.)

protein kinase C and the Na^+/H^+ exchanger in both the isolated papillary muscle and the in situ intact heart. In the latter, angiotensin II infusion increased LV systolic pressures by 50% while decreasing LV diastolic filling pressures. As an elevation of systolic LV pressure of such magnitude significantly increases LV diastolic pressure, it is not surprising that when the effects of angiotensin II on diastolic LV pressures were evaluated at matched systolic LV pressures a larger effect could be detected. In fact, in these circumstances, LV diastolic pressures decreased almost 50%. This means that angiotensin II might allow the ventricle to reach high filling volumes at almost half filling pressures, which is undoubtedly a quite powerful adaptation mechanism.

This compensatory effect of endothelin-1 and angiotensin II on myocardial distensibility in the acute setting might contribute, in the long term, to ventricular dilatation and remodeling. This potentially important pathophysiologic mechanism has not been studied in the failing heart so

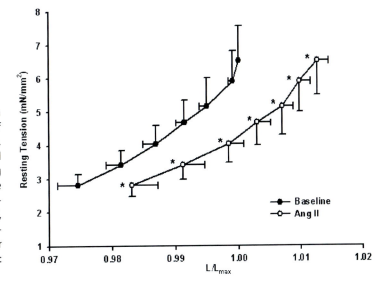

FIGURE 2.11. Diastolic length–tension relations at baseline and in the presence of angiotensin II (Ang II, 10^{-5} M) in rabbits. Angotensin II induced a rightward and downward shift of this relation, indicating a decrease in myocardial stiffness. Data are means ± SE; $p < 0.05$. *Ang II versus baseline. (Brunner F, Bras-Silva C, Cerdeira AS, Leite-Moreira AF. Cardiovascular endothelins: essential regulators of cardiovascular homeostasis. Pharmacol Ther 2006;111: 508–531.)

far and represents an interesting area for future investigations.

Ventricular Arterial Coupling and Diastolic Heart Failure

In order to understand DHF, we have to integrate loading conditions of the myocardium, myocardial relaxation disturbances, and passive stiffness of ventricle and myocardium. The heart is continuously interacting with the vessels, and this complex interaction determines cardiac load, hence the way the heart contracts and relaxes, ejects and fills.

Ventricular arterial coupling[60] can be described by the ratio of two parameters: effective arterial elastance (Ea = P_{es}/SV, where P_{es} is end-systolic pressure and SV is stroke volume) and systolic ventricular elastance or (slope of the ventricular end-systolic PV relation), or arterial contribution divided by ventricular contribution. From an energetic point of view, cardiac efficiency is maximal when Ea/Ees (end-systolic elastance) = 0.5. This is the situation in normal middle-aged healthy subjects[61] and corresponds to an EF = 0.65. The maximal external work is achieved when Ea/Ees = 1.0 and corresponds to an EF = 0.50. Arterial elastance is a simplified, lumped parameter of arterial stiffness. Both arterial elastance and end-systolic elastance can be approximately evaluated noninvasively.[62] Such a noninvasive approach may be used to characterize patient populations[63] or normal subjects,[61,64] keeping in mind the limitations of the method.

Diastolic heart failure or heart failure with preserved systolic function is a disease of both heart and vessels and can be more easily understood when considering alterations of heart and vessels as a global process[65] or as a coupling disorder.[10] Figure 2.12 schematically illustrates some of the processes that lead to diastolic dysfunction and failure. The LV undergoes structural and functional changes as a result of the increased vascular load presented by hypertension and loss of vascular compliance and elasticity due to arteriosclerosis, aging, and endothelial dysfunction. In addition, cardiac aging and, in some patients, episodic ischemia have direct effects on myocardial structure and function. These processes result in myocardial hypertrophy and fibrosis, with loss of myocardial compliance and, in some cases, impaired relaxation.[65]

In DHF, heart and vessels interact differently. An example of this different interaction is how myocardial relaxation responds to alterations of the systolic pressure pattern. If waves, reflected by the peripheral arterial tree, are delayed until after the aortic valve closure, such as in young subjects, the systolic pressure pattern is horizontal (control beat) or with an early peak similar to an early load clamp (Figure 2.13). These patterns do not significantly affect myocardial relaxation.[66] If reflected waves reach the heart before aortic closure, such as in elderly subjects, subjects with hypertension,

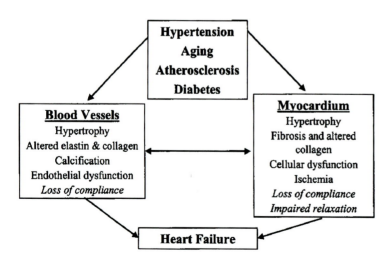

FIGURE 2.12. Some of the processes that lead to diastolic dysfunction and heart failure. (From Massie.[65])

2. Myocardial Relaxation and End-Diastolic Stiffness

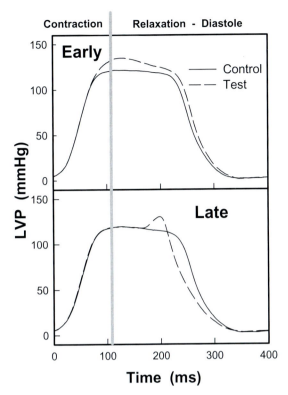

FIGURE 2.13. (Top) Early left ventricular pressure (LVP) elevation. The control heartbeat is displayed as a solid line. The solid vertical gray line indicates transition from contraction to relaxation. An elevation of systolic LVP (12 mm Hg) initiated during contraction and maintained throughout ejection (dashed line) delays the onset of LVP fall. Rate of LVP fall slightly accelerates. (Bottom) Late LVP elevation. An elevation of systolic LVP with a similar magnitude (12 mm Hg) but timed at mid ejection (dashed line) and is initiated during relaxation induces an early onset of LVP fall. The course of LVP fall is slower. (From Leite-Moreira and Gillebert.[3] © 1994 American Heart Association, Inc. All rights reserved. Reprinted with permission.)

or in general in subjects with a stiffening arterial tree, reflected waves will result in higher systolic pressures and in a systolic pressure pattern with a late peak, similar to a late-systolic load clamp.[67] This pressure waveform will delay myocardial relaxation[3,66] and will contribute to altered LV filling and elevated filling pressures.[4] A related issue is increased pulse pressure, characteristic for elderly subjects. Increased pulse pressure is a consequence of aortic stiffening and a loss of the windkessel capacity. During ventricular systole, the stroke volume ejected by the ventricle results in some forward blood flow to the organ beds, but part of the ejected volume is stored, buffered in the elastic arteries. This process represents the healthy pressure-equalizing or buffering function of the aorta. During ventricular diastole, the elastic recoil of the arterial wall maintains blood flow for the remaining part of the cardiac cycle. With aging, the stiffened aorta increases the systolic blood pressure, while the loss of elasticity decreases diastolic recoil so that the diastolic blood pressure falls.[68] The heart is overloaded during systole, whereas diastolic organ perfusion is at the lower limit or beyond.

Large cross-sectional studies have established age-dependent increases in vascular stiffening.[64,69,70] This vascular stiffening is accompanied by changes in the LV that increase end-systolic stiffness.[10,64] These changes can already be observed at an early stage of the disease in a subgroup of a normal middle-aged population (35–55 years old).[61] This combined ventricular arterial stiffening alters the way in which the cardiovascular system can respond to changes in pressures and volumes, hence to stress and physical exercise.

Figure 2.14 depicts the concept of age-dependent adaptations in two situations.[10] The left illustrates ventricular arterial coupling in a young and healthy subject. The right illustrates an elderly healthy subject. The left is the reference with balanced end-systolic elastance (Ees) and arterial elastance (Ea), normal ventricular and arterial

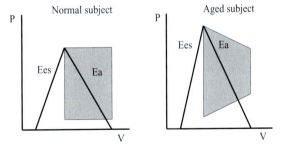

FIGURE 2.14. With increasing age, ventricular end-systolic elastance (Ees) and arterial elastance (Ea) both increase. Pressure (P)–volume (V) loops from young (left) and aged (right) subjects show increases in Ees that match increases in arterial loading indexed by arterial elastance (Ea). The coupling Ea/Ees remains close to optimal efficiency, somewhat higher than 0.5. The pressure–volume loop of the aged subject is distorted, trapezoidal. See text for further discussion.

elastances, and normal coupling with Ea/Ees close to 0.5. In the elderly subject we notice increased end-systolic elastance and increased arterial elastance. Both elastances are higher (slopes are steeper) but the coupling Ea/Ees remains unaltered. The heart adapts to increased arterial elastance by developing a matched increase in ventricular elastance so that coupling remains close to optimal efficiency. This preservation of ventricular arterial coupling is still present in patients with DHF[63] but not in patients with severe SHF, where uncoupling is observed.

What are the underlying mechanisms of the "coupling disorder" of the elderly and of the patient with DHF? Some information may be derived from the illustration. The PV loop is distorted. Instead of being roughly rectangular, such as in the young subject, the loop of the elderly subject is trapezoidal. During diastolic LV filling, pressure rises according to diastolic dysfunction. In addition, systolic pressure increases during ejection according to elevated pulse pressure (stiffening of the aorta) and to a late peaking systolic pressure waveform (prematurely reflected waves). Increased systolic pressure and altered systolic pressure waveform will delay myocardial relaxation and contribute to elevated filling pressures.[3,66] The elderly subject presents an adequate adaptation to vascular stiffening from an energetic point of view. However, this adaptation threatens his diastolic function and filling pressures, making him vulnerable for any additional load on the LV.

The patient with heart failure and preserved systolic function has an altered response to fluctuations in cardiovascular volume, to stress, and to physical exercise. A slight increase in cardiovascular volume will result in elevated systolic pressures. This will lead to elevated diastolic LV pressures and pulmonary congestion. An extreme example is the flash pulmonary edema of the hypertensive patient with preserved systolic function, as described earlier.[11] A slight decrease in cardiovascular volume will result in lower systolic blood pressures but also in lower diastolic blood pressures and organ perfusion pressures. The delicate balance between pulmonary congestion and organ failure (mainly renal failure) is in part the direct consequence of ventricular arterial stiffening. The responses to all sorts of stressors will be similar with development of increased systolic and diastolic pressures. The response to exercise and increased venous return will again result in similar alterations, resulting in marked elevations of diastolic pressures in response to limited increases in venous return and end-diastolic volumes.

Summary

From a pathophysiologic point of view, diastolic dysfunction of the heart may be considered as an early stage of a more global dysfunction of the heart. It is, however, a stage in which stress and exercise may elicit abnormal cardiovascular responses leading to limitations and symptoms.

When we face advanced heart failure with reduced EF, diastolic dysfunction with disturbances of myocardial relaxation and of end-diastolic LV properties inevitably contribute to an important extent to symptoms and signs of forward and backward failure. There is, however, a distinct disease of ventricular arterial stiffening in which diastolic dysfunction is the leading pathophysiologic mechanism. The main features of this disease are the following:

- Impaired LV filling. In order to understand this impairment we have to critically review possible causes of delayed myocardial relaxation, diastolic stiffness, and other causes that might interfere with filling.
- Impaired contractile function of the LV. Instead of using longitudinal shortening and twisting–untwisting of the ventricle, a merely linear type of mechanical activity is substituted, with emphasis on a piston-type radial inward–outward motion.
- Increased systolic LV elastance matched with an increased arterial elastance.
- Impaired diastolic Frank-Starling reserve due to alterations of passive end-diastolic properties.
- Impaired response to fluctuations in cardiovascular volume, to stress, and to exercise.

References

1. Guyton AC. Determination of cardiac output by equating venous return curves with cardiac response curves. Physiol Rev 1955;35:123–129.

2. De Hert SG, Gillebert TC, Ten Broecke PW, Moulijn AC. Length-dependent regulation of left ventricular function in coronary surgery patients. Anesthesiology 1999;91:379–387.

3. Leite-Moreira AF, Gillebert TC. Nonuniform course of left ventricular pressure fall and its regulation by load and contractile state. Circulation 1994;90:2481–2491.

4. Leite-Moreira AF, Correia-Pinto J, Gillebert TC. Afterload induced changes in myocardial relaxation: A mechanism for diastolic dysfunction. Cardiovasc Res 1999;43:344–353.

5. Warner JG, Metzger DC, Kitzman DW, Wesley DJ, Little WC. Losartan improves exercise tolerance in patients with diastolic dysfunction and a hypertensive response to exercise. J Am Coll Cardiol 1999;33:1567–1572.

6. De Hert SG, Gillebert TC, Ten Broecke PW, Mertens E, Rodrigus IE, Moulijn AC. Contraction–relaxation coupling and impaired left ventricular performance in coronary surgery patients. Anesthesiology 1999;90:748–757.

7. Gillebert TC, Leite-Moreira AF, De Hert SG. Relaxation-systolic pressure relation. A load-independent assessment of left ventricular contractility. Circulation 1997;95:745–752.

8. Swynghedauw B. Molecular mechanisms of myocardial remodeling. Physiol Rev 1999;79:215–262.

9. Eichhorn EJ, Willard JE, Alvarez L, Kim AS, Glamann DB, Risser RC, Grayburn PA. Are contraction and relaxation coupled in patients with and without congestive-heart-failure? Circulation 1992;85:2132–2139.

10. Kass DA. Ventricular arterial stiffening: integrating the pathophysiology. Hypertension 2005;46:185–193.

11. Gandhi SK, Powers JC, Nomeir AM, Fowle K, Kitzman DW, Rankin KM, Little WC. The pathogenesis of acute pulmonary edema associated with hypertension. N Engl J Med 2001;344:17–22.

12. Leite-Moreira AF, Correia-Pinto J, Gillebert TC. Diastolic dysfunction and hypertension. N Engl J Med 2001;344:1401.

13. Little WC. Enhanced load dependence of relaxation in heart-failure — clinical implications. Circulation 1992;85:2326–2328.

14. Little WC. Diastolic dysfunction beyond distensibility: adverse effects of ventricular dilatation. Circulation 2005;112:2888–2890.

15. Gillebert TC, Leite-Moreira AF, De Hert SG. Load dependent diastolic dysfunction in heart failure. Heart Fail Rev 2000;5:345–355.

16. Wiggers CJ. Studies on the consecutive phases of the cardiac cycle: I. The duration of the consecutive phases of the cardiac cycle and the criteria for their precise determination. Am J Physiol 1921;56:415–438.

17. Brutsaert DL, Declerck NM, Goethals MA, Housmans PR. Relaxation of ventricular cardiac-muscle. J Physiol (Lond) 1978;283:469–480.

18. Shintani H, Glantz SA. The left ventricular pressure–volume relation, relaxation and filling. In Gaasch WH, Lewinter MM, eds. Left Ventricular Diastolic Function and Heart Failure. Philadelphia: Lea & Febiger; 1994:103–117.

19. Grossman W. Evaluation of systolic and diastolic function of the ventricles and myocardium. In Baim SB, ed. Grossman's Cardiac Catheterisation, Angiography and Intervention, 7th ed. Philadelphia: Lippincott Williams & Wilkins; 2006:315–332.

20. Leite-Moreira AF, Correira-Pinto J. Load as an acute determinant of end-diastolic pressure-volume relation. Am J Physiol Heart Circ Physiol 2001;280:H51–H59.

21. Weisfeldt ML, Frederiksen JW, Yin FC, Weiss JL. Evidence of incomplete left ventricular relaxation in the dog: prediction from the time constant for isovolumic pressure fall. J Clin Invest 1978;62:1296–1302.

22. Glantz SA, Parmley WW. Factors which affect the diastolic pressure–volume curve. Circ Res 1978;42:171–180.

23. Paulus WJ, Grossman W, Serizawa T, Bourdillon PD, Pasipoularides A, Mirsky I. Different effects of two types of ischemia on myocardial systolic and diastolic function. Am J Physiol 1985;248:H719–H728.

24. Paulus WJ, Vantrimpont PJ, Shah AM. Acute effects of nitric oxide on left ventricular relaxation and diastolic distensibility in humans. Assessment by bicoronary sodium nitroprusside infusion. Circulation 1994;89:2070–2078.

25. Grossman W. Diastolic dysfunction in congestive heart failure. N Engl J Med 1991;325:1557–1564.

26. Weiss JL, Frederiksen JW, Weisfeldt ML. Hemodynamic determinants of the time-course of fall in canine left ventricular pressure. J Clin Invest 1976;58:751–760.

27. Matsubara H, Takaki M, Yasuhara S, Araki J, Suga H. Logistic time constant of isovolumic relaxation pressure–time curve in the canine left ventricle. Better alternative to exponential time constant. Circulation 1995;92:2318–2326.

28. Gaasch WH, Blaustein AS, Andrias CW, Donahue RP, Avitall B. Myocardial relaxation. II. Hemodynamic determinants of rate of left ventricular

isovolumic pressure decline. Am J Physiol 1980;239:H1–H6.

29. Correia-Pinto J, Henriques-Coelho T, Magalhaes S, Leite-Moreira AF. Pattern of right ventricular pressure fall and its modulation by afterload. Physiol Res 2004;53:19–26.

30. Brutsaert DL, Sys SU. Relaxation and diastole of the heart. Physiol Rev 1989;69:1228–1315.

31. Leite-Moreira AF, Correia-Pinto J, Gillebert TC. Load dependence of left ventricular contraction and relaxation. Effects of caffeine. Basic Res Cardiol 1999;94:284–293.

32. Leite-Moreira AF, Correia-Pinto J, Henriques-Coelho T. [Interaction between load and beta-adrenergic stimulation in the modulation of diastolic function.] Rev Port Cardiol 2001;20:57–62.

33. Correia-Pinto J, Henriques-Coelho T, Oliveira SM, Leite-Moreira AF. Distinct load dependence of relaxation rate and diastolic function in *Oryctolagus cuniculus* and *Ratus norvegicus*. J Comp Physiol [B] 2003;173:401–407.

34. Correia PJ, Henriques-Coelho T, Roncon-Albuquerque R Jr, Leite-Moreira AF. Differential right and left ventricular diastolic tolerance to acute afterload and NCX gene expression in Wistar rats. Physiol Res 2006;55:513–526.

35. Takimoto E, Soergel DG, Janssen PML, Stull LB, Kass DA, Murphy AM. Frequency- and afterload-dependent cardiac modulation in vivo by troponin I with constitutively active protein kinase a phosphorylation sites. Circ Res 2004;94:496–504.

36. Kass DA, Bronzwaer JG, Paulus WJ. What mechanisms underlie diastolic dysfunction in heart failure? Circ Res 2004;94:1533–1542.

37. Bers DM. Cardiac excitation–contraction coupling. Nature 2002;415:198–205.

38. Leite-Moreira AF. Current perspectives in diastolic dysfunction and diastolic heart failure. Heart 2006;92:712–718.

39. Cartwright EJ, Schuh K, Neyses L. Calcium transport in cardiovascular health and disease — the sarcolemmal calcium pump enters the stage. J Mol Cell Cardiol 2005;39:403–406.

40. Zile MR, Brutsaert DL. New concepts in diastolic dysfunction and diastolic heart failure. Part II: causal mechanisms and treatment. Circulation 2002;105:1503–1508.

41. Gaasch WH, Zile MR. Left ventricular diastolic dysfunction and diastolic heart failure. Annu Rev Med 2004;55:373–394.

42. Angeja BG, Grossman W. Evaluation and management of diastolic heart failure. Circulation 2003;107:659–663.

43. Badke FR, Boinay P, Covell JW. Effects of ventricular pacing on regional left ventricular performance in the dog. Am J Physiol 1980;238:H858–H867.

44. Gaasch WH, Blaustein AS, Bing OH. Asynchronous (segmental early) relaxation of the left ventricle. J Am Coll Cardiol 1985;5:891–897.

45. Lew WY, Rasmussen CM. Influence of nonuniformity on rate of left ventricular pressure fall in the dog. Am J Physiol 1989;256:H222–H232.

46. Gillebert TC, Lew WY. Nonuniformity and volume loading independently influence isovolumic relaxation rates. Am J Physiol 1989;257:H1927–H1935.

47. Leite-Moreira AF, Gillebert TC. Myocardial relaxation in regionally stunned left ventricle. Am J Physiol 1996;270:H509–H517.

48. Granzier HL, Labeit S. The giant protein titin: a major player in myocardial mechanics, signaling, and disease. Circ Res 2004;94:284–295.

49. Borbely A, van der Velden J., Papp Z, Bronzwaer JG, Edes I, Stienen GJ, Paulus WJ. Cardiomyocyte stiffness in diastolic heart failure. Circulation 2005;111:774–781.

50. Little WC, Zile MR, Kitzman DW, Hundley WG, O'Brien TX, Degroof RC. The effect of alagebrium chloride (ALT-711), a novel glucose cross-link breaker, in the treatment of elderly patients with diastolic heart failure. J Card Fail 2005;11:191–195.

51. Paulus WJ, Shah AM. NO and cardiac diastolic function. Cardiovasc Res 1999;43:595–606.

52. Leite-Moreira AF, Bras-Silva C, Pedrosa CA, Rocha-Sousa AA. ET-1 increases distensibility of acutely loaded myocardium: a novel ETA and Na^+/H^+ exchanger–mediated effect. Am J Physiol Heart Circ Physiol 2003;284:H1332–H1339.

53. Yamasaki R, Wu Y, McNabb M, Greaser M, Labeit S, Granzier H. Protein kinase A phosphorylates titin's cardiac-specific N2B domain and reduces passive tension in rat cardiac myocytes. Circ Res 2002;90:1181–1188.

54. Leite-Moreira AF, Castro-Chaves P, Pimentel-Nunes P, Lima-Carneiro A, Guerra MS, Soares JB, Ferreira-Martins J. Angiotensin II acutely decreases myocardial stiffness: a novel AT1, PKC and Na+/H+ exchanger–mediated effect. Br J Pharmacol 2006;147:690–697.

55. Brown RD, Ambler SK, Mitchell MD, Long CS. The cardiac fibroblast: therapeutic target in myocardial remodeling and failure. Annu Rev Pharmacol Toxicol 2005;45:657–687.

56. Brunner F, Bras-Silva C, Cerdeira AS, Leite-Moreira AF. Cardiovascular endothelins: essential regulators of cardiovascular homeostasis. Pharmacol Ther 2006;111:508–531.

57. Clozel M, Salloukh H. Role of endothelin in fibrosis and anti-fibrotic potential of bosentan. Ann Med 2005;37:2–12.

58. McElmurray JH, III, Mukherjee R, New RB, Sampson AC, King MK, Hendrick JW, Goldberg A, Peterson TJ, Hallak H, Zile MR, Spinale FG. Angiotensin-converting enzyme and matrix metalloproteinase inhibition with developing heart failure: comparative effects on left ventricular function and geometry. J Pharmacol Exp Ther 1999;291:799–811.

59. Grossman W, Barry WH. Diastolic pressure–volume relations in the diseased heart. Fed Proc 1980;39:148–155.

60. Westerhof N, Stergiopoulos N, Noble MIM. Snapshots of Hemodynamics. New York: Springer Science; 2005.

61. Claessens TE, Rietzschel ER, De Buyzere ML, De Bacquer D, De Backer G, Gillebert TC, Verdonck PR, Segers P. Noninvasive assessment of left ventricular and myocardial contractility in middle-aged men and women: disparate evolution above the age of 50? Am J Physiol Heart Circ Physiol 2007;292:H856–865.

62. Chen CH, Fetics B, Nevo E, Rochitte CE, Chiou KR, Ding PA, Kawaguchi M, Kass DA. Noninvasive single-beat determination of left ventricular end-systolic elastance in humans. J Am Coll Cardiol 2001;38:2028–2034.

63. Kawaguchi M, Hay I, Fetics B, Kass DA. Combined ventricular systolic and arterial stiffening in patients with heart failure and preserved ejection fraction: implications for systolic and diastolic reserve limitations. Circulation 2003;107:714–720.

64. Redfield MM, Jacobsen SJ, Borlaug BA, Rodeheffer RJ, Kass DA. Age- and gender-related ventricular-vascular stiffening: a community-based study. Circulation 2005;112:2254–2262.

65. Massie BM. Natriuretic peptide measurements for the diagnosis of "nonsystolic" heart failure — good news and bad. J Am Coll Cardiol 2003;41:2018–2021.

66. Gillebert TC, Lew WYW. Influence of systolic pressure profile on rate of left-ventricular pressure fall. Am J Physiol 1991;261:H805–H813.

67. Murgo JP, Westerhof N, Giolma JP, Altobelli SA. Aortic input impedance in normal man: relationship to pressure wave forms. Circulation 1980;62:105–116.

68. Kaplan NM, Opie LH. Controversies in cardiology 2 — controversies in hypertension. Lancet 2006;367:168–176.

69. Segers P, Rietzschel ER, De Buyzere ML, Vermeersch SJ, De Bacquer D, Van Bortel LM, De Backer G, Gillebert TC, Verdonck PR; Asklepios investigators. Noninvasive (input) impedance, pulse wave velocity, and wave reflection in healthy middle-aged men and women. Hypertension 2007;49:1248–1255.

70. Safar ME, Levy BI, Struijker-Boudier H. Current perspectives on arterial stiffness and pulse pressure in hypertension and cardiovascular diseases. Circulation 2003;107:2864–2869.

3
Ventricular Interaction via the Septum and Pericardium

Israel Belenkie, Eldon R. Smith, and John V. Tyberg

Introduction

The key to understanding ventricular interaction is to have an appreciation of how constraint to left ventricular (LV) filling can affect the true LV distending pressure (i.e., LV transmural pressure) and how the diastolic position and systolic function of the ventricular septum is affected by the relationship between LV and right ventricular (RV) end-diastolic pressures (i.e., the end-diastolic transseptal pressure gradient).

Transmural Pressure

The pericardium is effectively nondistensible acutely, the relation between stretch and tension being J-shaped.[1] Therefore, when the volume of the heart increases to the point where pericardial pressure begins to increase, further increases in cardiac volume are dramatically limited by the pericardium. Effective distending pressure[2] is the pressure difference across the chamber wall, that is, transmural pressure. This principle is rarely important with respect to systolic pressures,[3] but it may be critical with respect to diastolic pressures.[4] During diastole, the ventricles fill in proportion to transmural pressure, not intracavitary pressure; this is frequently overlooked because changes in intracavitary pressure often (but not always) reflect changes in transmural pressure (i.e., both will change in the same direction) and it is easy to measure.

It had been thought that the relationship between LV end-diastolic pressure and volume, so-called diastolic compliance,[5] was practically invariant. This assumption was the basis for Sarnoff's ventricular function curve analysis in which LV end-diastolic pressure was used to reflect LV end-diastolic volume, or LV preload.[6] However, diastolic compliance was believed to change rapidly, for example, by giving nitroglycerin in heart failure.[7] It was later suggested that this was due to unappreciated decreases in pericardial pressure,[8] but many believed this was unlikely because pericardial pressure had been thought to be negative and unchanging, even as RV end-diastolic pressure was raised to high values.[9] It was then shown that an artifact of the measurement technique for pericardial pressure accounted for that misconception. When pericardial pressure was more accurately measured,[10,11] such as with a flat, liquid-containing balloon transducer, it became clear that an open catheter seriously underestimates pericardial pressure unless there is an increased amount of fluid in the pericardial space. It is important to note that, fortuitously, pericardial pressure is similar to mean right atrial pressure and that both increase in parallel during volume loading.[12,13] Thus, pericardial pressure is changeable acutely and is approximately equal to RV end-diastolic pressure in most circumstances (transmural RV end-diastolic pressure, which is RV end-diastolic pressure minus pericardial pressure, is very low).[14,15] Without an excess of liquid, pericardial pressure is fundamentally a compressive contact stress.[11] Because of the normally thin wall of the right atrium, right atrial pressure also reflects external constraint during mechanical ventilation as well, as shown in both animal and clinical studies.[14,16]

The similarities between right atrial and pericardial pressures[12,17] and between pulmonary capillary wedge and LV end-diastolic pressures allows (in most circumstances) for a clinically useful estimate of LV transmural pressure and its equivalent, the transseptal pressure gradient. Because changes in right atrial pressure parallel changes in pericardial pressure and pulmonary capillary wedge pressure is usually similar to LV end-diastolic pressure, the difference between right atrial and pulmonary capillary wedge pressures approximates transmural LV end-diastolic pressure (and the transseptal pressure gradient as well).[18] Thus, as Smiseth et al.[19] have shown, measurement of pulmonary capillary and right atrial pressures in mechanically ventilated patients can provide reliable estimates of changes in LV end-diastolic volume during volume manipulation. It should be noted, however, that because small changes in transmural pressure may be hemodynamically important,[20] it is important that the pressure measurements be as precise as possible to provide reliable estimates of changes in LV preload.

Figure 3.1 shows data from a patient with severe congestive heart failure due to cardiomyopathy and atrial fibrillation. The top panel shows the beat-to-beat relations between pulmonary capillary wedge pressure and LV end-diastolic volume (estimated by the planimetered echo minor-axis view on a cycle-by-cycle basis). There is no clear relation present. In the bottom panel, estimated transmural LV end-diastolic pressure (pulmonary capillary wedge minus RA pressure) has a clear relationship with LV end-diastolic volume, as it should. In this case, the wedge pressure was clearly misleading as a predictor of LV end-diastolic volume (see later discussion of congestive heart failure).

One of several excellent demonstrations of how the pericardium affects intracavitary pressure and the LV pressure–volume (PV) relation is a study by Smiseth et al.[21] in which pericardial pressure, vascular capacitance, and diastolic PV relations were correlated in dogs. Angiotensin decreased abdominal vascular capacitance, increased pericardial pressure, and shifted the PV curve upward and to the right. Sodium nitroprusside had the opposite effects. These observations might be interpreted as a change in myocardial compliance. However, there was no shift of the diastolic

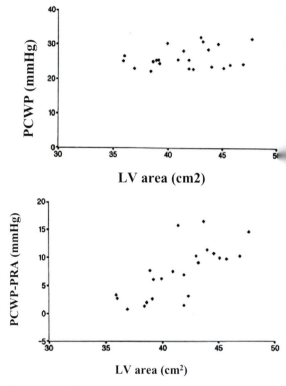

FIGURE 3.1. Left ventricular (LV) cross-sectional area, minor-axis area (echo). PCWP, pulmonary capillary wedge pressure; PRA, right atrial pressure. See text for further discussion.

PV relations when the pericardium was removed, indicating that myocardial compliance had, in fact, not changed. Similar results were observed during acute ischemia caused by balloon inflation during angioplasty and after induced ischemia in dogs (see later).

In practical terms, if one is to assess changes in LV preload indirectly using pressure measurements, it is necessary to consider how both LV intracavitary and the surrounding pressures might change. Pressure–volume relations observed in the dog clearly show how the pericardium can alter the curves, the differences in the y-axis being due to pericardial constraint.[22] For example, if LV end-diastolic pressure is 12 mm Hg, it is 12 mm Hg greater than atmospheric pressure. However, if pericardial pressure is 4 mm Hg, transmural LV end-diastolic pressure, which is the real or effective distending pressure, is 8 mm Hg. If intracavitary pressure increases to 15 mm Hg and pericardial pressure increases to 7 mm Hg, transmural pressure is still 8 mm Hg and LV end-diastolic volume will not have changed. As shown in Figure 3.2, as intracavitary pressure is increased during volume loading, LV end-diastolic volume usually increases (as long as the increase in intracavitary pressure is greater than that surrounding the LV) to a point where further increases are limited by the pericardium. The difference between intracavitary and transmural pressures is the pericardial pressure. In the top panel, the increase in intracavitary pressure is greater than the increase in pericardial pressure so that trans-

mural pressure is increased during volume loading. If the increase in intracavitary pressure is less than the increase in the surrounding pressure, as illustrated in the bottom panel, transmural pressure has actually decreased despite the fact that the intracavitary pressure has increased. Examples of how intracavitary and transmural pressure can change in opposite directions are presented later. Therefore, although the use of changes in intracavitary pressure to reflect changes in preload is often accurate, it can also be misleading.

There are similar issues regarding the interpretation of studies of diastolic function by Doppler echocardiography. Although the pericardium may contribute substantially to what is generally considered to be LV myocardial compliance, it is most often ignored. Loading conditions can clearly affect Doppler indices of diastolic function; the pericardial contribution to compliance is most often not considered in that context so that the implication is that myocardial compliance alone is being assessed. That this is not necessarily true is supported by a number of studies. For example, volume loading, inferior vena cava occlusion, head-up tilting, as well as lower-body negative and positive pressures result in changes in the Doppler assessment of diastolic function, indicating that loading conditions can substantially alter diastolic function despite the fact that *myocardial distensibility* per se must have remain unchanged.[23–27] As heart failure improves with various forms of treatment in patients, there are distinct changes in the Doppler measurements in both ventricles over short periods of time during which changes in myocardial compliance are unlikely to have occurred to account for those changes.[27–29] Similarly, administration of sodium nitroprusside and head-up tilting caused changes in the Doppler measurements in both normal and abnormal subjects that could not be explained by myocardial changes.[30,31] It is possible that longer term changes in these measurements reflect changes in the myocardium, but this has not been adequately studied.[28] Even during acute ischemia, shifts in the diastolic PV relations may be largely accounted for by pericardial constraint and not by changes in myocardial compliance.[32,33] Inferior vena occlusion or removal of the pericardium obliterates the apparent shifts in the curves during

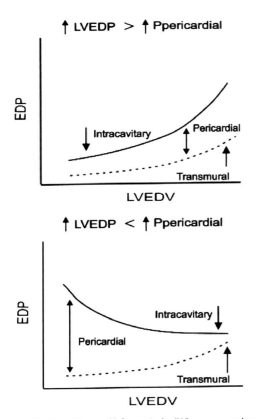

FIGURE 3.2. **(Top)** The usual left ventricular (LV) pressure–volume relation. As intracavitary pressure is increased (e.g., by volume loading), the increase in intracavitary pressure (the solid line) is greater than the increase in pericardial pressure so that the difference between the two, transmural pressure, also increases. **(Bottom)** The transmural pressure–volume relation is unchanged. However, if pericardial pressure increases more than the intracavitary pressure during volume loading, transmural pressure will decrease despite increased intracavitary pressure. In this situation, changes in intracavitary pressure do not reflect changes in volume. EDP, end-diastolic pressure; LVEDV, LV end-diastolic volume; $P_{pericardial}$, pericardial pressure.

diastole. That direct ventricular interaction is closely related to the restrictive filling pattern in congestive heart failure provides additional evidence that the pericardium contributes to Doppler indices of diastolic function; patients with a restrictive filling pattern are more likely to exhibit direct ventricular interaction (see later).[34]

Ventricular Septum

The septum is compliant and shifts leftward or rightward with small changes in the difference between LV and RV pressures during diastole (i.e., end-diastolic transseptal pressure gradient = LV minus RV end-diastolic pressure). Therefore, small changes in the transseptal pressure gradient can shift the septum in either direction (more positive to the right and more negative to the left), thereby affecting the volumes of both ventricles.[35] Figure 3.3 shows data from an animal experiment in which small thrombi were repeatedly injected intravenously (lodging in the lungs) with volume loading between injections. As the transseptal gradient decreased, the septum-to-RV free wall diameter increased and the septum-to-LV free wall diameter decreased. Leftward septal shift can be considerable and result in septal flattening or even inversion. During systole, when the septum is considerably less compliant, a similar, but steeper transseptal gradient–septal position relation exists.[36] When the difference between LV and RV systolic pressures is small, the septum will be flattened during systole as well.

Ventricular Interaction

Ventricular interaction includes both series and direct interaction. Series interaction is defined by the simple relation between RV and LV outputs; transit time through the lungs and other aspects of heart–lung interaction account for beat-to-beat differences in output, but the outputs must be equal over any substantial interval of time. Direct ventricular interaction can be defined as the instantaneous, complementary changes in RV and LV end-diastolic volumes such that, when RV end-diastolic volume increases, LV end-diastolic volume decreases and vice versa. This (direct) interaction is modulated by external constraint, either pericardial or that due to other mediastinal structures. Because the pericardium is, in the short term, effectively nondistensible, RV end-diastolic volume can increase only "at the expense" of LV end-diastolic volume in the presence of pericardial constraint. When the pericardium is opened and the lungs held back from the heart, direct ventricular interaction is substantially less[37,38] and similar to the limited interaction that occurs when pericardial pressure is very low.[39]

The complementary change in RV and LV end-diastolic volumes in the presence of pericardial constraint occurs most frequently by septal shift

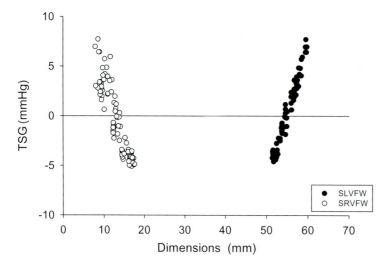

FIGURE 3.3. Data from an animal experiment in which small thrombi were repeatedly injected intravenously, with volume loading between injections. SLVFW, septum-to-left ventricular free wall diameter; SRVFW, septum-to-right ventricular free wall diameter; TSG, end-diastolic transseptal pressure gradient.

3. Ventricular Interaction

alone, effected by the transseptal pressure gradient. Therefore, changes in the transseptal gradient are a convenient indicator of ventricular interaction in these circumstances. Mirsky and Rankin[40] noted that the LV is surrounded by the pericardium over approximately two-thirds of its surface and by the RV over the remaining third. Therefore, when changes in RV and pericardial pressure are not similar,[41] it is best to modify the definition of transmural pressure to better account for these differences in constraint around the LV (= 1/3 RV end-diastolic pressure + 2/3 pericardial pressure).[38]

Pulmonary Hypertension — The Common Denominator

Let us first consider ventricular interaction in acute and chronic pulmonary hypertension and in chronic, severe congestive heart failure. In these conditions, direct ventricular interaction may contribute substantially to the hemodynamic responses to disease or therapeutic interventions. The common denominator is the presence of pulmonary hypertension — because of the increased RV afterload, there is the potential for LV and RV end-diastolic pressures and volumes to change by different amounts in response to a change in the condition or during volume manipulation. In the presence of pericardial constraint, changes in the transseptal pressure gradient may cause substantial septal shift, which can result in significant changes in both LV and RV end-diastolic volumes; when this happens, intracavitary pressures may not reflect the true preload, and the two may actually change in opposite directions. It is important to keep in mind that direct ventricular interaction is largely dependent on the presence of external constraint (most often pericardial unless the effect of the lungs is increased as during mechanical ventilation[42]) such that the total volume of the ventricles cannot be significantly increased.

Acute Pulmonary Hypertension

Acute pulmonary hypertension is the best-studied example of direct ventricular interaction. The most commonly employed experimental model has been pulmonary artery constriction. When the artery is constricted, RV output is decreased as would be predicted, and, as a consequence, LV output also decreases by the series mechanism. In addition, RV end-diastolic pressure increases while LV end-diastolic pressure usually decreases. Thus, the transseptal pressure gradient is decreased and may even become negative with severe constriction. As a result, the septum shifts leftward and either flattens or inverts.[43] Right ventricular end-diastolic volume increases, and LV end-diastolic volume (and transmural pressure) decreases; because the LV anteroposterior diameter does not change in this model, the decreased LV end-diastolic volume is due to leftward septal shift.

It has long been believed (and still is by many) that volume loading in acute RV failure due to acute pulmonary embolism would be beneficial via the Frank-Starling mechanism. Logic suggested that if the RV is failing, increased RV preload would improve RV preload and output and thus LV output. This was supported by measurements of filling pressures — both RV and LV end-diastolic pressures increase as fluid is administered, suggesting that preload is increased in both ventricles. However, this is an excellent illustration of the importance of understanding all aspects of ventricular interaction.[20,44,45] As illustrated in Figure 3.4, with the pericardium intact, the LV end-diastolic pressure–LV end-diastolic volume and LV stroke work–LV end-diastolic pressure relations suggest that pulmonary embolism and subsequent volume loading decreased LV compliance and contractility.[20] However, when diastolic compliance and contractility were more appropriately evaluated using transmural instead of intracavitary pressure (and also by LV dimensions measured by sonomicrometry), it is clear that LV myocardial compliance and contractility were unaffected by the embolism, that is, there was no shift in the transmural PV or transmural pressure–stroke work relations.[46] Despite the increased LV end-diastolic pressure during volume loading after the injections of clot, *transmural LV end-diastolic pressure and volume (as well as LV dimensions) actually decreased* and resulted in decreased stroke work and worsening hypotension. In these circumstances, that is, after inappropriate volume loading, volume removal

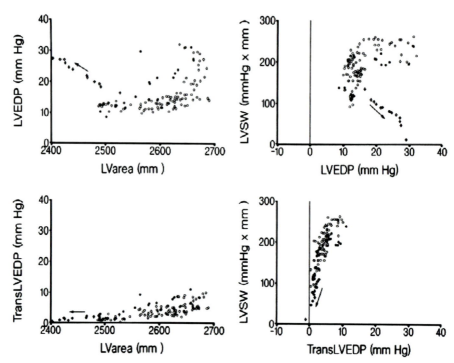

FIGURE 3.4. (Top) In the left panel, the left ventricular (LV) end-diastolic pressure (LVEDP)–LV cross-sectional area (our LV end-diastolic volume index) relation suggests that LV compliance has changed after multiple embolizations and subsequent volume loading. The arrow shows what occurred when the animal was very hypotensive. As LVEDP increased, LV end-diastolic volume (LVarea) decreased. Similarly, the right panel suggests that LV contractility has decreased; as LVEDP increased, stroke work (LVSW) decreased. (Bottom) However, when transmural pressure (transLVEDP) was used to correctly reflect LV preload, LV end-diastolic volume and stroke work were closely related, and single relations described both compliance and contractility (both were unchanged). The arrows depict the same cardiac cycles as those shown in the upper panels.

increased transmural LV pressure and volume and stroke work, despite the decreased intracavitary pressure. In the absence of external constraint, this apparent paradoxical response to volume manipulation was not observed.[45] Volume loading increased RV and LV outputs after embolism caused hemodynamic deterioration, provided the embolism was not quickly fatal. Thus, in these experimental models, embolism was better tolerated with the pericardium open, and subsequent volume loading also improved output. This demonstrated that external constraint to LV filling is responsible for some of the decreased cardiac output — the pericardium and leftward shifted septum constrained LV filling and triggered hemodynamic deterioration. When constraint was absent, the RV was able to increase stroke output in response to volume loading as opposed to what occurred when LV filling was limited by external constraint (when volume loading decreased LV preload).

These observations suggest that, although RV failure is important, the trigger for hemodynamic deterioration during embolism and subsequent volume loading is constraint to LV filling. The importance of this constraint was also demonstrated by opening the pericardium during acute pulmonary artery constriction; intracavitary pressures decreased, but LV transmural pressure increased and resulted in a substantially increased stroke work.[37] Although systematic clinical confirmation of these principles is still lacking, we have anecdotal experiences that are completely in keeping with these concepts. A clinical study of volume loading in acute pulmonary embolism did suggest that volume loading was actually beneficial in most cases.[47] However, the patients studied had a mean systemic arterial pressure of approxi-

Chronic Pulmonary Hypertension

It is clear that direct ventricular interaction is also relevant in chronic pulmonary hypertension. Diastolic flattening of the ventricular septum, frequently observed in patients with significant pulmonary hypertension, indicates that the end-diastolic transseptal pressure gradient is low or negative because of increased RV relative to LV end-diastolic pressure. Systolic septal flattening is an indication of near-systemic RV systolic pressure. Diastolic flattening of the septum should not be considered diagnostic of pulmonary hypertension per se, because it is the reduced transseptal pressure gradient that causes the septum to shift leftward and flatten. Septal flattening is also seen in nonpulmonary hypertensive conditions such as atrial septal defect (LV and RV end-diastolic pressures are similar, and the transseptal gradient is therefore approximately zero) and tricuspid regurgitation (increased RV compared with LV end-diastolic pressure).

Jardin et al.,[48] using flow-directed pulmonary artery catheters and echocardiography, have shown that the paradoxical response to volume loading described earlier can also occur in patients with chronic obstructive lung disease, presumably in those patients with significant pulmonary hypertension. An infusion of saline caused a decrease in LV end-diastolic volume and stroke work in some of the patients in association with a greater increase in right atrial than pulmonary capillary wedge pressure. The implied mechanism underlying this response is the greater increase in RV compared with LV end-diastolic pressure during volume loading, resulting in a decreased transseptal pressure gradient and thus a leftward septal shift. The decreased LV end-diastolic volume occurred despite the increased intra-cavitary pressure. Clearly, transmural LV end-diastolic pressure decreased in those patients with the decreased LV end-diastolic volume.

In an intraoperative study of patients with severe pulmonary hypertension due to chronic thromboembolic disease, opening the pericardium resulted in no significant chamber dimension or hemodynamic changes, which suggests that pericardial pressure was not increased much because of chronic remodeling.[49] This interpretation of the data appears to be correct for the patients studied; however, the mean RV end-diastolic pressure of 8 mm Hg suggests that the patients were not volume overloaded when studied. This study did not address the effects of pericardial constraint in decompensated patients; the study by Jardin et al.[48] suggests that, when right-sided filling pressures are acutely increased, pericardial pressure would be more important.

Congestive Heart Failure

It is commonly believed that there is a descending limb of the Starling curve in congestive heart failure, that is, with excessive myocardial fiber stretch, myocardial contractility decreases. Among the data supporting this concept are reports of improved cardiac function during phlebotomy,[50] during nitroglycerin infusion,[51] or with tailored therapy.[52] In the latter study, stroke work improved substantially when pulmonary capillary wedge pressure was reduced in response to treatment. The increased stroke work associated with the decreased filling pressure could not be attributed to changes in systemic vascular resistance, but perhaps decreased mitral regurgitation (not assessed) played a role. That this may not fully explain their results is suggested by the responses to nitroglycerin in some patients with severe heart failure in another study; LV end-diastolic volume increased, and in those patients stroke work also tended to increase.[51] The increased LV end-diastolic volume cannot be explained by reduced mitral regurgitation so that some other mechanism(s) must have contributed to the improved stroke work. However, as explained earlier in the section discussing LV transmural pressure, the use of filling pressures to reflect preload, while often appropriate, occasionally is misleading. This was already apparent in the preceding discussions of pulmonary hypertension. A descending limb of the Starling curve has not been

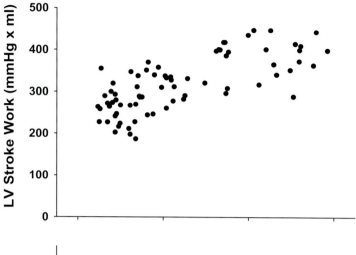

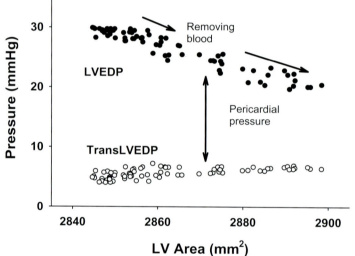

FIGURE 3.5. **(Top)** The rapid-pacing model of congestive heart failure showing the predicted left ventricular (LV) stroke work–end-diastolic volume relation. **(Bottom)** As blood was removed, intracavitary LV pressure decreased, but transmural LV end-diastolic pressure (TransLVEDP) increased, the difference being pericardial pressure. (From Kohl P, Sachs F, Franz MR. Cardiac Mechano-Electric Feedback and Arrhythmias. Philadelphia: WB Saunders; 2005. ©2005, with permission from Elsevier.)

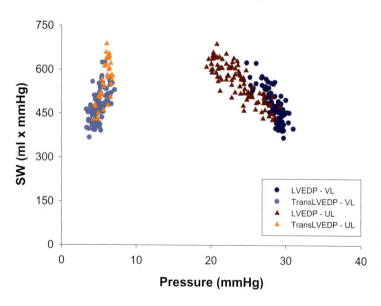

FIGURE 3.6. Transmural left ventricular (LV) end-diastolic pressure (LVEDP)–LV stroke work (SW) relation. TransLVEDP, transmural LVEDP; UL, removal of volume; VL, volume load. (From Moore et al.[55])

demonstrated in mammalian hearts in which ventricular volume measurements were used to reflect LV preload. Experimental work has shown that, in the mammalian heart, attempts to passively stretch myocardium beyond a sarcomere length of 23 μm tears rather than lengthens the fibers.[53]

In chronic, severe congestive heart failure, clinical deterioration is often associated with very high pulmonary artery pressure, with systolic pulmonary artery pressures as high as 70–90 mm Hg. The increased RV afterload simulates the conditions described earlier, and therefore there is the potential for LV and RV end-diastolic pressures to change by different amounts in response to volume manipulation; that is, RV end-diastolic pressure may increase more than LV end-diastolic pressure. Atherton et al.[54] used lower body negative pressure to test for direct ventricular interaction in patients with severe heart failure who had already been optimally treated. In all the control subjects, LV end-diastolic volume decreased when lower body negative pressure was applied. However, in approximately 40% of the patients, LV end-diastolic volume increased despite the presumed decrease in intracavitary pressure (not measured). Pulmonary artery and capillary wedge pressures were higher in those patients in whom LV end-diastolic volume increased than in those in whom it decreased. It is interesting that lower body negative pressure increased LV end-diastolic volume in most patients with a restrictive filling pattern on the Doppler studies but rarely in those without restrictive filling patterns.[34] Given that direct ventricular interaction is modulated by pericardial constraint, these results are in keeping with the suggested contribution of the pericardium to the Doppler assessment of diastolic function.

Subsequently, Moore et al.[55] clearly showed that direct ventricular interaction was the mechanism by which the apparently paradoxic changes in LV end-diastolic volume occurred in a rapid pacing model of congestive heart failure; septal shift accounted for the responses to volume manipulation just as it did in the acute pulmonary embolism model. As shown in Figure 3.5, as intracavitary pressure decreased during volume removal, transmural LV end-diastolic pressure (and LV end-diastolic volume) increased (bottom panel) just as stroke work increased (top panel) in parallel. The difference between the intracavitary and transmural pressures is pericardial pressure. In Figure 3.6, although a descending limb of the Frank-Starling curve was suggested when LV end-diastolic pressure is used to reflect LV end-diastolic volume during volume loading and unloading, the transmural LV end-diastolic pressure–stroke work relation was positive (as were the relations between transmural pressure and myocardial segment length), indicating that the apparent descending limb was an artifact and reflecting the fact that intracavitary pressure did not reflect LV preload accurately in this model.

Janicki[56] has demonstrated that pericardial constraint may also play an important role during exercise in chronic congestive heart failure. He showed that when stroke volume increased, the increase in pulmonary capillary wedge pressure was two to three times greater than the increase in right atrial pressure (which implies that transmural LV end-diastolic pressure and therefore LV preload increased) and that when the two pressures changed similarly (implying no change in transmural LV pressure), stroke volume also did not change.

Ventricular Interaction During Mechanical Ventilation

Heart–lung interaction during mechanical ventilation is complex, and a detailed discussion is beyond the scope of this chapter. However, elements of the phasic hemodynamic changes that occur during mechanical lung inflation and deflation imply that septal shift likely contributes to the hemodynamic responses to changes in airway pressure. Because increased airway pressure can also substantially constrain ventricular filling, the effects of changing airway pressure on septal position and external constraint deserve specific consideration.

During mechanical ventilation, constraint by the increased airway pressure decreases the sum of RV and LV end-diastolic volumes, and cardiac output decreases. Positive end-expiratory pressure also adds to the potentially important constraint and thus usually decreases cardiac output further — another example of reduced preload and output despite increased diastolic intracavitary pressure. Some studies suggest that the leftward septal shift associated with positive end-expiratory pressure (thought to be caused by increased pulmonary vascular resistance at higher lung volumes) may decrease LV end-diastolic volume more than that caused by constraint alone.[48,57] Positive pressure inspiration transiently decreases systemic venous return and RV output, with the reverse occurring during expiration.[57–60] Simultaneously, positive pressure inspiration tends to express blood from the pulmonary vasculature. The opposite effects on RV and LV inflow cause the transseptal pressure gradient to change with the potential result of phasic septal shifts during the ventilation cycle. Therefore, RV and LV end-diastolic volumes may be modulated by direct ventricular interaction as well as by other mechanisms that are not considered further here. The consequences of these changes on LV function vary. In some circumstances, LV end-diastolic volume and output decrease during positive pressure inspiration,[61] and in others both end-diastolic volume and output increase.[57,60] A synthesis of available data suggests that during mechanical ventilation pulmonary vascular resistance increases more at lower LV end-diastolic pressures (zone 2 conditions), which tends to result in a decreased transseptal pressure gradient and leftward septal shift during positive pressure inspiration, and that pulmonary vascular resistance increases little during positive pressure inspiration at higher LV end-diastolic pressures (zone 3 conditions) with little or no leftward septal shift. The decreased RV end-diastolic volume that occurs during positive pressure inspiration then allows for increased filling of the LV (despite a decreased total volume of the ventricles as airway pressure increases) and, therefore, LV output. The reverse occurs during expiration.

Conclusion

It is clear that pericardial constraint and septal displacement play important roles in various disease states, as well as during mechanical ventilation. It would also appear from the preceding discussion that there are many circumstances in which it would be easy to use the phrase "diastolic function" in an ambiguous manner. In the presence of external constraint, an assessment of compliance or preload should include consideration of the effects of that constraint on ventricular filling. Certainly, the pericardium contributes to ventricular filling pressures and also to various measures of diastolic function. Although the phrase "diastolic dysfunction" is most often used to describe myocardial characteristics, it is clear that ventricular filling pressures may be substantially changed by changes in external pressure without necessarily changing the myocardial contribution to overall compliance. That this may merit more consideration and systematic study is highlighted by the effects of different loading conditions on measurements that are used to assess diastolic function.

References

1. Lee MC, LeWinter MM, Freeman G, et al. Biaxial mechanical properties of the pericardium in normal and volume overload dogs. Am J Physiol Heart Circ Physiol 1985;249:H222–H230.
2. Henderson Y, Barringer TBJ. The relation of venous pressure to cardiac efficiency. Am J Physiol 1913;13: 352–369.
3. Haykowsky M, Taylor D, Teo K, et al. Left ventricular wall stress during leg-press exercise performed with a brief valsalva maneuver. Chest 2001;119:150–154.
4. Katz LN. Analysis of the several factors regulating the performance of the heart. Physiol Rev 1955;35:91–106.
5. Braunwald E, Ross J Jr. Editorial: The ventricular end-diastolic pressure. Am J Med 1963;34:147–150.
6. Sarnoff SJ, Berglund E. Ventricular function. 1. Starling's law of the heart studied by means of simultaneous right and left ventricular function curves in the dog. Circulation 1954;9:706–718.
7. Ludbrook PA, Byrne JD, Kurnik PB, et al. Influence of reduction of preload and afterload by nitroglycerin on left ventricular diastolic pressure–volume relations and relaxation in man. Circulation 1977; 56:937–943.
8. Tyberg JV, Misbach GA, Glantz SA, et al. A mechanism for the shifts in the diastolic, left ventricular, pressure-volume curve: the role of the pericardium. Eur J Cardiol 1978;7(Suppl):163–175.
9. Kenner HM, Wood EH. Intrapericardial, intrapleural, and intracardiac pressures during acute heart

failure in dogs studied without thoracotomy. Circ Res 1966;19:1071–1079.

10. Smiseth OA, Frais MA, Kingma I, et al. Assessment of pericardial constraint in dogs. Circulation 1985; 71:158–164.

11. Hamilton DR, deVries G, Tyberg JV. Static and dynamic operating characteristics of a pericardial balloon. J Appl Physiol 2001;90:1481–1488.

12. Tyberg JV, Taichman GC, Smith ER, et al. The relationship between pericardial pressure and right atrial pressure: an intraoperative study. Circulation 1986;73:428–432.

13. Boltwood CM Jr, Skulsky A, Drinkwater DC Jr, et al. Intraoperative measurement of pericardial constraint: role in ventricular diastolic mechanics. J Am Coll Cardiol 1986;8:1289–1297.

14. Boltwood CM, Skulsky A, Drinkwater DC, et al. Intraoperative measurement of pericardial constraint: role in ventricular diastolic mechanics. J Am Coll Cardiol 1986;8:1289–1297.

15. Traboulsi M, Scott-Douglas NW, Smith ER, et al. The right and left ventricular intracavitary and transmural pressure-strain relationships. Am Heart J 1992;123:1279–1287.

16. Fauchere JC, Walker AM, Grant DA. Right atrial pressure as a measure of ventricular constraint arising from positive end-expiratory pressure during mechanical ventilation of the neonatal lamb. Crit Care Med 2003;31:745–751.

17. Smiseth OA, Refsum H, Tyberg JV. Pericardial pressure assessed by right atrial pressure: a basis for calculation of left ventricular transmural pressure. Am Heart J 1983;108:603–605.

18. Belenkie I, Kieser TM, Sas R, et al. Evidence for left ventricular constraint during open heart surgery. Can J Cardiol 2002;18(9):951–959.

19. Smiseth OA, Thompson CR, Ling H, et al. A potential clinical method for calculating transmural left ventricular filling pressure during positive end-expiratory pressure ventilation: an intraoperative study in humans. J Am Coll Cardiol 1996;27:155–160.

20. Belenkie I, Dani R, Smith ER, et al. Ventricular interaction during experimental acute pulmonary embolism. Circulation 1988;78:761–768.

21. Smiseth OA, Manyari DE, Lima JA, et al. Modulation of vascular capacitance by angiotensin and nitroprusside: a mechanism of changes in pericardial pressure. Circulation 1987;76:875–883.

22. Janicki JS, Weber KT. The pericardium and ventricular interaction, distensibility and function. Am J Physiol Heart Circ Physiol 1980;238:H494–H503.

23. Lavine SJ. Genesis of the restrictive filling pattern: pericardial constraint or myocardial restraint. J Am Soc Echocardiogr 2004;17:152–160.

24. Nakatani S, Beppu S, Miyatake K, et al. Effect of pericardium on left ventricular early filling assessed by pulsed Doppler echocardiography. J Am Soc Echocardiogr 1991;4:29–34.

25. Pepi M, Guazzi M, Maltagliati A, et al. Diastolic ventricular interaction in normal and dilated heart during head-up tilting. Clin Cardiol 2000;23:665–672.

26. Guazzi M, Pepi M, Maltagliati A, et al. How the two sides of the heart adapt to graded impedance to venous return with head-up tilting. J Am Coll Cardiol 1995;26:1732–1740.

27. Takahashi T, Iizuka M, Sato H, et al. Doppler echocardiographic–determined changes in left ventricular diastolic filling flow velocity during the lower body positive and negative pressure method. Am J Cardiol 1990;65:237–241.

28. Temporelli PL, Corra U, Imparato A, et al. Reversible restrictive left ventricular diastolic filling with optimized oral therapy predicts a more favorable prognosis in patients with chronic heart failure. J Am Coll Cardiol 1998;31:1591–1597.

29. Ohta T, Nakatani S, Izumi S, et al. Serial assessment of left and right ventricular filling in patients with congestive heart failure. Jpn Circ J 2001;65:803–807.

30. Pozzoli M, Traversi E, Cioffi G, et al. Loading manipulations improve the prognostic value of Doppler evaluation of mitral flow in patients with chronic heart failure. Circulation 1997;95:1222–1230.

31. Pepi M, Guazzi M, Maltagliati, A et al. Diastolic ventricular interaction in normal and dilated heart during head-up tilting. Clin Cardiol 2000;23:665–672.

32. Kass DA, Midei M, Brinker J, et al. Influence of coronary occlusion during PTCA on end-systolic and end-diastolic pressure-volume relations in humans. Circulation 1990;81:447–460.

33. Yamamoto K, Masuyama T, Tanouchi J, et al. Decreased and abnormal left ventricular filling in acute heart failure: role of pericardial constraint and its mechanism. J Am Soc Echocardiogr 1992;5:504–514.

34. Atherton JJ, Moore TD, Thomson HL, et al. Restrictive left ventricular filling patterns are predictive of diastolic ventricular interaction in chronic heart failure. J Am Coll Cardiol 1998;31:413–418.

35. Kingma I, Tyberg JV, Smith ER. Effects of diastolic transseptal pressure gradient on ventricular septal position and motion. Circulation 1983;68:1304–1314.

36. Smith ER, Tyberg JV. Ventricular interdependence. In Konstam MA, Isner JM, eds. The Right Ventricle. Kluwer Academic Publishers: Dordrecht, Netherlands 1988:37–51.

37. Belenkie I, Sas R, Mitchell J, et al. Opening the pericardium during pulmonary artery constriction improves cardiac function. J Appl Physiol 2004;96:917–922.
38. Baker AE, Belenkie I, Dani R, et al. Quantitative assessment of the independent contributions of the pericardium and septum to direct ventricular interaction. Am J Physiol Heart Circ Physiol 1998;275: H476–H483.
39. Gibbons-Kroeker CA, Shrive NG, Belenkie I, et al. Pericardium modulates left and right ventricular stroke volumes to compensate for sudden changes in atrial volume. Am J Physiol Heart Circ Physiol 2003;284:H2247–H2254.
40. Mirsky I, Rankin JS. The effects of geometry, elasticity, and external pressures on the diastolic pressure–volume and stiffness-stress relations. How important is the pericardium? Circ Res 1979;44:601–611.
41. Smiseth OA, Scott-Douglas NW, Thompson CR, et al. Nonuniformity of pericardial surface pressure in dogs. Circulation 1987;75:1229–1236.
42. Smiseth OA, Thompson CR, Ling H, et al. Juxtacardiac pleural pressure during positive end-expiratory pressure ventilation: an intraoperative study in patients with open pericardium. J Am Coll Cardiol 1994;23:753–758.
43. Dong S-J, Smith ER, Tyberg JV. Changes in the radius of curvature of the ventricular septum at end diastole during pulmonary arterial and aortic constrictions in the dog. Circulation 1992;86:1280–1290.
44. Belenkie I, Dani R, Smith ER, et al. Effects of volume loading during experimental acute pulmonary embolism. Circulation 1989;80:178–188.
45. Belenkie I, Dani R, Smith ER, et al. The importance of pericardial constraint in experimental pulmonary embolism and volume loading. Am Heart J 1992;123:733–742.
46. Glantz SA, Parmley WW. Factors which affect the diastolic pressure–volume curve. Circ Res 1978;42:171–180.
47. Mercat A, Diehl JL, Meyer G, et al. Hemodynamic effects of fluid loading in acute massive pulmonary embolism. Crit Care Med 1999;27:540–544.
48. Jardin F, Gueret P, Prost JF, et al. Two-dimensional echocardiographic assessment of left ventricular function in chronic obstructive pulmonary disease. Am Rev Respir Dis 1984;129:135–142.
49. Blanchard DG, Dittrich HC. Pericardial adaptation in severe chronic pulmonary hypertension. Circulation 1992;85:1414–1422.
50. Howarth S, McMichael J, Sharpey-Schafer EP. Effects of venesection in low output heart failure. Clin Sci 1946;6:41–50.
51. Dupuis J, LaLonde G, Lebeau R, et al. Sustained beneficial effect of a seventy-two hour intravenous infusion of nitroglycerin in patients with severe chronic congestive heart failure. Am Heart J 1990;120:625–637.
52. Stevenson LW, Tillisch JH. Maintenance of cardiac output with normal filling pressures in patients with dilated heart failure. Circulation 1986;74:1303–1308.
53. ter Keurs HEDJ, Rijnsburger WH, van Heuningen R, et al. Tension development and sarcomere length in rat cardiac trabeculae: evidence of length-dependent activation. In Baan J, Arntzenius AC, Yellin EL, ed. Cardiac Dynamics. The Hague: Martinus Nijhoff; 1980:25–36.
54. Atherton JJ, Moore TD, Lele SS, et al. Diastolic ventricular interaction in chronic heart failure. Lancet 1997;349:1720–1724.
55. Moore TD, Frenneaux MP, Sas R, et al. Ventricular interaction and external constraint account for decreased stroke work during volume loading in CHF. Am J Physiol 2001;281(6):H2385–H2391.
56. Janicki JS. Influence of the pericardium and ventricular interdependence on left ventricular diastolic and systolic function in patients with heart failure. Circ. 1990;81:III15–III20.
57. Mitchell JR, Sas R, Zuege DJ, et al. Ventricular interaction during mechanical ventilation in closed-chest anesthetized dogs. Can J Cardiol 2005;21:73–81.
58. Pinsky MR. Determinants of pulmonary arterial flow variation during respiration. J Appl Physiol 1984;56:1237–1245.
59. Pinsky MR. Instantaneous venous return curves in an intact canine preparation. J Appl Physiol 1984;56:765–771.
60. Mitchell JR, Whitelaw WA, Sas R, et al. RV filling modulates LV function by direct ventricular interaction during mechanical ventilation. Am J Physiol Heart Circ Physiol 2005;289:H549–H557.
61. Denault AY, Gorcsan J, III, Pinsky MR. Dynamic effects of positive-pressure ventilation on canine left ventricular pressure–volume relations. J Appl Physiol 2001;91:298–308.

4
Role of the Left Atrium

Sergio Macciò and Paolo Marino

Introduction

There is currently a general consensus in the literature about the definitions of diastolic dysfunction and diastolic failure, even though these concepts have only relatively recently been introduced into the clinical arena. The key to their definitions, as discussed in other chapters, is the central and predominant role played by the ventricular chamber in terms of its ability to accommodate adequate filling volume at reasonably low pressure through its capacity to rapidly relax while maintaining chamber elastic properties.[1] More marginal, if not completely neglected, is the role of the atrial chamber within the clinical scenario of diastolic dysfunction and failure. Recently, however, several studies have demonstrated how the left atrium plays a primary role not only in modulating ventricular filling and function through the atrioventricular interaction mechanism but also in providing important prognostic clues for the risk stratification of patients with diastolic dysfunction.[2,3]

Basic Mechanical Function of the Left Atrium

The main function of the left atrium is to connect the pulmonary circulation with the left ventricle, acting as a reservoir during atrial filling when the mitral valve is closed or as a booster when the atrial contraction ensues, but especially acting as a conduit during diastasis. Accordingly, the atrial cavity has at times been assigned the minimal role of being a "transit chamber" devoted exclusively to collecting and redirecting the reflux blood from the pulmonary district toward the systemic circulation. It would be wrong to deduce from this "pipeline" function that the left atrium is a passive player in the complex scenario of the cardiac cycle; on the contrary, it performs multiple tasks either in direct interaction with the underlying ventricle, or by paracrine modulation of the systemic circulation.

Its interaction with the ventricular cavity, which is not restricted to the ventricular filling phase in diastole, is discussed later. It should be emphasized at the outset, however, that, in addition to this relation with the underlying chamber, the left atrium can also interact with general systemic homeostasis, acting as a true "control" center. It is now well known, in fact, that the left (as well as the right) atrium also acts as a volume sensor.

The Atrium as a Control Center

Blood Volume Regulation

The control of flow volume is effected by the left atrium through the production of neurohormonal substances.[4] Among these substances, a major role is played by the natriuretic peptides, including atrial natriuretic peptide (ANP), brain natriuretic peptide (BNP) of predominantly ventricular origin, and endothelial peptide (C-type natriuretic peptide [CNP]), which also has a regulatory function in the renin-angiotensin-aldosterone system.[5]

Whenever a load of volume, salts or vasoconstricting drugs, stimulates the atrial mechanoreceptors, ANP performs its vasodilatory action either directly or indirectly, inhibiting sympathetic activity.[6] It also induces natriuresis, inhibits the renin-angiotensin-aldosterone system, increases capillary permeability, and antagonizes the proliferation of smooth muscle cells.[7] With the progression of cardiac insufficiency, plasmatic concentration of this peptide increases in proportion to the severity of the pathology.[8] In patients with cardiac disorders, then, ANP may be produced not only by the atrium but also by the ventricle, a typical feature of the fetal heart that is lost in adult life.[9] Brain natriuretic peptide has a structure similar to that of ANP, but BNP is secreted mostly by the ventricles when they dilate, even though small quantities are released at the atrial level.[10] For BNP, as for ANP, there is a correlation between the severity of the disorder and the amount of peptide produced.[11]

Because of the presence of ANP and BNP in the serum of patients suffering from asymptomatic left ventricular (LV) dysfunction, natriuretic peptides have been proposed as markers targeted to an early diagnosis of ventricular dysfunction.[12] There is evidence that in the advanced stages of diastolic dysfunction the negative reshaping of the atrial cavity can cause, over time, increased concentrations of natriuretic peptides mostly ascribed to ANP.[13,14] In addition to the stimulus that follows stretching of the walls, the atrium may also react to other stimuli, such as levels of angiotensin II[15] and endothelin[16] by secreting ANP.

Mechanoreceptors and Signaling Mechanisms

A second mechanism of interaction between the atrial cavity and the cardiovascular system is due to the presence of receptors for the afferent paths of various reflexes.[17,18] Among the most important of these receptors are the mechanoreceptors disseminated throughout the atrial walls: in case of increased venous backflow (such as during physical stress), the relaxation of the walls causes the activation of these receptors, with the final consequence of accelerating the discharge frequency of

the cells of the sinus node (stress-induced tachycardia, the Bainbridge reflex).[19]

Structural Characteristics

To analyze the role played by the left atrium in the various progressive stages of diastolic dysfunction, it is obviously necessary to consider, last but not least, the histologic and structural properties of this chamber. Both atria show, in fact, peculiar morphologic and structural characteristics different, to some extent, from those characterizing the ventricular cavities. These include peculiar reactions and behaviors of the atrial wall in response to hemodynamic alterations associated with the progressive dysfunction of the underlying cavity. At the histologic level, the atrial chambers show myocytes of smaller dimensions than those of the corresponding ventricular myocytes and are characterized by the presence of chains of myosin with fetal type expressions (in the case of both light and heavy chains), which are associated with a shorter duration of the action potential.[20]

As mentioned earlier, we know that the atrium is particularly sensitive not only to the physical stretching of its walls but also to surrounding levels of angiotensin II. This is explained by the fact that the atrium depends largely on phosphatidylinositol for signal translation,[21] and this dependence may explain why the positive inotropic angiotensin-mediated effect is sensibly greater at the atrial than at the ventricular level.[22]

These peculiar histologic and physiologic features may derive, in part, from the fact that the atrial chambers do not need to exert a particularly strong contractile activity, as they do not have to generate high intracavity pressures, although they must be capable of responding, rather quickly, to changes in the surrounding volume while maintaining a pumping capacity able to guarantee adequate ventricular filling.

How the Atrium Interacts with Ventricular Filling

Left atrial function is intimately related to ventricular function throughout the whole cardiac cycle.[23] During ventricular systole, longitudinal fiber shortening forces the descent of the cardiac base, contributing to atrial filling from the pulmonary veins,[24] while, during diastole, the left atrium passively and actively contributes to ventricular filling. Because the left atrium, during diastole, is directly exposed to the ventricular pressure through the open mitral valve, the atrial emptying pattern is obviously strongly influenced by LV diastolic properties.[25]

Atrial function can best be described by the relation between pressure and volume.[26] Gathering this information, however, implies the use of a pressure micromanometer in the atrial chamber, a maneuver that is rarely performed in everyday clinical practice. An easier way to describe atrial function is to rely on the atrial volume curve. Noninvasive assessment of the left atrial volume curve, based on the concept that the instantaneous atrial volume can be defined as the net difference between the forward flow from the pulmonary veins and the flow leaving the atrium through the mitral valve, has been shown to be feasible in the noninvasive laboratory,[27] although not routinely performed (Figure 4.1).

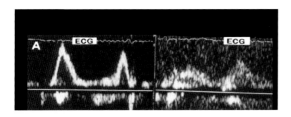

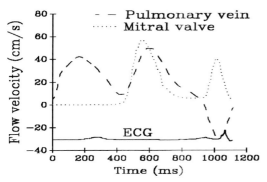

FIGURE 4.1. (Top) Original mitral (left) and pulmonary vein (right) flow velocity profiles. (Bottom) Digitized Doppler mitral and pulmonary venous flow velocity profiles. The two digitized tracings have been superimposed according to the end of the QRS complex.

It has been shown, in fact, that the LV volume curve can be derived from the Doppler-determined mitral flow velocity integral × the mitral cross-sectional area[28] and that the results thus obtained correlate, at a reasonable level of statistical significance, with the estimate of LV volume obtained by thermodilution.[29] Alternatively, given that the effective mitral valve area is known to vary over time,[30] filling volume can be calibrated to the two-dimensional echocardiographic stroke volume.[31] A similar approach can be applied also to pulmonary vein velocities, defining the pulmonary venous flow as the product of the pulmonary veins' integral × the pulmonary veins' area and obtaining the left atrial volume curve as the difference between the forward-flowing blood from the lungs and the blood flowing through the mitral valve. The two-dimensional echocardiographic ventricular volume at end systole and the atrial volume at early diastole are then used to quantify the volume of the ventricular and the atrial cavities at the beginning of their respective filling curves (Figures 4.1 and 4.2).

As ventricular systole begins, the left atrial volume progressively increases, reaching a maximum in the vicinity of end systole, after which it decreases, rapidly at first, and then slightly refilling during diastasis. At the end of the diastasis period the left atrium begins to contract actively, expelling blood into the left ventricle and thus allowing refilling of the cavity with the next beat.

It must be emphasized, however, that the atrial volume curve does not provide an exact measure of the amount of blood entering the left ventricle from the atrium during diastole. In the phase of passive atrial emptying and atrial diastasis, in fact, blood also flows from the pulmonary veins to the ventricle (see Figure 4.2). Furthermore, during active atrial emptying, some blood may flow back into the pulmonary veins. It is only the simultaneous availability of the left atrial and LV volume curves that allows a precise definition of the contribution of the left atrium to the ventricular filling process. The approach described, which links the continuous flow of the pulmonary veins to the intermittent diastolic filling of the ventricle through the atrioventricular orifice, underlines the complex role that the left atrial cavity exerts in the ventricular filling process.

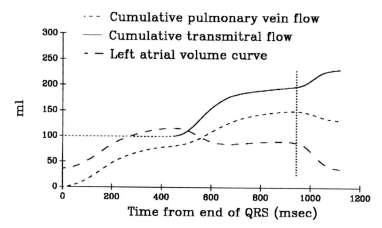

FIGURE 4.2. Output of the flow velocity pattern analysis as described by Marino et al.[27,28] Cumulative transmitral flow, cumulative pulmonary vein flow, and derived left atrial volume curve. The two-dimensional echocardiographic estimates of ventricular volume at end systole and of atrial volume at end diastole are used to quantify the ventricular and atrial volumes at the beginnings of the respective volume curves. The dotted vertical line indicates timing of atrial systole (defined according to the peak of cumulative pulmonary vein flow). (From Prioli et al.[33] © 1998, with permission of Elsevier.)

Thus, contrary to superficial thinking, the atrium is an "active agent" for most of the ventricular filling process. It is possible, in fact, to identify three phases in which the atrium actually interacts with LV filling that correspond to the triple action of the atrial cavity during the cardiac cycle: reservoir, conduit, and pump.[32] The reservoir function can be defined as the difference between the maximum and minimum volumes minus the volume of the backward flow into the pulmonary veins during atrial contraction. The pump function can be defined as the blood volume pushed into the left ventricle during atrial systole. Finally, the conduit function can be defined as the filling volume of the left ventricle minus the sum of the left atrial reservoir plus the volume ejected during atrial systole. These three functions can be quantified and expressed in the form of a fraction of the filling volume of the ventricle.[33]

Reservoir

The reservoir phase of the left atrium takes place during ventricular systole, and we can identify two periods within it. In the first, just after atrial systole and following the closure of the mitral valve, there is a relaxation phase that basically modulates flow from the pulmonary veins; this phase is characterized by a rapid increase in atrial volume.[34] The second phase, with left atrial volume increasing more slowly, is dominated by systolic longitudinal shortening of the ventricle, which causes the descent of the cardiac base, "sucking" blood into the atrium,[35] and by right ventricular systolic contraction, which contributes to atrial filling by determining the transpulmonary wave propagation that "pushes" blood into the atrial cavity.[36]

The active part of the filling process is due to the intracellular reuptake drive of calcium ions from cytosol toward the sarcoplasmic reticulum, which allows the myofibrils to start the relaxation phase.[37,38] This active phase is followed by a passive period in which the flow from the pulmonary veins enters the atrium according to the driving pressure gradient modulated by the elastic characteristics of the atrial wall and its structural composition. Such characteristics can, through an increase in parietal stiffness, effect important modifications to the atrial filling process, leading to a rise and a final value for intraatrial pressure that is mostly a function of the passive characteristics of the cavity (Figure 4.3).[39]

The atrial filling volume that accumulates within the cavity in this way will subsequently prove to be responsible for about 40% of the stroke volume of the left ventricle. Thus, similarly to what happens for the ventricle, relaxation con-

4. Role of the Left Atrium

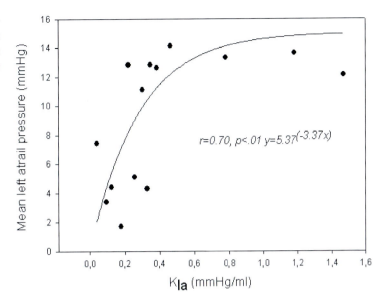

FIGURE 4.3. Plot of mean left atrial pressure versus operative atrial stiffness (K_{la}) in a group of 15 patients undergoing open heart surgery. (Reprinted with permission from Marino et al.[39])

trols the early filling phase of the atrium, whereas chamber material properties, together with cavity stretching and elongation due to concomitant ventricular contraction, affect late atrial diastolic filling.

Conduit

The conduit phase sees the atrium acting as a simple conduit that transits blood toward the underlying ventricle. This function, which is generated by a deviation from the constant-volume state of the left heart that assumes that the total volume of the four-chambered heart remains invariant throughout the cardiac cycle, can be correctly quantified only if the left atrial and LV volume curves are simultaneously available, as was confirmed very recently with a combined magnetic resonance imaging–echocardiographic approach, which allows precise definition of the contribution of the left atrium to the ventricular filling process.[40] The conduit function is reciprocal to the other two functions at the various stages of diastolic ventricular dysfunction (Figure 4.4).

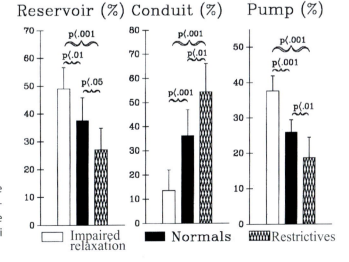

FIGURE 4.4. Percentages of contributions of the atrial reservoir, conduit, and pump function to ventricular filling, arranged according to progressive degrees of ventricular filling impairment (From Prioli et al.[33] © 1998, with permission of Elsevier.)

Unlike the reservoir and pump functions, in fact, the conduit function makes little contribution to ventricular stroke volume in the initial stages of diastolic derangement, but this contribution gains importance in the advanced stages of diastolic dysfunction, while the role of the other two functions diminishes.

The Pump

The pump phase, or atrial systole, is responsible for the fast ventricular filling at the end of diastole. In normal subjects and in patients with an impaired relaxation type of ventricular filling, the pump function is closely related to the precontraction volume of the atrial cavity in accordance with a Starling mechanism, which loses its effectiveness by end-stage ventricular dysfunction when the limits of the atrial preload are reached. This relationship, in fact, is blunted in advanced diastolic dysfunction, when intrinsic depression of atrial contractility, or an afterload mismatch due to high ventricular filling resistance, impairs the atrial booster pump function (see later discussion). A loss of atrial contraction because of atrial fibrillation or ventricular pacing reduces cardiac output by approximately 15%–20%.[41]

It is interesting that experimental and clinical studies have shown that an episode of atrial fibrillation, even if very brief, may cause serious impairment of atrial contractility.[42] In this case, the loss of atrial function is thought to be triggered by Ca^{2+} overload during atrial fibrillation and may be mediated by a decrease in the release of Ca^{2+} from the sarcoplasmic reticulum.[43] The kind of ionic atrial remodeling seen in the atrioventricular afterload mismatch situation seems to be very similar to that caused by atrial fibrillation. In fact, high intraatrial pressure and the resulting increased wall stress may cause calcium overload. Many studies have shown that atrial contractile dysfunction is related to the downregulation of the L-type Ca^+ channel,[44,45] Alternatively, atrial contractile dysfunction may be linked to an impaired β-adrenergic response, which has been demonstrated in both canine[46] and human models of heart failure.[47–49] Reduced density of β-adrenoceptors and upregulation of the inhibitory G protein could explain the altered response of the reshaped atrium to sympathetic tone.[46,50]

Pathophysiology of Ventricular Filling and Involvement of the Left Atrium in Diastolic Dysfunction

The mutual relationship among these three distinct components of atrial activity — reservoir, conduit, and pump — can be appreciated not only in the context of diastolic dysfunction but also in the physiologic response to physical exercise during which, along with an unchanged conduit phase, an increase in the reservoir and/or in the pump function is observed.[51] In this situation, indeed, the increase in volume that can be accommodated during the reservoir phase makes it possible to improve the fast filling volume of the left ventricle in early diastole because of a higher pressure gradient at the moment of the opening of the mitral valve. Similarly, greater relaxation of the atrial walls during the reservoir phase produces, in accordance with a Frank-Starling mechanism, a stronger contraction exerted by the atrial muscle system during the atrial kick.[51]

Profound changes in left atrial mechanics can be detailed in response to progressive degrees of LV filling impairment. In light of what has been said so far, it is evident that changes in ventricular relaxation have direct repercussions on the atrioventricular pressure gradient at the beginning of ventricular filling. Deranged ventricular relaxation induces a slower reduction of the intraventricular pressure and, consequently, a decrease in early transmitral flow, which is related to the pressure difference between the two chambers; this is reflected in the transmitral Doppler flow velocity, with a reduction in the peak E wave velocity profile.[52] As a consequence, the atrial conduit function, which takes effect at this time, is minimized, while the reservoir/pump complex is variously enhanced in order to maintain ventricular stroke volume (see Figure 4.4).[33]

It becomes evident, therefore, how the atrium, in the early stage of diastolic dysfunction, exerts a sort of compensatory action in order to support the deficient ventricle. The upregulation of the reserve function, with an increase in atrial volume at the end of ventricular systole, together with stronger pump activity, makes it possible to compensate, in the second half of diastole, for what, in terms of ventricular filling, is lost in the first half. Areas of different distensibility within the left atrium, particularly at the level of the auricula, may further act on the reservoir function, increasing the capacity of the cavity to deal with an excess of load because they are less resistant to distension than the rest of the chamber.[53,54]

Such compensatory mechanisms are well evident by Doppler analysis of the transmitral flow in which, along with a reduction in the peak E wave velocity, an increased A wave is a sign of the intensified contribution of atrial systole. In the initial phases, this mechanism has proved to be effective in maintaining adequate ventricular filling and, therefore, effective stroke volume. However, the worsening of ventricular diastolic dysfunction, which is linked to progressive structural alterations of the myocardial wall, complicates the initial problem of an impaired relaxation with the condition associated with increased ventricular stiffness. Although the left ventricle is initially capable of accommodating the flow from the atrium at a normal pressure, at a later stage of ventricular disease this is no longer possible, given the marked increase in resistance to filling that characterizes worsening ventricular dysfunction. The increased pump activity, which so far has been able to compensate for impaired ventricular relaxation, now becomes inadequate. It is in this phase that the Doppler image of the transmitral flow shows "pseudonormalization."[52]

As mentioned earlier, it has been suggested that impaired atrial function in end-stage diastolic ventricular dysfunction is functionally related to an afterload mismatch because of increased ventricular stiffness and diastolic pressure.[55] In patients with hypertrophic cardiomyopathy, for example, a close inverse relation between atrial ejection fraction and LV stiffness has been found.[56] However, changes in the atrial booster pump function may be the result of altered loading conditions and/or impaired contractility of the atrial musculature. In a comparison between patients with aortic stenosis and dilated cardiomyopathy, the atrial systolic pump appeared to be more compromised in those with myopathic disease, even for an equivalent level of atrial afterload, suggesting that an atrial myopathic process might contribute to the depression of contractility at this level.[57]

In the advanced stages of diastolic dysfunction, because of the increase in late diastolic pressure, greater importance is attributed to the ventricular fast filling early diastolic phase, with a shortening of the filling period and an increase of the early peak E wave velocity. It is hardly surprising, therefore, that the mitral E wave, in its peak and deceleration time, correlates so well, in these advanced stages, with the level of operative ventricular stiffness.[58] At this point, the reservoir/pump function is clearly exhausted, while the conduit function takes prevalence.

In normal subjects and in patients with an impaired relaxation type of filling, the amount of blood pumped into the ventricle with the atrial kick is a function of the atrial volume before contraction (Figure 4.5).

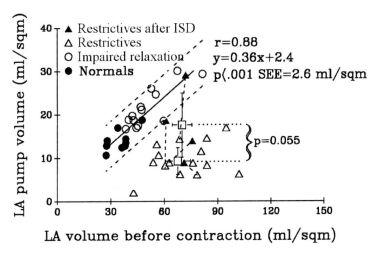

FIGURE 4.5. Regression of the left atrial (LA) pump volume versus the volume of the cavity before its contraction. There is a linear significant relation for pooled normal and impaired relaxation patients. In those with a restrictive type of filling, in contrast, this relation is poor. For any degree of atrial preload, the atrial pump is less in this group than in the other two. Isosorbide dinitrate (ISD) sublingually given to four restrictive patients moves these patients toward the lower 95% confidence interval of the aforementioned regression line. (From Marino, unpublished data, reproduced with permission from Rossi et al.[59])

In patients with a restrictive type of filling, in contrast, this relation is poor. For any atrial cavity volume, in fact, the atrial pump volume is lower in this last group than in the other two. Manipulation of systemic blood pressure and, probably, left atrial afterload (i.e., ventricular end-diastolic pressure) using nitrates can improve atrial pump function significantly, moving these patients toward the lower 95% confidence interval of the regression line relating pump volume to the volume of the atrial cavity before contraction for the other two groups combined.[59] Interestingly, this can be achieved with no detectable changes in atrial cavity volume (Figure 5), a finding potentially consistent with the resolution of some baseline constraint, if LV end-diastolic pressure is assumed to decrease with administration of the drug.[60] Thus, a pericardium-mediated afterload mismatch might contribute significantly to the reduced atrial pump activity that characterizes the restrictive filling of cardiomyopathic patients. This consideration, as mentioned earlier, does not exclude intrinsic atrial dysfunction as a potential contributor to such an impairment. Increased atrial preload in restrictives, in fact, might suggest overdistension of the atrial fibers to a critical point beyond which contraction deteriorates.[61] This would imply impaired atrial contractility, which, in turn, could contribute to the depression of atrial pump performance for any given loading condition.

According to the results of the Pearson product moment correlations (Table 4.1), ventricular filling volume appears, in the initial stages of diastolic dysfunction (impaired relaxation pattern), to be strongly linked to the combined effects of the atrial reservoir (r = 0.89, p = 0.00006) and pump functions (r = 0.84, p = 0.0003). This is similar to what has been shown in the initial grades of diastolic dysfunction that characterize hypertensive heart disease, with conduit function minimized and unrelated to ventricular filling.[62] When more marked diastolic dysfunction develops, stroke volume appears to be related mainly to the conduit function (r = 0.85, p = 0.00007), with a weaker, albeit significant, association with the reservoir/pump complex (r = 0.73, p = 0.002 and r = 0.60, p = 0.018, respectively). At this stage, only a limited proportion of ventricular filling proves to be associated with any active contribution by the atrium.

Elasticity, Stiffness, and Atrial Remodeling

The physiologic significance of atrial stiffness is not completely understood, but some indirect evidence does suggest that it is important in hemodynamics. It is well known, in fact, that the addition of a flexible atrium to the inlet of an artificial heart substantially improves the heart's output.[63] Conversely, an increase in atrial stiffness should reduce stroke volume and cardiac output.[64] In a recent study average atrial operative stiffness, computed as Δpressure/Δvolume during the reservoir phase and excluding the suction-initiated (negative stiffness) portion of early filling, was inversely related to cardiac index (r = −0.69, p < 0.01) and stroke volume (r = −0.55, p < 0.05)

TABLE 4.1. Results of the Pearson product moment correlations between ventricular filling volume and atrial reservoir, conduit, and pump functions, respectively.

	Reservoir	Conduit	Pump
Normal pattern	0.57	0.15	0.58
(n = 9)	(p = NS)	(p = NS)	(p = NS)
Impaired relaxation	0.89	0.21	0.84
pattern (n = 13)	(p = 0.00006)	(p = NS)	(p = 0.0003)
Restrictive pattern	0.73	0.85	0.60
(n = 15)	(p = 0.002)	(p = 0.00007)	(p = 0.018)

Note: NS, not significant.
Source: From Prioli et al.[33]

and directly related to mean atrial pressure (r = 0.70, $p < 0.01$; see Figure 4.3).[39]

It has been suggested that the shift in the pattern of LV filling that occurs during the process of normal aging, represented by a prolongation of the isovolumic relaxation time, a marked reduction in the early diastolic filling rate associated with a more gradual deceleration of early filling, and an augmentation of the atrial component (the so-called impaired relaxation type of filling), might be ascribed not to a slowing of the rate of LV pressure decline but rather to a reduced early diastolic left atrial pressure due to changes in active or passive properties of the atrium.[65] Indeed, left atrial passive compliance might change with advancing age. Aging, in fact, is associated with a progressive fragmentation and rupture of elastic fibers that could make the atrial wall flaccid at low volume because of loss of elasticity but stiff at high volume because of the fibrosis of the endocardial cavity layer that takes place between the third and ninth decades of life.[66] Thus, at low volume, left atrial pressure might be low because of flaccidity, but at high volume the pressure might be high because of increased stiffness. This hypothesis would explain the reduced peak E velocity of normal older adults and the increased propensity to "pseudonormalize" with volume overload.[65] Unfortunately, very little data on human invasively assessed atrial stiffness are available, and noninvasive data for the same parameter are currently lacking. Thus, the hypothetical changes in atrial stiffness due to aging await confirmation.

Recently, some attempts have been made to apply to the atrial chamber a method of evaluation of wall deformation similar to what was already used for evaluating ventricular chamber properties. One example comes from the study of Inaba et al.,[67] who assessed left atrial function in relation to both age and the process of cavity dilatation that takes place during atrial fibrillation. Peak strain rate was measured for each atrial wall (septum, lateral, rear, front, and lower walls). Mean peak systolic strain rate and late diastolic strain rate were measured as well. In a population of 50 control subjects, both peak systolic strain rate and late diastolic strain rate appeared to correlate inversely with age, atrial dimensions, and the data obtained from the transmitral flow. Peak

systolic strain rate, however, was consistently lower in 27 persistent atrial fibrillation patients than in age-matched controls (1.7 + 0.8 vs. 2.9 + 0.9 s −1; $p < 0.01$). Other investigators looked at strain of the interatrial wall in patients who underwent electrical cardioversion.[68] In that study, 65 patients with lone atrial fibrillation underwent echocardiographic strain and strain rate imaging before successful external electrical cardioversion. Maintenance of sinus rhythm was assessed over a 9-month follow-up. Atrial strain and strain rate parameters alone were confirmed to be independent predictors of sinus rhythm maintenance by multivariate analysis, with patients with the highest values for strain and strain rate at baseline before cardioversion having the greatest likelihood of maintaining sinus rhythm over time (Figure 4.6).

This evidence might suggest the possibility of making a direct evaluation of atrial deformation properties that could reflect the structural changes that characterize the fibrillating atrium. Studies on a large, multicenter population are necessary to confirm the reproducibility, the sensitivity, and the specificity of such a method. The problem of the poor sensitivity of atrial volume for identifying the initial stages of diastolic dysfunction might perhaps be solved in future because of the introduction of more refined methods and technologies for the analysis of tissue deformation of the atrial walls after their effectiveness in describing derangements in atrial function has been confirmed.

Finally, it must be remembered that a problem of electrical reshaping arises along with the stiffening of the atrial walls. As demonstrated by Sanders et al.,[69] patients with congestive cardiac disorders exhibit, in addition to the enlargement of the atrial chambers, an evident loss of atrial musculature, with regions displaying altered voltages and scarlike areas. Several studies have demonstrated the presence of such areas of nonhomogeneity in patients affected by recurrent atrial tachyarrhythmias.[70,71] These scar areas, which are partially linked to the fibrotic process secondary to long-standing wall stretching, would act as barriers around which some reentry phenomena may take place, with the low voltage areas behaving like a slow circuit path, further delaying activation of the left atrium.[69]

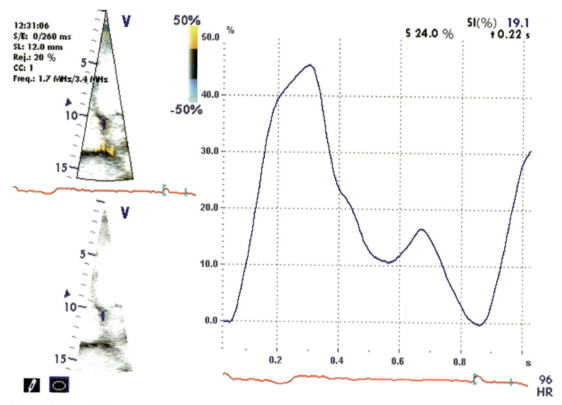

FIGURE 4.6. Normal left atrial strain curve obtained by placing the sample volume in the basal segment of the interatrial septum. Left ventricular end-diastole is the starting point of the cycle.

Cellular Pathophysiology of Atrial Remodeling

As reported above, the left atrium responds to ventricular diastolic dysfunction by up-regulating its contractile contribution. With time, this causes a "work mismatch" followed by an increase in atrial operative stiffness.[72] According to several experimental findings, the increased wall stress induces[73] an overexpression of β-myosin heavy chain at the atrial level; such isoform would be responsible for a slowing down of the contraction speed.

Along with alterations existing at the tissue level, it is possible to identify and explain diastolic alterations of the left atrium at a cellular level. There are many proteins that contribute to the active and passive tensions of the atrial walls. Atrial cardiomyocytes have a cytoskeleton made of microtubules, intermediate filaments (desmin), microfilaments (actin) and endosarcomeric proteins (titin, nebulin, α-actin, myomesin, and M protein), alterations that have direct repercussions on diastolic function.[74,75] Among these molecules, titin appears to be the most important; its role at the sarcomeric level is crucial (through the presence of several isoforms) in determining the modulation of passive tension, as demonstrated by the experimental work of Wu et al.[76]

The atrium that is chronically exposed to a pressure or volume overload reacts initially with an increased contractile status partly mediated by the Frank-Starling mechanism. However, such status impacts on the homeostasis of intracellular calcium and its reuptake. In this condition, in fact, there is an overload of cytosolic calcium (calcium overload) that the proteins assigned to the reuptake of the sarcoplasmatic grid (among which the

4. Role of the Left Atrium

phospholambans are particularly significant) cannot overcome.[77] The high intracytosolic concentrations of calcium in diastole are partly responsible for enhanced atrial stiffness and explain, in the later stages of diastolic dysfunction, the loss both in reservoir function and in contractile capacity.

A significant contribution to atrial stiffness also comes from the extracellular matrix and from its variations following the changes in volume and pressure that the cavity undergoes.[78] The main components are the fibril proteins such as collagen (type I, type III, and elastin), the proteoglycans and proteins of the basement membrane such as type IV collagen.[79,80] Among these proteins, collagen is one of the major contributors to passive stiffness of the muscle fibers and wall stiffness. Indeed, it is possible to identify several types of collagen according to their different capacities to resist stretching. Type I, for example, because of its well-structured spatial conformation, offers a higher resistance to traction than type III, which is more compliant[81]; it is evident, therefore, how a certain "rigid" conformation of the extracellular matrix may heavily influence atrial deformation and, finally, ventricular volume by negatively modulating the atrial reservoir.[82,83]

Experimental studies have demonstrated how scenarios of chronic ventricular diastolic dysfunction are associated with pathologic parietal fibrosis due to an abnormal turnover of collagen[84,85]; the renin-angiotensin-aldosterone tissue system appears to have a significant role in collagen genesis also at the atrial leve.l[86] Several conditions may be responsible for altered expression of these proteins. Structural alterations of collagen may, indeed, take place either because of protracted parietal stress caused by volume overload or, more rapidly, in response to disorders in electrical atrial conduction, as in the case of atrial fibrillation or of pacing-related cardiomyopathies.[87] In this regard several authors have underlined the active role, in the phenomena of both ventricular and atrial remodeling, of the metalloproteinase and proteolytic enzymes, whose main purpose is to degrade collagen fibers.[88,89] A faulty balance between substances stimulating collagen formation and degrading substances may lead to an overproduction of collagen, as happens in conditions of advanced heart failure.[90]

Importance of Left Atrial Volume as a Prognostic Index

The literature includes many references to the prognostic role of atrial dimension measurement (diameter and/or area) or atrial volume computation.[91,92] The presence of an enlarged atrium (>45 mm) in subjects with dilated cardiomyopathy of nonischemic etiology was associated, in one observational study with a follow-up of 155 ± 20 months, with a cardiac mortality rate (54%) that was about double that (29%) of patients having an atrial dimension <45 mm.[93] Similar results were shown in another study of patients with LV dysfunction of mixed etiology. Using a bivariate Cox model, the researchers showed that left atrial volume, even if evaluated in only one apical four-chamber projection, was capable of predicting the prognosis independently of variables such as LV volume, E/A ratio, or the degree of mitral regurgitation.[94]

Although this last study highlighted the significant relationship that links the extent of atrial remodeling to the level of diastolic dysfunction of the underlying ventricular chamber,[76] it also stressed the apparent predictive capacity of the atrium — independently of ventricular diastolic parameters evaluated using Doppler echocardiography — in stratifying patients. Indeed, the difficulty of accurate evaluation of LV diastolic function in contrast to the relative ease of the measurement of atrial parameters suggested the idea that dimensional or volumetric measurement of the atrium might represent, in everyday clinical practice, a strong and easier estimate of cardiovascular risk than the noninvasive but time-consuming evaluation of the diastolic characteristics of the ventricle.[95]

Not everybody agrees on the value of simple atrial dimensions, as compared with other atrial parameters, in stratifying patients. For example, according to Tsang et al.,[96] atrial volume has a prognostic value that is definitely stronger than the simple evaluation of the M-mode–derived parasternal diameter or the cavity area as measured in four-chamber apical view. Wherever the truth lies, a fact that appears to emerge is the poor prognostic significance of any traditional atrial dimension parameter in identifying the very early forms of diastolic heart failure. It is possible to imagine an explanation for this progressively increasing prognostic capacity of the left atrium only in the more advanced stages of diastolic dysfunction. As we know, there are three functions with which the left atrium regulates and interacts with the process of ventricular filling: the reservoir, conduit, and pump functions. The percentage contributions of these three components vary considerably with the worsening of the degree of ventricular diastolic dysfunction. In particular, the atrial stroke volume, a direct expression of the pump capacity of the atrial cavity, appears to be linearly related, at least initially, to its reservoir or preload (see Figure 5.5). It is therefore likely that, in this phase, atrial volume may respond to load variations with fast changes that may make atrial volume a relatively "volatile" parameter and as such not very dissimilar from the indexes of diastolic function deducible from Doppler transmitral and transvenous pulmonary profiles. In other words, it is possible that only in this early phase is atrial volume modifiable by loading changes. In the presence of more severe grades of ventricular dysfunction, however, the above-described relationship could be lost. In patients with moderate congestive heart failure, in fact, the unloading obtained with ultrafiltration induces quite substantial modifications of the E wave deceleration time compared with atrial size, which does not decrease substantially.[97] One explanation for this phenomenon could be the presence of a reduced elastic recoil of the atrial walls secondary to a process of fibrosis that ensues from long-standing parietal distension[98] or from some pericardium-mediated interaction effect that characterizes the restrictive filling stage of cardiomyopathic patients.[59]

According to some researchers this characteristic could make it possible to "read," through atrial volumetric and structural alterations, the history of a patient's diastolic dysfunction. This aspect might, then, allow the diagnosis in patients who are asymptomatic at the time of the examination and in stable hemodynamic conditions of previously "hidden" or silent episodes of LV dysfunction. With this perspective, Pamela Douglas[99] goes so far as to propose for volumetric alterations of the left atrium a role similar to that of glycated hemoglobin in diabetes as a marker of the chronic, cumulative effects of dysfunction of the underlying cavity.

Atrial Fibrillation, Left Atrium, and Diastolic Dysfunction

Atrial fibrillation is an electrical disorder that can profoundly affect the mechanics of the atrium and, because of the loss of pumping capacity, can impact negatively on the ventricular filling process. As reported earlier, the lost contribution of the atrial booster function in late diastole produces a reduction of about 20%–25% in stroke volume. This loss, which is not significant in conditions of physiologic filling, can become dramatically important in situations of advanced diastolic impairment, when such a contribution can become fundamental given the markedly increased resistance to ventricular filling. The sudden onset of atrial fibrillation is also associated with increasing intraatrial pressure. This increment initially represents a compensation mechanism that induces, by means of an increased atrioventricular pressure gradient, a larger contribution to filling through an increase in flow during the conduit phase.[100]

The association of a fibrillating atrium with the condition of ventricular diastolic dysfunction creates an autosourcing mechanism in which the atrial cavity, either because of increased intracavitary pressures or because of the atrial fibrillation itself, undergoes a process of progressive enlargement.[101,102] This process affects the compliance of the atrium, minimizing the chance of reestablishing a stable sinus rhythm, given the negative relation existing between such a possibility and increasing atrial cavity dimensions.[103] The electrical disorder negatively affects atrial compliance not only through a mechanism of expansion and structural alteration of the walls but also through an overload of intracellular calcium. The problem is comparable to what has been reported in patients subjected to atrial pacing at very high rates in whom intracellular calcium overload impairs ventricular function.[104]

The presence, in a fibrillating patient, of a concurrent diastolic dysfunction imposes a more articulated approach toward the electrical cardioversion procedure. It is true that several studies, such as the AFFIRM trial, point to the substantial parity between "the rhythm versus the rate control" strategy in this condition.[105] However, it is obvious that in patients affected by significant diastolic dysfunction and with already high filling pressures at rest, a strategy aiming to preserve a rhythm versus a rate control will definitely be more efficacious than in a population that is not affected by irreversible ventricular structural alterations. The study by Ito et al.[106] demonstrates that, 3 months after electrical cardioversion, not only is there an almost complete recovery of the atrial contractile state to the original level (provided that the relaxation of atrial myofibrils has not been irreversibly damaged) but also that a significant improvement in the reservoir and conduit function takes place. The study also shows how the recovery of normal electrical atrial activation is capable of positively remodeling the cavity, similar to what has been described for the ventricle.

A couple of studies have underlined some differences that exist between pharmacologic and electrical cardioversion.[107,108] The electrical procedure would appear, in fact, to be associated with a slower recovery of the contractile state and of resynchronization between the auricola and the rest of the atrium. Among the different hypotheses proposed, the most plausible relates to a possible increase in intracellular calcium (calcium overload produced by the passage of the current and by the resulting rapid atrial depolarization) that, inadequately compensated by the mechanisms of re-uptake at the sarcoplasmatic reticulum level, would produce a situation of "stunning" and of "slowly regressing delayed relaxation" that is not generated by pharmacologic cardioversion.[108,109]

Relationships Among Mitral Insufficiency, Left Atrial Cavity, and Ventricular Dysfunction

The presence of mitral regurgitation, of either structural or functional origin, imposes hemodynamic alterations at both the atrial and the ventricular levels. Increasing amounts of mitral insufficiency modify the atrial volume curve and might cause misinterpretation of parameters of systolic and diastolic ventricular function. The reduced impedance of the atrial low-pressure chamber allows LV systolic wall stress to be normalized, thereby concealing a condition of potential initial ventricular dysfunction.[110] The presence of mitral regurgitation also interferes with the noninvasive interpretation of LV diastolic function. Increased E wave velocity, reduced E wave deceleration time, increased E/A ratio, and blunted systolic pulmonary vein velocity are considered hallmarks of LV diastolic impairment,[111] with mitral regurgitation modifying these parameters in the same direction.

The consequences of mitral regurgitation on the left atrium are even more striking, given that the regurgitant volume fills the atrium during ventricular systole so that mitral regurgitation is a main determinant of the atrial volume curve.[112] The volume variation of the atrial chamber during ventricular systole, in fact, is the sum of blood filling the atrium from the pulmonary veins and from the mitral leak. This volume overload, which initially exerts an important compensatory mechanism in the case of excessive central blood volume by buffering pressure rise in the atrium through a progressive decrement of atrial chamber stiffness,[113] leads in time to structural alterations of the walls, to a reduction in atrial compliance, and to loss of contractile force.[114] Even if, in this condition, it contributes to reduction of the atrial pumping capacity through chronic stretching of the cavity walls, mitral insufficiency does not necessarily impact negatively on ventricular diastolic function, which is actually improved, at least in the early stages of mitral incompetence.[115,116]

Conclusion

Left atrial function is an important determinant of the ventricular filling process. Assessment of the complex role that the atrial cavity plays in such a process, while tracking the mechanical adaptations to increasing degrees of ventricular filling impairment, can be done noninvasively. Parameters of left atrial function may offer additional information on stratifying prognostically patients with LV dysfunction while contributing to a better understanding the pathophysiology of cardiac failure.

References

1. Zile MR, Brutsaert D. New concepts in diastolic dysfunction and diastolic heart failure. Part I. Circulation 2002;105:1387–1393.
2. Tsang TSM, Barnes ME, Gersh BJ, Bailey KR, Seward JB. Left atrial volume as a morphophysiologic expression of LV diastolic dysfunction and relation to cardiovascular risk burden. Am J Cardiol 2002;90:1284–1289.
3. Pritchett AM, Mahoney DW, Jacobsen SJ, Rodeheffer RJ, Karon BL, Redfield MM. Diastolic dysfunction and left atrial volume. J Am Coll Cardiol 2005;45:87–92.
4. McGrath MF, Kuroski de Bold ML, de Bold AJ. The endocrine function of the heart. Trends Endocrinol Metab 2005;16:469–477.
5. Kasama S, Toyama T, Kumakura H, et al. Effects of intravenous atrial natriuretic peptide on cardiac sympathetic nerve activity in patients with decompensated congestive heart failure. J Nucl Med 2004;45:1108–1113.
6. Arlt J, Jahn H, Kellner M, Strohle A, Yassouridis A, Wiedemann K. Modulation of sympathetic activity by corticotropin-releasing hormone and atrial natriuretic peptide. Neuropeptides 2003;37:362–368.
7. Angelis E, Tse MY, Pang SC. Interactions between atrial natriuretic peptide and the renin-angiotensin system during salt-sensitivity exhibited by the proANP gene-disrupted mouse. Mol Cell Biochem 2005;276:121–131.
8. Brandt RR, Wright RS, Redfield MM, Burnett JC Jr. Atrial natriuretic peptide in heart failure. J Am Coll Cardiol 1993;22:86–93.
9. Arbustini E, Pucci A, Grasso M, et al. Expression of atrial natriuretic peptide in ventricular myocardium of failing human hearts and its correlation with the severity of clinical and hemodynamic impairment. Am J Cardiol 1990;66:973–980.
10. De Bold AJ, Kuroski de Bold ML Determinants of natriuretic peptide production by the heart: basic and clinical implications. J Invest Med 2005;53:371–377.
11. Vanderheyden M, Goethals M, Verstreken S, et al. Wall stress modulates brain natriuretic peptide production in pressure overload cardiomyopathy. J Am Coll Cardiol 2004;44:2349–2354.
12. Latour-Perez J, Coves-Orts FJ, Abad-Terrado C, Abraira V, Zamora J. Accuracy of B-type natriuretic peptide levels in the diagnosis of left ventricular dysfunction and heart failure: a systematic review. Eur J Heart Fail 2006;8:390–399.
13. Tabata T, Oki T, Yamada H, Abe M, Onose Y, Thomas JD. Relationship between left atrial appendage function and plasma concentration of atrial natriuretic peptide. Eur J Echocardiogr 2000;1:130–137.
14. Takeichi N, Fukuda N, Tamura Y, Oki T, Ito S. Relationship between atrial function and plasma level of atrial natriuretic peptide in patients with heart disease. Cardiology 1998;90:13–19.
15. Focaccio A, Volpe M, Ambrosio G, et al. Angiotensin II directly stimulates release of atrial natriuretic factor in isolated rabbit hearts. Circulation 1993;87:192–198.
16. Fyhrquist F, Sirvio ML, Helin K, et al Endothelin antiserum decreases volume-stimulated and basal plasma concentration of atrial natriuretic peptide. Circulation 1993;90:1172–1176.
17. Longhurst JC. Cardiac receptors: their function in health and disease. Prog Cardiovasc Dis 1984;27:201–222.
18. Hainsworth R. Reflex from the heart. Physiol Rev 1991;71:617–658.
19. Hakumaki MO. Seventy years of the Bainbridge reflex. Acta Physiol Scand 1987;130:177–185.
20. Reiser PJ, Portman MA, Ning XH, Schomisch Moravec C. Human cardiac myosin heavy chain isoforms in fetal and failing adult atria and ventricles. Am J Physiol Heart Circ Physiol 2001;280: H1814–H1820.
21. Mouton R, Lochner JDV, Lochner A. New emphasis on atrial cardiology. S Afr Med J 1992;82:222–223.
22. Rogg H, de Gasparo M, Graedel E, et al. Angiotensin II receptor subtypes in human atria and evidence for alterations in patients with cardiac dysfunction. Eur Heart J 1996;17:1112–1120.
23. Braunwald E, Frahm CJ. Studies on Starling's law of the heart. IV. Observations on the hemodynamic functions of the left atrium in man. Circulation 1961;24:633–642.
24. Castello R, Pearson AC, Lenzen P, Labovitz AJ. Evaluation of pulmonary venous flow by transesophageal echocardiography in subjects with a normal heart: comparison with transthoracic echocardiography. J Am Coll Cardiol 1991;18:65–71.
25. Kono TK, Sabbah HN, Rosman H, Alam M, Stein PD, Goldstein S. Left atrial contribution to ventricular filling during the course of evolving heart failure. Circulation 1992;86:1317–1322.

26. Payne RM, Stone HL, Engelken EJ. Atrial function during volume loading. J Appl Physiol 1971;31:326–331.
27. Marino P, Prioli MA, Destro G, LoSchiavo I, Golia G, Zardini P. The left atrial volume curve can be assessed from pulmonary vein and mitral valve velocity tracings. Am Heart J 1994;127:886–898.
28. Marino P, Destro G, Barbieri E, Zardini P. Early left ventricular filling: an approach to its multifactorial nature using a combined hemodynamic–Doppler technique. Am Heart J 1991;122:132–141.
29. Choong CY, Herrman HC, Weyman AE, Fifer MA. Preload dependence of Doppler-derived indexes of left ventricular diastolic function in humans. J Am Coll Cardiol 1987;10:800–808.
30. Bowman AW, Frihauf PA, Kovacs SJ. Time-varying effective mitral valve area: prediction and validation using cardiac MRI and Doppler echocardiography in normal subjects. Am J Physiol Heart Circ Physiol 2004;287:H1650–H1657.
31. Marino P, Little WC, Rossi A, et al. Can left ventricular diastolic stiffness be measured noninvasively? J Am Soc Echocardiogr 2002;15:935–943.
32. Hitch DC, Nolan SP. Descriptive analysis of instantaneous left atrial volume with special references to left atrial function. J Surg Res 1981;30:110–120.
33. Prioli A, Marino P, Lanzoni L, Zardini P. Increasing degrees of left ventricular filling impairment modulate left atrial function in humans. Am J Cardiol 1998;82:756–761.
34. Barbier P, Solomon SB, Schiller NB, Glantz SA. Left atrial relaxation and left ventricular systolic function determine left atrial reservoir function. Circulation 1999;100:427–436.
35. Fujii K, Ozari M, Yamagishi T, et al. Effect of left ventricular contractile performance on passive left atrial filling: clinical study using radionuclide angiography. Clin Cardiol 1994;17:258–262.
36. Smiseth OA, Thompson CR, Lo K, et al. The pulmonary venous systolic flow pulse — its origin and relationship to left atrial pressure. J Am Coll Cardiol 1999;34:802–809.
37. Ingwall JS. Energetics of the normal and failing human heart: focus on the creatine kinase reaction. Adv Org Biol 1998;4:117–141.
38. Solaro RJ, Wolska BM, Westfall M. Regulatory proteins and diastolic relaxation. In Lorell BH, Grossman W, eds. Diastolic Relaxation of the Heart. Boston: Kluwer Academic Publishers; 1988: 43–54.

39. Marino P, Faggian G, Bertolini P, Mazzucco A, Little WC. Early mitral deceleration and atrial stiffness. Am J Physiol Heart Circ Physiol 2004;287: H1172–H1178.
40. Bowman AW, Kovacs SJ. Left atrial conduit volume is generated by deviation from the constant-volume state of the left heart: a combined MRI-echocardiographic study. Am J Physiol Heart Circ Physiol 2004;286:H2416–H224.
41. Stefanadis C, Dernellis J, Toutouzas P. Evaluation of the left atrial performance using acoustic quantification. Echocardiography 1998;82:756–761.
42. Altemose GT, Zipes DP, Weksler J, et al. Inhibition of the Na^+/H^+ exchanger delays the development of rapid pacing induced atrial contractile dysfunction. Circulation 2001;103:762–768.
43. Sun H, Chartier D, Leblanc N, et al. Intracellular calcium changes and tachycardia-induced contractile dysfunction in canine atrial myocytes. Cardiovasc Res 2001;49:751–761.
44. Yuel L, Feng J, Gaspo R, Li GR, Wang Z, Nattel S. Ionic remodeling underlying action potential changes in a canine model of atrial fibrillation. Circ Res 1997;81:512–525.
45. Schotten U, Ausma J, Stellbrink C, et al. Cellular mechanism of depressed atrial contractility in patients with chronic atrial fibrillation. Circulation 2001;103:691–698.
46. Marzo KP, Frey MJ, Wilson JR, et al. Beta-adrenergic receptor G-protein–adenylate cyclase complex in experimental canine congestive heart failure produced by rapid ventricular pacing. Circ Res 1991;69:1546–1556.
47. Nagata K, Iwase M, Sobue T, Yokota M. Differential effects of dobutamine and a phosphodiesterase inhibitor on early diastolic filling in patients with congestive heart failure. J Am Coll Cardiol 1995;25:295–304.
48. Parker JD, Landzberg JS, Bittl JA, Mirsky I, Colucci WS. Effects of beta-adrenergic stimulation with dobutamine on isovolumic relaxation in the normal and failing human left ventricle. Circulation 1991;84:1040–1048.
49. Bristow MR, Ginsburg R, Umans V, et al. Beta1 and beta2 adrenergic receptor subpopulations in non-failing and failing human ventricular myocardium: coupling of both receptor subtypes to muscle contraction and selective beta1-receptor downregulation in HF. Circ Res 1986;59:297–309.
50. Bristow MR, Ginsburg R, Minobe W, et al. Decreased catecholamine sensitivity and beta-adrenergic receptor density in failing human hearts. N Engl J Med 1982;307:205–211.

51. Toutouzas K, Trikas A, Pitsavos C, et al. Echocardiographic features of left atrium in elite male athletes. Am J Cardiol 1996;78:1314–1317.
52. Appleton CP, Hatle LK. The natural history of left ventricular filling abnormalities: assessment by two-dimensional and Doppler echocardiography. Echocardiography 1992;9:437–457.
53. Hoit BD, Walsh RA. Regional atrial distensibility. Am J Physiol Heart Circ Physiol 1992;262:H1356–H1360.
54. Tabata T, Oki T, Yamada H, et al. Role of the left atrial appendage clamping during cardiac surgery. Am J Cardiol 1998;81:327–332.
55. Marino P, Barbieri E, Prioli MA, Zardini P. Does prostaglandin E1 infusion affect the left ventricular filling pattern of end-stage dilated cardiomyopathy? A combined hemodynamic–echo Doppler study. J Card Pharm 1998;29:188–195.
56. Briguori C, Betocchi S, Losi MA, et al. Noninvasive evaluation of left ventricular diastolic function in hypertrophic cardiomyopathy. Am J Cardiol 1998;81:180–187.
57. Triposkiadis F, Pitsavos C, Boudoulas H, Trikas A, Toutouzas P. Left atrial myopathy in idiopathic dilated cardiomyopathy. Am Heart J 1994;128:308–315.
58. Little WC, Ohno M, Kitzman DW, Thomas JD, Cheng CP. Determinants of left ventricular chamber stiffness from the time for deceleration of early left ventricular filling. Circulation 1995;92:1933–1939.
59. Rossi A, Zardini P, Marino P. Modulation of left atrial function by ventricular filling impairment. Heart Fail Rev 2000;5:325–331.
60. Atherton JJ, Moore TD, Thomson HL, Frenneaux MP. Restrictive left ventricular filling patterns are predictive of diastolic ventricular interaction in chronic heart failure. J Am Coll Cardiol 1998;31:413–418.
61. Dernellis JM, Stefanadis CI, Zacharoulis AA, Toutouzas PK. Left atrial mechanical adaptation to long-standing hemodynamic loads based on pressure-volume relations. Am J Cardiol 1998;81:1138–1143.
62. Matsuda Y, Toma Y, Moritani K, et al. Assessment of left atrial function in patients with hypertensive heart disease. Hypertension 1986;8:779–785.
63. Suga H. Importance of atrial compliance in cardiac performance. Circ Res 1974;35:39–43.
64. Ishida Y, Meisner JS, Tsujioka K, et al. Left ventricular filling dynamics: influence of left ventricular relaxation and left atrial pressure. Circulation 1986;74:187–196.
65. Hees PE, Fleg JL, Dong SJ, Shapiro EP. MRI and echocardiographic assessment of the diastolic dysfunction of normal aging: altered LV pressure decline or load? Am J Physiol Heart Circ Physiol 2004;286:H782–H788.
66. Masugata H, Mizushige K, Kenda S, et al. Evaluation of left atrial wall elasticity using acoustic microscopy. Angiology 1999;50:583–590.
67. Inaba Y, Yuda S, Kobayashi N, et al. Strain rate imaging for noninvasive functional quantification of the left atrium: comparative studies in controls and patients with atrial fibrillation. J Am Soc Echocardiogr 2005;18:729–736.
68. Di Salvo G, Caso P, Lo Piccolo R, et al. Atrial myocardial deformation properties predict maintenance of sinus rhythm after external cardioversion of recent-onset lone atrial fibrillation. Circulation 2005;112:387–395.
69. Sanders P, Morton JB, Davidson NC, et al. Electrical remodeling of the atria in congestive heart failure — electrophysiological and electroanatomic mapping in humans. Circulation 2003;108:1461–1468.
70. Ausma J, Wijffels M, Thone F, Wouters L, Allessie M, Borgers M. Structural changes of atrial myocardium due to sustained atrial fibrillation in the goat. Circulation 1997;96:3157–3163.
71. Boldt A, Wetzel U, Lauschke J. Fibrosis in left atrial tissue of patients with atrial fibrillation with and without underlying mitral valve disease. Heart 2004;90:400–405.
72. Kono T, Sabbah HN, Rosman H, Alam M, Stein PD, Goldstein S. Left atrial contribution to ventricular filling during the course of evolving heart failure. Circulation 1992;86:1317–1322.
73. Hoit BD, Shao Y, Gabel M, Walsh RA. Left atrial mechanical and biochemical adaption to pacing induced heart failure. Cardiovasc Res 1995;29:469–474.
74. Cooper G 4th. Cardiocyte cytoskeleton in hypertrophied myocardium. Heart Fail Rev 2000;5:187–201.
75. Kostin S, Klein S, Amon E, Scholz D, Schaper J. The cytoskeleton and related proteins in the human failure heart. Heart Fail Rev 2000;5:271–280.
76. Wu Y, Cazorla O, Labeit D. Changes in titin and collagen underlie diastolic stiffness diversity of cardiac muscle. J Mol Cell Cardiol 2000;32:2151–2161.
77. Gwathmey JK, Copelas L, McKinnon R, et al. Abnormal intracellular calcium handling in myocardium from patients with end-stage heart failure. Circ Res 1987;61:70–76.

78. Granzier H, Irving T. Passive tension in cardiac muscle: contribution of collagen, titin, microtubules, and intermediate filaments. Biophys J 1995;68:1027–1044.

79. Borg TK, Caulfield JB. The collagen matrix of the heart. Fed Proc 1981;40:2037–2041.

80. Weber KT. Cardiac interstitium in health and disease: the fibrillar collagen network. J Am Coll Cardiol 1989;13:1637–1652.

81. Medugorac I. Characterization of intramuscular collagen in the mammalian left ventricle. Bas Res Cardiol 1982;77:589–598.

82. Coker M, Thomas C, Clair M, et al. Myocardial matrix metalloproteinase activity and abundance with congestive heart failure. Am J Physiol Heart Circ Physiol 274:H1516–H1523.

83. Cleutjens J. The role of matrix metalloproteinase in heart disease. Cardiovasc Res 1996;32:816–821.

84. Villari B, Campbell SE, Hess OM, et al. Influence of collagen network on left ventricular systolic and diastolic function in aortic valve disease. J Am Coll Cardiol 1993;22:1477–1484.

85. Kato S, Spinale FG, Tanaka R, Johnson W, Cooper G 4th, Zile MR. Inhibition of collagen cross-linking: effects on fibrillar collagen and ventricular diastolic function. Am J Physiol Heart Circ Physiol 1995;269:H863–H868.

86. Weber KT, Sun Y, Tyagi SC, Cleutjiens JP. Collagen network of the myocardium: function, structural remodeling and regulatory mechanism. J Mol Cell Cardiol 1994;26:279–292.

87. Hoit BD, Shao Y, Gabel M, Pawloski-Dahm C, Walsh RA. Left atrial systolic and diastolic function after cessation of pacing in tachycardia-induced heart failure. Am J Physiol Heart Circ Physiol 1997;273:H921–H927.

88. Spinale FG, Coker ML, Krombach SR, et al. Matrix metalloproteinase inhibition during the development of congestive heart failure: effects on left ventricular dimensions and function. Circ Res 1999;85:364–376.

89. Nagatomo Y, Carabello BA, Coker ML, et al. Differential effects of pressure or volume overload on myocardial MMP levels and inhibitory control. Am J Physiol Heart Circ Physiol 2000;278:H151–H161.

90. Spinale FG, Coker ML, Bond BR, Zellner JL. Myocardial matrix degradation and metalloproteinase activation in the failing heart: a potential therapeutic target. Cardiovasc Res 2000;46:225–238.

91. Benjamin EJ, D'Agostino RB, Belanger AJ, Wolf PA, Levy D. Left atrial size and the risk of stroke and death. The Framingham Heart Study. Circulation 1995;92:835–841.

92. Tsang TS, Barnes ME, Bailey KR, et al. Left atrial volume: important risk marker of incident atrial fibrillation in 1,655 older men and women. Mayo Clinic Proc 2001;76:467–475.

93. Modena MG, Muia N, Sgura FA, Molinari R, Castella A, Rossi R. Left atrial size is the major predictor of cardiac death and overall clinical outcome in patients with dilated cardiomyopathy: a long term follow-up study. Clin Cardiol 1997;20:553–560.

94. Rossi A, Cicoria M, Zanolla L, et al. Determinants and prognostic value of left atrial volume in patients with dilated cardiomyopathy. J Am Coll Cardiol 2002;40:1425–1430.

95. Douglas PS. The left atrium: a biomarker of chronic diastolic dysfunction and cardiovascular disease risk. J Am Coll Cardiol 2003;42:1206–1207.

96. Tsang TSM, Barnes ME, et al. Prediction of risk for first age related cardiovascular events in an elderly population: the incremental value of echocardiography. J Am Coll Cardiol 2003;42:1199–1205.

97. Pepi M, Marenzi GC, Agostoni PG, et al. Sustained cardiac diastolic changes elicited by ultrafiltration in patients with moderate congestive heart failure: pathophysiological correlates. Br Heart J 1993;70:135–140.

98. Ohtani K, Yutani C, Nagata S, et al. High prevalence of atrial fibrosis in patients with dilated cardiomyopathy. J Am Coll Cardiol 1995;25:1162–1169.

99. Douglas PS. The left atrium: a biomarker of chronic diastolic dysfunction and cardiovascular disease risk. J Am Coll Cardiol 2003;42:1206–1207.

100. Leistad E, Christensen G, Ilebekk A. Significance of increased atrial pressure on stroke volume during atrial fibrillation in anaesthetized pigs. Acta Physiol Scand 1993;32:149–157.

101. Sanfilippo A, Abascal V, Sheehan M, et al. An atrial enlargement as a consequence of atrial fibrillation. A prospective echocardiographic study. Circulation 1990;82:792–797.

102. Sun H, Gaspo R, Leblanc N, Nattel S. Cellular mechanisms of atrial contractile dysfunction caused by sustained atrial tachycardia. Circulation 1998;98:719–727.

103. Psaty Bm, Manolio TA, Kuller LH, et al. Incidence of and risk factors for atrial fibrillation in older adults. Circulation 1997;96:2455–2461.

104. Shapiro EP, Effron MB, Lima S, Ouyang P, Siu CO, Bush D. Transient atrial dysfunction after cardio-

version of chronic atrial fibrillation to sinus rhythm. Am J Cardiol 1988;62:1202–1207.

105. Olshansky B, Rosenfled LE, Warner AL, et al. The Atrial Fibrillation Follow-up Investigation of Rhythm Management (AFFIRM) study: approaches to control rate in atrial fibrillation. J Am Coll Cardiol 2004;43:1201–1208.

106. Ito Y, Arakawa M, Noda T, et al. Atrial reservoir and active transport function after cardioversion of chronic atrial fibrillation. Heart Vessels 1996; 11:30–38.

107. Leistad E, Aksnes G, Verburg E, Christensen G. Atrial contractile dysfunction after short-term atrial fibrillation is reduced by verapamil but increased by BAY. Circulation 1996;93:1747–1754.

108. Harjai KJ, Mobarek S, Cheirif J, Boulos LM, Murgo JP, Abi-Samra F. Clinical variables affecting recovery of left atrial mechanical function after cardioversion from atrial fibrillation. J Am Coll Cardiol 1997;30:481–486.

109. Louie EK, Liu D, Reynertson SI, Loeb HS, McKiernan TL, Scanlon PJ, Hariman RJ. Stunning of the left atrial atrium after spontaneous conversion of atrial fibrillation to sinus rhythm: demonstration by transesophageal Doppler techniques in a canine model. J Am Coll Cardiol 1998; 32:2081–2086.

110. Urschel CW, Covell JW, Sonnenblick EH. Myocardial mechanics in aortic and mitral valvular regurgitation: the concept of instantaneous impedance as a determinant of the performance of the intact heart. J Clin Invest 1968;47:867–883.

111. Nishimura RA, Tajik AJ. Evaluation of diastolic filling of left ventricle in health and disease: Doppler echocardiography is the clinician's Rosetta stone. J Am Coll Cardiol 1997;30:8–18.

112. Ren JF, Kotler MN, DePace NL, et al. Two-dimensional echocardiographic determination of left atrial emptying volume: a noninvasive index in quantifying the degree of nonrheumatic mitral regurgitation. J Am Coll Cardiol 1983;2:729–736.

113. Kihara Y, Sasayama S, Miyazaki S, et al. Role of the left atrium in adaptation of the heart to chronic mitral regurgitation in conscious dogs. Circ Res 1988;62:543–553.

114. Stefanadis C, Dernellis J, Toutouzas P. A clinical appraisal of left atrial function. Eur Heart J 2001; 22:22–36.

115. Zile Mr, Tomita M, Nakano K, et al. Effects of left ventricular volume overload produced by mitral regurgitation on diastolic function. Am J Physiol Heart Circ Physiol 1991;261:H1471–H1480.

116. Corin WJ, Murakami T, Monrad ES, Hess OM, Krayenbuehl HP. Left ventricular passive diastolic properties in chronic mitral regurgitation. Circulation 1991;83:797–807.

5
Role of Neurohormones and Peripheral Vasculature

Gretchen L. Wells and William C. Little

Introduction

Heart failure is a complex syndrome involving both cardiac and noncardiac abnormalities. For example, patients with systolic heart failure (SHF; heart failure in association with a reduced left ventricular ejection fraction) have a dilated, hypocontractile left ventricle (LV). In addition, neurohormonal activation, inflammation, renal dysfunction, and anemia also play important roles in the clinical syndrome of SHF. Similarly, diastolic dysfunction is almost invariably present in diastolic heart failure (DHF)[1]; however, other factors also importantly contribute to DHF. This chapter specifically addresses the role of neurohormonal activation and vascular effects in DHF.

Role of Neurohormonal Activation

Much more is known about the role of neurohormones in SHF than in DHF. However, the syndrome of heart failure is similar in SHF and DHF with similar degrees of neurohormonal activation.[2] Thus, knowledge of the role of neurohormones in SHF may also be applicable to DHF.

Neurohormonal activation (including the renin-angiotensin-aldosterone system, sympathetic nervous system, endothelins, and natriuretic peptides) plays a pivotal role in the development and progression of SHF. While these neurohormonal changes are initially compensa-tory, with progression of heart failure, the neurohormonal activation becomes deleterious. Such adverse consequences of prolonged neurohormonal activation include vasoconstriction, increased afterload, excessive fluid retention, adverse ventricular remodeling, and arrhythmias. The severity of neuroendocrine activation correlates with the onset of SHF, symptomatic status, progression, survival, and response to therapy.[3,4] Agents that block neurohormonal activation (e.g., angiotensin-converting enzyme [ACE] inhibitors, angiotensin receptor blockers, β-adrenergic blockers, and aldosterone antagonists) can slow and/or reverse the progression of SHF.

Renin-Angiotensin-Aldosterone System

The renin-angiotensin-aldosterone system is activated when there is inadequate renal perfusion. Angiotensin II is produced from its inactive substrate angiotensin I by ACE. Angiotensin II is a potent vasoconstrictor, and through renal effects and stimulation of aldosterone it promotes fluid retention. Chronic activation of the renin-angiotensin-aldosterone system increases cardiac extracellular matrix fibrillar collagen and is associated with increased myocardial stiffness. In addition to promoting fibroblast growth, angiotensin II stimulates cardiac myocyte hypertrophy and activates other neurohormonal pathways, including aldosterone, endothelin, and the sympathetic nervous system. The importance of the renin-angiotensin-aldosterone system in the pathophysiology of heart failure is underscored by the effectiveness of antagonists of this system

TABLE 5.1. Potential neurohormonal effects in diastolic heart failure.

	Structural effects	Functional effects
Angiotensin II	Left ventricular (LV) hypertrophy fibrosis	Slow relaxation, decreased distensibility
Aldosterone	LV fibrosis	?
Norepinephrine	LV hypertrophy	Chronic: impaired filling
		Acute: enhanced relaxation
Endothelin-1	LV hypertrophy	Slow relaxation, decreased distensibility

in reducing mortality,[5] improving symptoms,[6] and delaying the progression of asymptomatic LV systolic dysfunction to heart failure.[7]

Renin-angiotensin systems are present not only in the circulation but also in the tissues, including the heart.[8] The tissue production of angiotensin II may occur by pathways not dependent on ACE (i.e., the chymase pathway). It has been suggested that this pathway is of major importance, particularly when the levels of renin and angiotensin I are increased by the use of ACE inhibitors.

The renin-angiotensin-aldosterone system has important effects in the setting of cardiac changes associated with diastolic dysfunction, both on cardiac structure and function (Table 5.1). Angiotensin II stimulates the development of LV hypertrophy and fibrosis, both directly and by stimulating the formation of aldosterone. The development of myocardial hypertrophy and fibrosis impairs diastolic distensibility. The renin-angiotensin-aldosterone system also has adverse functional consequences both by producing vasoconstriction that increases systolic arterial pressure and by direct effects on the myocardium.

There is an alteration in the cardiac response to angiotensin II in the presence of LV hypertrophy. In animals with LV hypertrophy, administration of angiotensin I results in an increase in cardiac ACE activity and a subsequent increase in angiotensin II, but this increase in both cardiac ACE and angiotensin II is not observed in animals without LV hypertrophy. Furthermore, this increase in ACE and angiotensin II results in altered diastolic properties in hypertrophied hearts.[9] This finding suggests that ACE inhibitors would be beneficial for patients with LV hypertrophy and diastolic dysfunction. Consistent with this concept, human subjects with LV hypertrophy due to hypertension had an improvement in LV relaxation in response to intracoronary enalaprilat. This improvement in active relaxation was directly proportional to the severity of LV hypertrophy.[10]

The cardiac effects of angiotensin II are also altered by the presence of heart failure. In dogs studied before pacing-induced heart failure, angiotensin II produced only a load-dependent slowing of LV relaxation; however, after pacing-induced heart failure, angiotensin II severely depressed LV contraction and relaxation (Figure 5.1).[11] These effects are mediated through angiotensin I (AT$_1$) receptors. A follow-up study of dogs with pacing-induced heart failure demonstrated augmentation of the normal exercise-induced increase in angiotensin II (Figure 5.2A). Associated with this rise in angiotensin II were elevations in LV diastolic pressure, left atrial pressure, and slowed LV relaxation (Figure 5.2B).[12] Treatment with the AT$_1$ receptor antagonist, losartan, blunted this abnormal exercise response in heart failure.

Other animal models of DHF have demonstrated the activation of the renin-angiotensin-aldosterone system and endothelin-1 resulting in progressive myocardial stiffening.[13] This effect is blunted by either an AT$_1$ receptor antagonist or an endothelin type A (ET$_A$) receptor antagonist.[14] Similarly, the use of an angiotensin II receptor blocker reduced myocardial fibrosis and improved diastolic LV stiffness in patients with hypertension, LV hypertrophy, and marked myocardial fibrosis.[15]

Patients with DHF may experience symptoms only with exertion as they are able to augment their cardiac output only with an abnormal elevation in the LV filling pressures (i.e., left atrial pressure). Furthermore, systolic blood pressure normally increases with exercise, and this increase

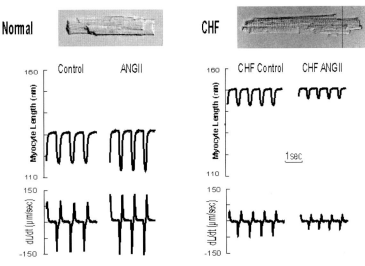

FIGURE 5.1. The effect of angiotensin II (ANGII) on myocytes obtained from the canine left ventricle. In normal myocytes, the infusion of angiotensin II increased the extent of myocyte shortening as well as the rate of shortening and the rate of relengthening (dL/dt). After congestive heart failure (CHF), the myocytes were longer with a reduced extent of shortening. The infusion of angiotensin II decreased the extent of shortening as well as the speed of shortening and relaxation. (Data from Cheng et al.[11])

may be exaggerated in elderly and hypertensive patients, even when the blood pressure is well-controlled at rest. Hypertension is known to exacerbate diastolic dysfunction. The angiotensin II receptor blocker, losartan, blunts the hypertensive response to exercise and increases exercise tolerance in elderly hypertensive patients with diastolic dysfunction (Figure 5.3).[16] Further studies demonstrated that the angiotensin II receptor blockers, losartan and candesartan, improved exercise tolerance; whereas, verapamil and hydrochlorothiazide did not.[17,18]

Despite the similar pathophysiologies of DHF and SHF, there have been few studies of ACE inhibitors and AT$_1$ receptor antagonists in patients with DHF. The Candesartan in Heart Failure-Assessment of Reduction in Mortality and Morbidity (CHARM) Preserved arm (one of three arms of the broader CHARM program) is the only large trial published to date of patients with DHF.[19] This trial did not find a significant mortality benefit of the AT$_1$ receptor antagonist, candesartan, in DHF. The primary endpoint of cardiovascular death occurred in 333 (22%) patients in the candesartan arm and in 366 (24%) of those in the placebo arm (hazard ratio, 0.89; 95% CI, 0.77–1.03; $p = 0.12$) (Figure 5.4). However, the mean age of this study group was only 67 years, and only 40% of the participants were women (as opposed to most series in which patients are aged 75 years or older and more than 60% are women).

Observational studies following the postdischarge outcomes of patients hospitalized with DHF have reached conflicting conclusions regarding the use of ACE inhibitors and angiotensin receptor antagonists in this population. Two studies have suggested a mortality benefit in patients treated with these agents;[20,21] whereas, another study demonstrated no difference with a trend toward poorer outcomes.[22]

Aldosterone, the final product of the renin-angiotensin-aldosterone system, is released from the adrenal glands in response to stimulation by angiotensin II. Aldosterone is also released independent of angiotensin II in response to an increase in serum potassium, catecholamines, or endothelin. Aldosterone is a potent stimulant of myocardial fibrosis and hypertrophy. Blocking

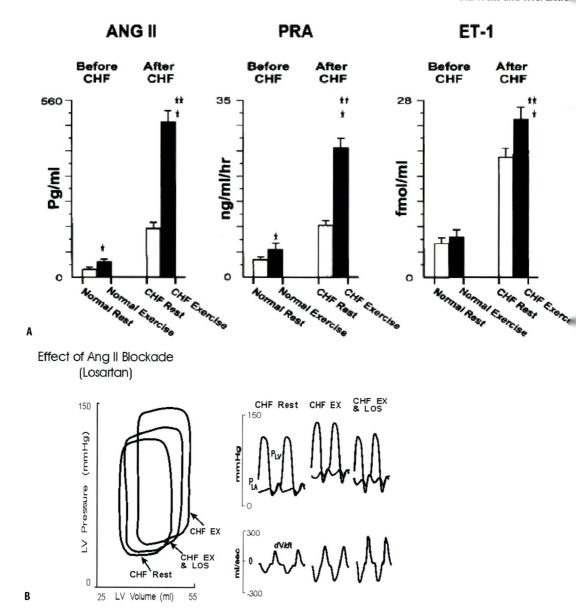

FIGURE 5.2. **(A)** Serum levels of angiotensin II (ANG II), plasma renin activity (PRA), and endothelin-1 (ET-1). All three increased during normal exercise. After the development of congestive heart failure (CHF), the baseline levels of all three increased, and they increased to even higher levels during heart failure exercise. (Reprinted from Cheng et al.,[12] with permission of The American Physiological Society.) **(B)** Effect of exercise after heart failure. There is an upward shift in the diastolic portion of the LV pressure–volume loop with heart failure exercise (CHF EX). This is accompanied by an increase in left atrial pressure. The angiotensin receptor blocker losartan (LOS) blunted the upward shift of the diastolic portion of the pressure–volume loop as well as the increase in left atrial pressure. In addition, there was an increase in the maximum rate of LV filling (dV/dt). (Data from Cheng et al.[12])

aldosterone's actions with spironolactone or the aldosterone receptor antagonist, eplerenone, is effective in improving the outcome in selected patients with SHF.[23] The National Heart, Lung and Blood Institute has approved funding for a large, randomized, placebo-controlled trial of the aldosterone blocker, spironolactone, in patients with DHF.

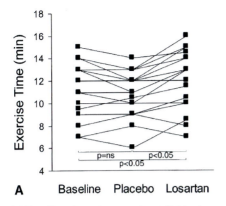 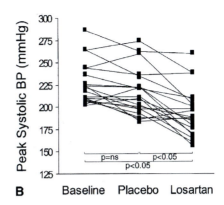

FIGURE 5.3. **(A)** The effect of exercise on peak systolic blood pressure (BP) and exercise time in a randomized, double-blind, crossover study. Placebo did not decrease peak systolic BP, but losartan did. **(B)** The decrease in peak systolic BP with losartan was associated with an increase in exercise time. (Reprinted from Warner et al.,[16] with permission of the American College of Cardiology Foundation.)

Endothelin

There is also considerable evidence to support the role of endothelin-1 in disease progression in heart failure. Endothelin-1 is a potent vasoconstrictor and a stimulus for the renin-angiotensin-aldosterone system and the sympathetic nervous system.[24] Endothelin-1 levels are elevated in heart failure, and the magnitude of elevation correlates with disease severity.[25] In addition to the increase in angiotensin II levels with exercise in animals with heart failure, there is a concomitant increase in endothelin-1 that is not seen normally with exertion (see Figure 5.2A). In an animal model of pacing-induced heart failure, treatment with L-754,142, a potent endothelin-1 antagonist, decreased this abnormal response (Figure 5.5).[12] Combined treatment with both the AT_1 receptor

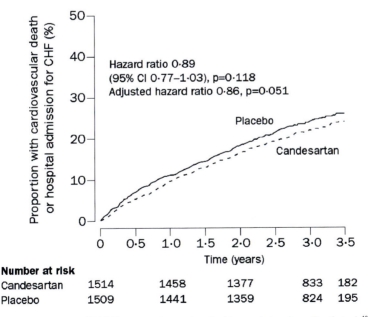

FIGURE 5.4. Results of the CHARM Preserved Trial. The proportion of patients with cardiovascular death or hospital admission was reduced by candesartan. CHF, congestive heart failure. (Reproduced with permission from Yusuf et al.,[19] with permission of Elsevier.)

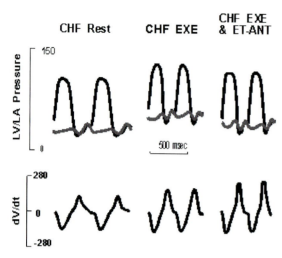

FIGURE 5.5. The effect of exercise (EXE) after congestive heart failure (CHF). With exercise, there is an increase in left atrial pressure. After treatment with an endothelin antagonist (ET-ANT), the increase in left atrial pressure with exercise is reduced. (Data from Cheng et al.[12])

antagonist and the endothelin-1 antagonist was more effective at blocking the abnormal exercise response than either agent alone.

Clinical trials of endothelin receptor antagonism have shown no benefit in acute or chronic SHF.[26] However, endothelin receptor antagonists may be beneficial in DHF, but no studies of patients with DHF have been completed.

Sympathetic Activation

In conjunction with the renin-angiotensin-aldosterone system, the sympathetic nervous system is activated in heart failure. Long-term exposure of the heart to norepinephrine causes not only downregulation of cardiac β-adrenoceptors but also cardiac hypertrophy, ischemia, arrhythmias, and direct myocyte toxicity with necrosis and apoptosis.[27] Levels of circulating catecholamines increase in patients with heart failure in proportion to the severity of disease, and those with the highest plasma levels of norepinephrine have the most unfavorable prognosis.[28] Most clinical trials of β-blockers in the treatment of SHF have established a survival benefit.[29,30] However, a class effect with β-blockers has not been established, as survival was not affected by the more β_2-adrenreceptor–selective antagonist, bucindolol.[31]

β-Blockers have a favorable effect on diastolic function in patients with systolic dysfunction. In patients with idiopathic dilated cardiomyopathy, transmitral Doppler indices of diastolic function improved within the first 3 months of treatment with the β-receptor antagonist, metoprolol, predating the improvement in systolic function.[32] Later invasive studies of 14 patients with an idiopathic cardiomyopathy treated with metoprolol had a decrease in LV end-diastolic pressure associated with faster LV relaxation, a decrease in the LV chamber stiffness constant, and an improvement in LV elastance.[33] No studies of long-term use of β-blockers have been completed in DHF.

Natriuretic Peptides

Natriuretic peptides are a family of hormones that are activated in heart failure in response to ventricular dilatation and pressure overload.[34] Plasma levels of brain (B-type) natriuretic peptide (BNP) are elevated in patients with congestive heart failure and increase in proportion to the severity of heart failure symptoms and degree of LV dysfunction.[35] The actions of BNP include natriuresis, vasodilatation, and inhibition of the renin-angiotensin-aldosterone system and sympathetic nervous system.[36] Intravenous administration of BNP (nesiritide) improved cardiac hemodynamic parameters acutely in patients with decompensated heart failure.[37] However, two post-hoc analyses have suggested that nesiritide may be associated with the development of renal dysfunction[38] and increased mortality.[39]

Measurement of neurohormones has become an accepted clinical practice to diagnose heart failure and to assess disease severity and response to therapy. Neurohormones are elevated in patients with DHF, although they have not been as extensively studied as in SHF. In a study comparing the pathophysiology of isolated DHF to SHF, Kitzman et al.[2] found that norepinephrine levels were similar in patients with DHF (306 [64] pg/ml) and SHF (287 [62] pg/ml) ($p = 0.56$), and both were increased in comparison to healthy controls (169 [80] pg/ml) ($p = 0.007$ and 0.03, respectively). B-type natriuretic peptide was only modestly elevated in DHF (56 [30] pg/ml) compared with SHF (154 [28] pg/ml); however, both groups were elevated in comparison to healthy

5. Neurohormones and Peripheral Vasculature

controls (3 [38] pg/ml) ($p = 0.02$ and 0.001, respectively). In a larger series of patients with diastolic dysfunction, elevation of plasma BNP correlated with the severity of diastolic abnormalities on echocardiography.[40]

Role of the Vascular System

Arterial System

Diastolic dysfunction is a common sequela of arterial hypertension. Normal aging is associated with an increase in systolic blood pressure at both rest and exertion. Hypertension, which is primarily a vascular disease, leads to increased arterial wall thickening and stiffness. In response to this pressure overload on the heart, the myocytes enlarge (hypertrophy) to maintain a normal cardiac output. Although LV hypertrophy allows the heart to maintain systolic function, this adaptive process becomes detrimental, leading to diastolic dysfunction. Early studies of hypertensive patients with LV hypertrophy demonstrated that reducing blood pressure reversed ventricular hypertrophy and improved diastolic function.[41]

The rise in systolic blood pressure in normal elderly patients is due to a decrease in aortic compliance. Studies have identified a relationship between exercise intolerance and increased vascular stiffness in healthy older individuals. Hundley et al.[42] assessed the proximal aorta with magnetic resonance imaging in older patients with DHF and found reduced distensibility of the aorta out of proportion to that associated with normal aging. The severity of exercise intolerance correlated with the decrease in aortic distensibility (Figure 5.6).

Patients with DHF also demonstrate combined systolic ventricular and arterial stiffening. Kawaguchi et al.[43] found elevated end-systolic elastance (stiffness) and arterial elastance in patients with DHF compared with age-matched controls and those patients with hypertension without heart failure. Such ventricular–vascular stiffening tightens the coupling between left ventricular pressure and systolic arterial pressure. Thus, these patients frequently have labile systolic blood pressure. Episodes of systolic hypertension may be associated with acute pulmonary edema.[44] The same patients may experience orthostatic hypotension when only slightly volume depleted. Redfield et al.[45] found that advancing age and female gender are associated with increases in vascular and ventricular systolic and diastolic stiffness, even in the absence of cardiovascular disease. This combined ventricular–vascular stiffening may contribute to the increase of CHF in elderly women. The increase in cardiac (systolic ventricular) stiffening and arterial stiffening has a number of adverse cardiovascular effects, including blunted contractile reserve, augmented systolic pressure, sensitivity to volume loading, and increased energy demand.

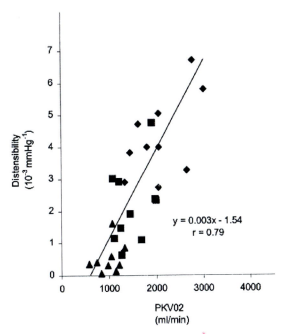

FIGURE 5.6. Relation between aortic distensibility and exercise tolerance measured by peak oxygen consumption (PKVO$_2$) in elderly subjects with and without diastolic heart failure. (Reprinted from Hundley et al.,[42] with permission of the American College of Cardiology Foundation.)

Venous System

In addition to increased arterial stiffness, patients with DHF may also have abnormalities of the venous system. Acute decreases in venous capacitance may shift blood into the lungs, contributing to the development of acute pulmonary edema.[46]

References

1. Zile MR, Gaasch WH, Carroll JD, et al. Heart failure with a normal ejection fraction: is measurement of diastolic function necessary to make the diagnosis of diastolic heart failure? Circulation 2001;104:779–782.
2. Kitzman DW, Little WC, Brubaker PH, et al. Pathophysiological characterization of isolated diastolic heart failure in comparison to systolic heart failure. JAMA 2002;288:2144–2150.
3. Benedict CR, Shelton B, Johnstone DE, et al. Prognostic significance of plasma norepinephrine in patients with asymptomatic left ventricular dysfunction. Circulation 1996;94:690–697.
4. Jourdain P, Funck F, Gueffet P, et al. Benefits of BNP plasma levels for optimizing therapy: the Systolic Heart Failure Treatment Supported by BNP Multicenter Randomised Trial (STARS-BNP) [abstr]. J Am Coll Cardiol 2005;45(Suppl A): 3A.
5. The CONSENSUS Trial Study Group. Effects of enalapril on mortality in severe congestive heart failure. N Engl J Med 1987;316:1429–1435.
6. The SOLVD Investigators. Effect of enalapril on survival in patients with reduced left ventricular ejection fractions and congestive heart failure. N Engl J Med 1991;325:293–302.
7. The SOLVD Investigators. Effect of enalapril on mortality and the development of heart failure in asymptomatic patients with reduced left ventricular ejection fractions. N Engl J Med 1992;327:685–691.
8. Dzau VJ. Cardiac renin-angiotensin system. Am J Med 1988;84(Suppl 3):22–27.
9. Schunkert H, Dzau VJ, Tang SS, et al. Increased rat cardiac angiotensin converting enzyme activity and mRNA expression in pressure overload left ventricular hypertrophy. Effects on coronary resistance, contractility, and relaxation. J Clin Invest 1990;86:1913–1920.
10. Haber HL, Powers ER, Gimple LW, et al. Intracoronary angiotensin-converting enzyme inhibition improves diastolic function in patients with hypertensive left ventricular hypertrophy. Circulation 1994;89:2616–2625.
11. Cheng CP, Suzuki M, Ohte N, et al. Altered ventricular and myocyte response to angiotensin II in pacing-induced heart failure. Circ Res 1996;78:880–892.
12. Cheng CP, Ukai T, Onishi K, et al. The role of ANG II and endothelin-1 in exercise-induced diastolic dysfunction in heart failure. Am J Physiol Heart Circ Physiol 2001;280:H1853–H1860.
13. Yamamoto K, Masuyama T, Sakata Y, et al. Local neurohumoral regulation in the transition to isolated diastolic heart failure in hypertensive heart disease: absence of AT1 receptor downregulation and "overdrive" of the endothelin system. Cardiovasc Res 2000;46:421–432.
14. Yoshida J, Yamamoto K, Mano T, et al. Angiotensin II type 1 and endothelin type A receptor antagonists modulate the extracellular matrix regulatory system differently in diastolic heart failure. J Hypertens 2003;21:437–444.
15. Diez J, Querejeta R, Lopez B, et al. Losartan-dependent regression of myocardial fibrosis is associated with reduction of left ventricular chamber stiffness in hypertensive patients. Circulation 2002;105:2512–2517.
16. Warner JG J., Metzger DC, Kitzman DW, et al. Losartan improves exercise tolerance in patients with diastolic dysfunction and a hypertensive response to exercise. J Am Coll Cardiol 1999;33:1567–1572.
17. Little WC, Wesley-Farrington D, Hoyle J, et al. Effect of candesartan and verapamil on exercise tolerance in diastolic dysfunction. J Cardiovasc Pharmacol 2004;43:288–293.
18. Little WC, Zile MR, Klein A, et al. Effect of losartan and hydrochlorothiazide on exercise tolerance in exertional hypertension and left ventricular diastolic dysfunction. Am J Cardiol 2006;98:383–385.
19. Yusuf S, Pfeffer MA, Swedberg K, et al. Effects of candesartan in patients with chronic heart failure and preserved left-ventricular ejection fraction: the CHARM Preserved Trial. Lancet 2003;362:777–781.
20. Sueta CA, Russo A, Schenck A, et al. Effect of angiotensin-converting inhibitor or angiotensin receptor blocker on one-year survival in patients ≥65 years hospitalized with a left ventricular ejection fraction ≥50%. Am J Cardiol 2003;91:363–365.
21. Philbin EF, Rocco TA, Jr. Use of angiotensin-converting enzyme inhibitors in heart failure with preserved left ventricular systolic function. Am Heart J 1997;134:188–195.
22. Dauterman KW, Go AS, Rowell R, et al. Congestive heart failure with preserved systolic function in a statewide sample of community hospitals. J Card Fail 2001;7:221–228.
23. Pitt B, Reichek N, Willenbrock R, et al. Effects of eplerenone, enalapril, and eplerenone/enalapril in patients with essential hypertension and left ventricular hypertrophy: the 4E-Left Ventricular Hypertrophy Study. Circulation 2003;108:1831–1838.

5. Neurohormones and Peripheral Vasculature

24. Haynes WG, Webb DJ. Endothelin as a regulator of cardiovascular function in health and disease. J Hypertens 1998;16:1081–1098.
25. Wei CM, Lerman A, Rodeheffer RJ, et al. Endothelin in human congestive heart failure. Circulation 1994;89:1580–1586.
26. Rich S, McLaughlin VV. Endothelin receptor blockers in cardiovascular disease. Circulation 2003;108:2184–2190.
27. Sackner-Bernstein JD, Mancini DM. Rationale for treatment of patients with chronic heart failure with adrenergic blockade. JAMA 1995;274:1462–1467.
28. Cohn JN, Levine TB, Olivari MT, et al. Plasma norepinephrine as a guide to prognosis in patients with chronic congestive heart failure. N Engl J Med 1984;311:819–823.
29. Packer M, Bristow MR, Cohn JN, et al. The effect of carvedilol on morbidity and mortality in patients with chronic heart failure. N Engl J Med 1996;334:1349–1355.
30. Goldstein S, Fagerberg B, Hjalmarson A, et al. Metoprolol controlled release/extended release in patients with severe heart failure: analysis of the experience in the MERIT-HF Study. J Am Coll Cardiol 2001;38:932–938.
31. The Beta-Blocker Evaluation of Survival Trial Investigators. A trial of the beta-blocker bucindolol in patients with advanced chronic heart failure. N Engl J Med 2001;344:1659–1667.
32. Andersson B, Caidahl K, Di Lenarda A, et al. Changes in early and late diastolic filling patterns induced by long-term adrenergic beta-blockade in patients with idiopathic dilated cardiomyopathy. Circulation 1996;94:673–682.
33. Kim MH, Devlin WH, Das SK, et al. Effects of beta-adrenergic blocking therapy on left ventricular diastolic relaxation properties in patients with dilated cardiomyopathy. Circulation 1999;100:729–735.
34. Levin ER, Gardner DG, Samson WK. Natriuretic peptides. N Engl J Med 1998;339:321–328.
35. Maisel A. B-type natriuretic peptide levels: a potential novel "white count" for congestive heart failure. J Card Failure 2001;7:183–193.
36. Stein BC, Levin RI. Natriuretic peptides: physiology, therapeutic potential, and risk stratification in

ischemic heart disease. Am Heart J 1998;135(5 Pt 1):914–923.
37. Mills RM, LeJemtel TH, Horton DP, et al. Sustained hemodynamic effects of an infusion of nesiritide (human B-type natriuretic peptide) in heart failure: a randomized, double-blind, placebo-controlled clinical trial. Natrecor Study Group. J Am Coll Cardiol 1999;34:155–162.
38. Sackner-Bernstein JD, Skopicki HA, Aaronson KD. Risk of worsening renal function with nesiritide in patients with acutely decompensated heart failure. Circulation 2005;111:1487–1491.
39. Sackner-Bernstein JD, Kowalski M, Fox M, et al. Short-term risk of death after treatment with nesiritide for decompensated heart failure: a pooled analysis of randomized controlled trials. JAMA 2005;293:1900–1905.
40. Lubien E, DeMaria A, Krishnaswamy P, et al. Utility of B-natriuretic peptide in detecting diastolic dysfunction: comparison with Doppler velocity recordings. Circulation 2002;105:595–601.
41. Trimarco B, DeLuca N, Rosiello G, et al. Effects of long-term antihypertensive treatment with tertatolol on diastolic function in hypertensive patients with and without left ventricular hypertrophy. Am J Hypertens 1989;2(11 Pt 2):278S–283S.
42. Hundley WG, Kitzman DW, Morgan TM, et al. Cardiac cycle–dependent changes in aortic area and distensibility are reduced in older patients. J Am Coll Cardiol 2001;38:796–802.
43. Kawaguchi M, Hay I, Fetics B, et al. Combined ventricular systolic and arterial stiffening in patients with heart failure and preserved ejection fraction: implications for systolic and diastolic reserve limitations. Circulation 2003;107:714–720.
44. Gandhi SK, Powers JC, Nomeir AM, et al. The pathogenesis of acute pulmonary edema associated with hypertension. N Engl J Med 2001;344:17–22.
45. Redfield MM, Jacobsen SJ, Borlaug BA, et al. Age- and gender-related ventricular–vascular stiffening: a community-based study. Circulation 2005;112:2254–2262.
46. Burkhoff D, Tyberg JV. Why does pulmonary venous pressure rise after onset of LV dysfunction: a theoretical analysis. Am J Physiol 1993;265:H1819–H1828.

6
Filling Velocities as Markers of Diastolic Function

Otto A. Smiseth

Introduction

Left ventricular (LV) filling velocities provide important insights into ventricular function and are useful clinical markers of diastolic dysfunction. Filling velocities can be measured at bedside by Doppler echocardiography and can be incorporated into everyday cardiology practice. Interpretation of filling velocities in a clinical context, however, requires insights into cardiac mechanics. The objective of this chapter is to review the essential physiology of filling and how changes in LV systolic and diastolic function can modify filling velocities as measured by Doppler echocardiography. This chapter addresses filling of the *left* ventricle only. Filling patterns for the *right* ventricle are of clinical importance for the diagnosis of restrictive cardiomyopathy and constrictive pericarditis and are addressed in Chapter 21.

The three hallmarks of diastolic dysfunction are (1) retarded LV relaxation, (2) reduced diastolic compliance, and (3) a compensatory elevation of LV diastolic pressure (Table 6.1). The latter is not a primary disturbance of cardiac function but is the result of regulatory mechanisms that seek to maintain stroke volume. Retarded relaxation and reduced compliance may occur in combination, or only one of the two may be disturbed. When one assesses diastolic function clinically, it is essential to interpret measurements with each of the three hallmarks in mind. Furthermore, one should understand that filling velocities are markers only and do not provide quantitative data regarding LV relaxation, chamber compli-

ance, or end-diastolic pressure. Filling patterns, however, provide indices of diastolic dysfunction that are very useful clinically and can be recorded at bedside in virtually every patient. Filling velocities can be measured in the pulmonary veins, in the mitral orifice, and in the LV cavity, and this chapter deals with each of these measurement sites separately.

Pulmonary Venous Flow Velocities

Introduction

Assessment of pulmonary venous flow velocities by Doppler echocardiography represents an important "window" into the physiology of cardiac filling. Pulmonary flow velocities provide insights into left atrial as well as LV mechanical function. The pulmonary venous flow velocity typically has three phases: a systolic wave (S wave), a diastolic wave (D wave), and a reversed flow wave during atrial contraction (Figure 6.1). Furthermore, as illustrated in Figure 6.2, in many patients the systolic flow pulse has an early systolic wave and a late systolic wave. The latter is usually the larger of the two waves. Figure 6.2 also demonstrates that the pulmonary venous flow trace looks like an approximately inverted left atrial pressure tracing, which means that flow accelerates when atrial pressure decreases and vice versa. An exception to this is during mid/late systole, when flow accelerates while pressure is rising, and this is discussed later in more detail.

TABLE 6.1. Key points in assessment of diastolic filling.

Markers of impaired left ventricular (LV) relaxation
- Reduced transmitral early (E) velocity: confounded by elevated left atrial pressure, which may increase the transmitral pressure gradient and E velocity
- Reduced LV lengthening velocity (E') by tissue Doppler imaging

Markers of reduced LV chamber compliance (increased stiffness)
- Abbreviated transmitral E deceleration time
- Reduced transmitral atrial (A) velocity

Markers of elevated LV end-diastolic pressure
- Duration of transmitral A much less than retrograde pulmonary venous A
- Elevated E/E' ratio
- Increased transmitral E/A ratio
- Enlarged left atrium

Markers of increased pericardial constraint
- Marked respiratory variation in mitral and tricuspid velocities
- Elevated jugular venous pressure indicates elevated pericardial pressure

Limitations of filling velocities
- Reduction of LV distensibility with no change in chamber compliance (parallel shift of pressure-volume curve) may not change E deceleration time or A velocity
- Filling velocities do not provide quantitative data on diastolic function

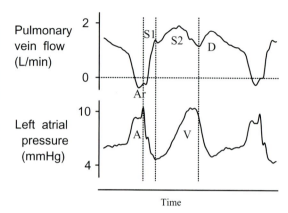

FIGURE 6.2. Representative recording of pulmonary vein flow and left atrial pressure. taken prior to cardiopulmonary bypass. Left ventricular pressure and electrocardiogram are included for timing. The letters indicate the atrial pressure waves and four pulmonary venous flow pulses, the Ar wave during atrial contraction, the S1 and S2 waves during ventricular systole, and the D wave in early diastole. (Modified from Smiseth OA, Thompson CR. Atrioventricular filling dynamics, diastolic function and dysfunction. Heart Fail Rev 2000;5:291–299.)

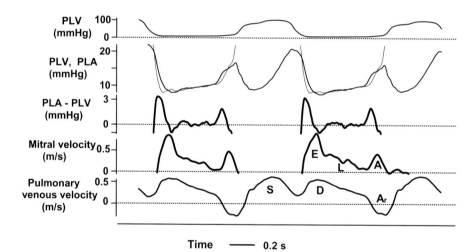

FIGURE 6.1. Intraoperative measurements of left atrial and left ventricular filling in a patient with coronary artery disease. Left ventricular ejection fraction was normal. Recordings were done prior to cardiopulmonary bypass. Left atrial and left ventricular pressures were measured with a single catheter with two pressure sensors 7 cm apart. Midway between the pressure sensors there was an electromagnetic velocity sensor that measured mitral blood flow velocity. Pressures were zero-referenced by comparison to pressure measured via a fluid-filled catheter in the left atrium. Pulmonary venous flow was measured by ultrasound transit time from a flow probe on the right lower pulmonary vein, and flow velocity was derived by dividing with the cross-section of the vein by transesophageal echocardiography. A, transmitral atrial-induced velocity; Ar, atrial-induced reversed velocity; D, diastolic velocity; E, transmitral early velocity; L, transmitral L-wave, PLA, left atrial pressure; PLA-PLV, the atrioventricular pressure difference; PLV, left ventricular pressure; S, systolic velocity.

Early and Mid-Diastolic Pulmonary Venous Flow

The early diastolic pulmonary venous flow is initiated by onset of transmitral filling, which leads to atrial emptying and a drop in left atrial pressure. This results in an increase in the pulmonary venous to left atrial pressure gradient. Therefore, the pulmonary venous D wave corresponds to the transmitral early filling velocity, and the peak D wave velocity is determined by many of the factors that determine peak early transmitral filling velocity.[1] Figure 6.1 illustrates the timings of pulmonary venous and mitral velocities. After the peak of the D wave, the pulmonary venous velocity decreases progressively until atrial contraction causes marked flow deceleration.

Late-Diastolic Pulmonary Venous Flow

The reversed late-diastolic pulmonary venous flow (Ar) is caused by atrial contraction, and its magnitude and duration are determined by atrial systolic function, by atrial preload, and by impedance to forward flow across the mitral valve and to retrograde flow into the pulmonary veins. Measurement of Ar in combination with transmitral flow is of clinical interest for estimation of LV diastolic pressure.[2,3]

The relative amount of blood that moves forward or backward during atrial contraction depends on the relative compliance of the LV and the pulmonary veins. When atrial mean pressure is elevated, there is an accompanying decrease in LV chamber compliance. This is a consequence of the curvilinear relationship between LV diastolic pressure and volume (see later). Therefore, at elevated LV diastolic pressure there is reduced atrial contribution to LV filling, which is reflected in a small and abbreviated transmitral A velocity.[4] The pulmonary vasculature appears to be more compliant than the left ventricle, and therefore markedly elevated preload is associated with a large Ar but a small and shortened transmitral A velocity.[2,3] This forms the basis for using the difference between duration of the transmitral A wave and Ar as a clinical index of LV diastolic pressure. This index functions best when atrial function is preserved and can generate a marked pressure rise in end diastole.

Heart rate should be taken into account when using Ar to assess diastolic function.[5] Thus, at slow heart rates the pulmonary venous flow rate approaches zero prior to atrial contraction. Therefore, inertial forces are small, and atrial contraction most often results in flow reversal. During tachycardia, however, atrial contraction starts early in diastole when antegrade flow is substantial and inertial forces are much stronger. Therefore, during tachycardia the Ar may be absent, although left atrial mean pressure is markedly elevated.[5]

Systolic Pulmonary Venous Flow

The etiology of the systolic pulmonary venous flow pulse (S wave) has been controversial.[6-14] One theory is that the S wave is caused by transpulmonary propagation of the right ventricular pressure pulse. The other theory is that the S wave is caused by the early systolic fall in left atrial pressure, which sucks blood from the pulmonary veins, caused by atrial relaxation and systolic descent of the atrioventricular plane. Differentiation between these two mechanisms has been possible by applying the principles of wave intensity analysis.[15,16] This analysis indicates that the early systolic flow wave is caused by atrial suction (a backward going wave), and the mid/late systolic flow wave is caused predominantly by the right ventricular pressure pulse (a forward going wave). These etiologies can be appreciated intuitively by considering simultaneous measurements of pulmonary venous pressure and velocity, as displayed in Figure 6.2. During early systole there is a decrease in pulmonary venous pressure along with an increase in velocity, as would be expected if somebody is "pulling" the blood forward.[16] During most of mid and late systole, however, there are simultaneous increases in pulmonary venous pressure and velocity, as if somebody is "pushing" the blood forward.[16] During this flow phase a "suction" effect from the left atrium may also contribute, but the dominant mechanism is the forward "pushing" effect caused by right ventricular contraction. In addition, reflected waves may contribute to the pulmonary venous flow pattern but do not appear to be of major importance.[17]

As shown by the wave intensity analysis, the pulsations in the pulmonary venous flow trace throughout most of the heart cycle, that is, diastole and early systole, are attributed to left-sided cardiac events.[16] The only time that right-sided events dominate is mid and late systole. Another important point is that LV systolic function is a determinant of the systolic flow pulse, because systolic descent of the atrioventricular plane contributes to the S-wave in both the early and late phases of systole.

It has been suggested to use the pulmonary venous systolic/diastolic velocity ratio as a marker of LV diastolic pressure. This is based on observations in patients with congestive heart failure and elevated LV diastolic pressure who tend to have reduced magnitude of the S wave.[18,19] When LV diastolic pressure is elevated acutely, however, there is on the contrary an increase in the S wave. This is demonstrated in Figure 6.3. It appears that the relationship between the systolic/diastolic velocity ratio and LV diastolic pressure in congestive heart failure reflects an association and not a causal relationship. Possibly, reduced LV contractility in heart failure attenuates the S wave by reducing LV long-axis shortening and hence the early systolic fall in left atrial pressure. Furthermore, right ventricular contractility may be reduced and contribute to the reduction of the S wave.

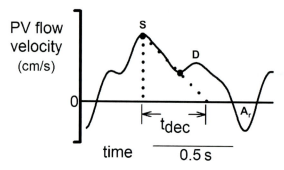

FIGURE 6.4. Calculation of deceleration time of systolic pulmonary venous flow (t_{dec}). A line was drawn between the point of peak systolic flow to the nadir between the systolic and early diastolic flow pulses, and the line was extrapolated to zero flow. The T_{dec} is the time interval between peak systolic flow and the zero flow intercept. Ar, atrial-induced reversed velocity.

Deceleration Time of Systolic Pulmonary Venous Flow — A Marker of Left Atrial Compliance and Pressure

As demonstrated recently, the deceleration time of systolic pulmonary venous flow reflects left atrial chamber compliance.[20] The principle for measuring deceleration time is illustrated in Figure 6.4. The mechanism behind this relation-

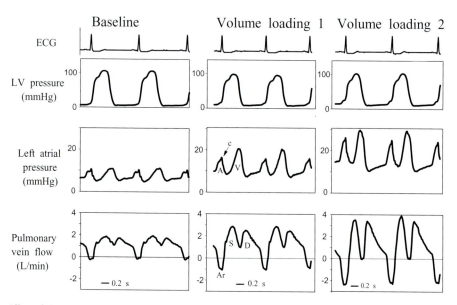

FIGURE 6.3. Effect of elevated left atrial pressure on pulmonary venous flow pattern. Intraoperative recordings prior to cardiopulmonary bypass. Left atrial pressure was increased in two steps by volume loading. There was an increase in the pulmonary venous S and D waves. (From Smiseth OA, Thompson CR. Atrioventricular filling dynamics, diastolic function and dysfunction. Heart Fail Rev 2000;5:291–299.)

ship is that filling of a stiff atrium is associated with a marked rise in atrial pressure, which leads to faster deceleration of atrial inflow. This principle is analogous to that used to assess LV diastolic compliance from deceleration time of early transmitral flow as addressed elsewhere in this chapter.

Because of the curvilinearity of the atrial diastolic pressure–volume (PV) relationship, elevation of left atrial pressure leads to a decrease in left atrial chamber compliance and therefore a short deceleration time. These principles explain why deceleration time provides an estimate of atrial pressure. Figure 6.5 illustrates how elevation of atrial pressure leads to a reduction in atrial compliance and a reduction in deceleration time.

The relationship between deceleration time and left atrial compliance suggests a new noninvasive approach for estimating left atrial passive elastic properties and left atrial pressure. It remains to be investigated how this principle may be utilized clinically. Importantly, deceleration time does not differentiate between "true" changes in left atrial compliance due to structural remodeling of the atrial wall and pressure-related changes in chamber compliance. When changes in deceleration time occur acutely, however, significant structural remodeling can be excluded, and it is likely that deceleration time reflects changes in left atrial compliance and pressure.

It has been proposed to use the deceleration time of PV diastolic flow to estimate left atrial pressure.[21] Whereas this method is quite promising, it may be limited by tachycardia, which may markedly abbreviate or abolish the PV diastolic flow wave. Furthermore, deceleration time measured from diastolic venous flow is determined by elastic properties of the left ventricle as well as the left atrium, while systolic deceleration time is determined predominantly by left atrial elastic properties.

Conclusion

The pulsations in pulmonary venous flow are attributed almost entirely to downstream events; that is, the D wave is caused by the decrease in left atrial pressure that results from LV relaxation, the Ar is caused by atrial systolic contraction, and the early systolic flow wave is caused by the decrease in atrial pressure due to atrial relaxation and systolic descent of the mitral ring. The only exception is the mid/late systolic flow, which is caused predominantly by an upstream event, that is, forward propagation of the right ventricular systolic pulse.

The pulmonary venous velocity pattern is primarily a reflection of pressure oscillations in the left atrium and therefore represents a noninvasive method for evaluating patients with potential diastolic dysfunction. It is important to be aware, however, that the pulmonary vein flow velocities are also influenced by left and right ventricular systolic function due to direct effects on the S wave. The deceleration time for systolic pulmonary venous flow appears to be a marker of atrial compliance and pressure level.

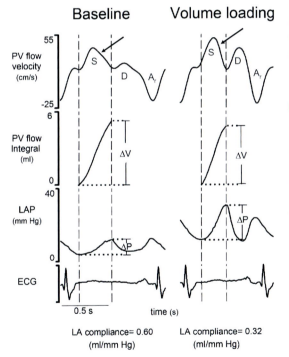

FIGURE 6.5. Reduction of left atrial (LA) compliance at elevated pressure. Recordings from a patient in an intraoperative study. Left atrial compliance was calculated as the time integral of systolic pulmonary venous flow (ΔV) divided by the increment in left atrial pressure (LAP) during ventricular systole (ΔP). Flow in one single pulmonary vein was assumed to represent a constant fraction of flow in all pulmonary veins. ECG, electrocardiogram; PV, pulmonary vein. The arrow points to the deceleration of systolic flow, which is much faster after volume loading. (From Hunderi et al.[20])

Transmitral Flow Velocities

Figure 6.6 illustrates the four phases of diastole: isovolumic relaxation, rapid early filling, diastasis, and atrial-induced filling. During isovolumic relaxation LV pressure falls rapidly, the mitral valve is closed, and no filling of the ventricle occurs. When ventricular pressure has declined to a level below atrial pressure, a pressure gradient is established between the atrium and the ventricle, the mitral valve opens, and the ventricle fills rapidly. During diastasis left atrial and LV pressures almost equilibrate, and transmitral flow occurs at a low rate. Subsequently, atrial contraction causes a pressure gradient, and late diastolic filling of the ventricle occurs.

Isovolumic Relaxation

The isovolumic relaxation time (IVRT) is defined as the time interval between aortic valve closure and mitral valve opening, and it can be measured by echocardiography (see Chapter 10). This time interval is determined by the decay rate of LV pressure, and therefore IVRT reflects the rate of LV relaxation. However, other determinants of valve movements will also influence IVRT, and this includes LV and left atrial pressures. For example, elevated LV systolic pressure will cause prolongation of IVRT because isovolumic relaxation starts from a higher pressure, whereas elevation of left atrial pressure will abbreviate the IVRT because of premature opening of the mitral valve.[22] Therefore, IVRT as an index of LV relaxation is confounded by changes in LV systolic and left atrial pressures, and these variables need to be taken into account when using IVRT in the evaluation of diastolic function.

Rapid Early Diastolic Filling

Relationship Between Filling Velocities and Pressure Gradient

The transmitral pressure gradient is the difference between left atrial and LV pressures. The Bernoulli equation is used clinically to calculate transvalvular pressure gradients from Doppler flow velocities.[23] The Bernoulli equation consists of a *convective term*, which relates the drop in pressure to the rise in kinetic energy as velocity increases because of narrowing at the valve orifice (convective acceleration), an *inertial term*, which expresses the pressure drop needed to accelerate the mass of blood through the valve (local acceleration), and a *viscous term*, which expresses the pressure loss caused by viscous drag along the walls.[24-26]

In mitral stenosis convective acceleration dominates, and the simplified Bernoulli equation ($\Delta P = 4v^2$) can be applied to calculate the transmitral gradient. In normal mitral valves, however, a relatively large volume of blood is contained within the valve, and a substantial fraction of the transmitral pressure gradient is needed to overcome inertia. Therefore, mitral velocity cannot be converted to pressure difference using the simplified Bernoulli equation, and the real pressure gradient is larger than predicted by the simplified Bernoulli equation. This is a systematic underestimation, and therefore peak transmitral filling rate correlates very well with the transmitral pressure gradient (see Figure 6.7).[27,28] Viscous friction is not important, because the blood is in contact with the walls only briefly.

The inertial effect also accounts for the marked delay in peak velocity relative to peak gradient. This is illustrated in Figure 6.1, which demonstrates that peak mitral flow velocity occurs when the pressure gradient is near zero. Transmitral flow velocity increases as long as there is a positive pressure gradient, that is, an accelerating force. When the pressure gradient reverses, it represents a decelerating force and causes velocity to decrease. This implies that timing of velocities cannot be used to define exact timing of gradient.

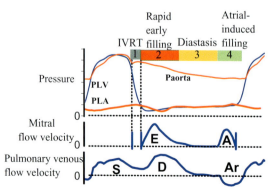

FIGURE 6.6. Schematic representation of the four phases of diastole. IVRT, isovolumic relaxation time; PLA, left atrial pressure; PLV, left ventricular pressure.

6. Filling Velocities

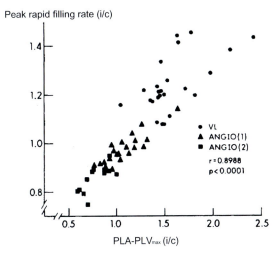

FIGURE 6.7. Relationship between normalized peak transmitral filling rate and peak transmitral pressure difference. Values during intervention are normalized relative to control (i/c); The interventions include intravenous volume loading (VL) and angiotensin II at two different doses (ANGIO 1 and ANGIO 2). PLA, left atrial pressure; PLV, left ventricular pressure. (Modified from Ishida et al.[27])

Despite these limitations, peak transmitral filling velocity is a very useful marker of peak mitral pressure gradient. For research studies, color M-mode Doppler echocardiography represents a means to calculate the instantaneous transmitral pressure gradient by taking the inertial component into account.[29] This methodology, however, is not needed in routine assessment of diastolic filling.

One should be aware of the confusion that may be created by using the terms *pressure gradient* and *pressure difference* interchangeably, as pressure gradient is pressure difference per distance (cm). In cardiology literature, however, it is customary to use gradient instead of pressure difference. The term *pressure gradient* is used in this chapter except when it is important to make the distinction. Because of regional pressure differences in the left ventricle during diastole, the transmitral pressure difference may vary depending on catheter position, but this theoretical problem does not limit the use of transmitral filling velocities in a clinical context.

Determinants of Peak Early Transmitral Pressure Gradient

The peak early diastolic transmitral pressure gradient is determined by rate of relaxation, by LV restoring forces (elastic recoil), by the diastolic PV relationship of the left ventricle and the left atrium, and by the operating pressure (e.g., slowing of relaxation leads to elevation of LV minimum diastolic pressure and therefore tends to reduce the transmitral pressure gradient and E velocity; Figure 6.8). Because minimum diastolic pressure depends on end-systolic volume, changes in systolic function will modify the transmitral pressure gradient and hence the peak E velocity. For instance, depression of systolic function with an increase in LV end-systolic volume leads to a higher minimum diastolic pressure, which tends to reduce peak early transmitral gradient and E velocity. Improvement in systolic function with a reduction in end-systolic volume has the opposite effect. Changes in blood volume can markedly modify the transmitral pressure gradient. Furthermore, left atrial reservoir function and compliance determine how rapidly atrial pressure declines after onset of LV filling. This means that factors other than true changes in LV diastolic function can modify the peak E wave.

The role of diastolic suction in LV filling is not entirely clear. In animal experiments, however, when end-systolic volumes are reduced below the unstressed LV volume, significant negative LV transmural pressures are generated, reflecting restoring forces that may contribute to LV filling. Furthermore, systolic LV twist (torsion) and subsequent early diastolic untwist may contribute to filling. The early diastolic untwist has been attributed to restoring forces and appears to be a function of LV end-systolic volume.[30] Figure 6.9 demonstrates that most of the untwist occurs in early diastole. Further studies are needed to define how diastolic suction and untwist may play a role in diastolic filling in the diseased heart.

Mid-Diastolic Filling

During diastasis left atrial and LV pressures almost equilibrate, and transmitral flow occurs at a low rate, that is, the L wave. The etiology and determinants of the L wave are not entirely clear. As illustrated in Figure 6.1, the L wave does not appear to be the result of atrial emptying, because there is a steady rise in left atrial pressure during diastasis, indicating increasing atrial volume. However, pulmonary venous flow continues throughout the period of diastasis, indicating that

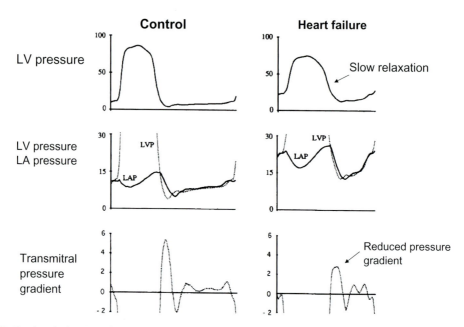

FIGURE 6.8. Slowing of relaxation in heart failure causes a reduction in peak transmitral pressure difference. Data from animal model of acute ischemic left ventricular failure. LA, left atrium; LAP, left atrial pressure; LV ventricle; LVP, left ventricular pressure. (Modified from Stugaard M, Risøe C, Ihlen H, Smiseth OA. Intracavitary filling pattern in the failing left ventricle assessed by color M-mode Doppler echocardiography. J Am Coll Cardiol 1994;24:663–670.)

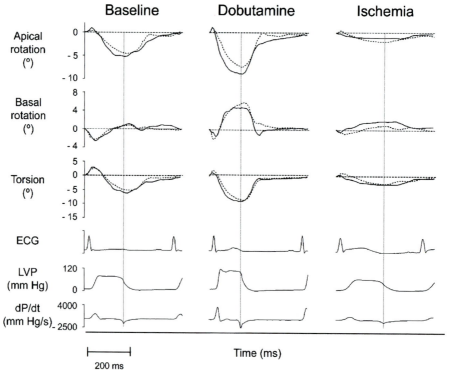

FIGURE 6.9. Left ventricular rotation and torsion measured by sonomicrometry and speckle tracking echocardiography in a dog model. The vertical lines define end systole (peak negative left ventricular dP/dt). Torsion (twist) is the difference in rotation at the apical and basal level. Both methodologies conform substantial untwist in early diastole. ECG, electrocardiogram; LVP, left ventricular pressure. (Modified from Helle-Valle T, Crosby J, Edvardsen T, Lyseggen E, Amundsen BH, Smith HJ, Rosen BD, Lima JA, Torp H, Ihlen H, Smiseth OA. New noninvasive method for assessment of left ventricular rotation: speckle tracking echocardiography. Circulation 2005;112(20):3149–3156.)

the L wave is attributed entirely to pulmonary venous return. The transmitral pressure difference during the L wave is very small, suggesting that transmitral flow during diastasis may be driven in part by the momentum of the blood that enters the atrium from the pulmonary veins.

Atrial-Induced Filling

The left atrium contracts in late diastole and sets up a pressure gradient that causes the transmitral A wave. As described for rapid early filling, there is flow acceleration when the gradient is positive and deceleration when it reverses (see Figure 6.1). The transmitral A velocity is determined by atrial function, LV function, and loading conditions. To interpret measurements of transmitral A velocity

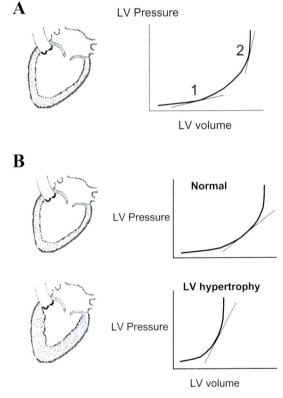

FIGURE 6.10. Left ventricular (LV) pressure–volume curves (curved lines) and LV chamber compliance (straight lines). **(A)** An increase in LV diastolic pressure from 1 to 2 causes a reduction in LV chamber compliance. Because the pressure–volume coordinates are moving along a single pressure–volume curve, there is no change in LV passive elastic properties. **(B)** Left ventricular hypertrophy leads to a shift in the LV pressure volume curve, indicating an increase in LV stiffness.

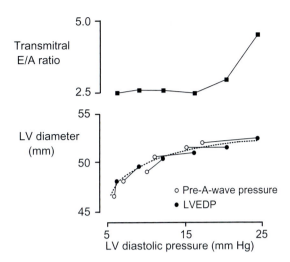

FIGURE 6.11. Relationship between atrial contribution to left ventricular (LV) filling and LV diastolic pressure. **(Top)** Progressive rise in transmitral E/A velocity ratio at elevated LV diastolic pressures. **(Bottom)** Atrial contribution to LV filling, measured as an increase in LV short axis diameter during atrial contraction, is reduced when diastolic pressure is elevated. Pre-A-wave pressure, LV pressure prior to atrial contraction; LVEDP, LV end-diastolic pressure. (From Myreng et al.[4])

it is essential to understand the meaning of *LV chamber compliance*, because this variable is an important determinant of magnitude and duration of transmitral A velocity.

Chamber compliance is the relationship between change in LV diastolic pressure and change in volume and is determined by myocardial compliance and by the extraventricular constraint exerted by pericardium and lungs. Furthermore, because the LV PV relationship is curvilinear, chamber compliance is a function of the operative LV diastolic pressure and consequently is markedly load dependent. Therefore, a change in LV chamber compliance does not necessarily mean there has been a change in myocardial elastic properties; it may just be a change in loading conditions, as illustrated schematically in Figure 6.10. Importantly, chamber compliance represents the effective compliance that faces the blood that flows into the ventricle in diastole and therefore has a major effect on LV filling velocities. Comprehensive invasive evaluation of diastolic function is outlined in Chapter 9.

Figure 6.11 illustrates how an acute increase in LV diastolic pressure causes a marked decrease in atrial contribution and therefore an increase in the transmitral E/A ratio. The reduced atrial contribution was due to a reduction in chamber compliance, which represents an increase in afterload for the left atrium.

Filling Patterns in Heart Failure

The transmitral filling pattern is determined by rate of LV relaxation, chamber compliance, and level of diastolic pressure, and each of these variables can be evaluated by Doppler echocardiography. Left ventricular relaxation can be evaluated by measuring myocardial early diastolic lengthening velocity by tissue Doppler imaging (see Chapter 10), chamber compliance by deceleration time of early transmitral filling velocity, and diastolic pressure by a number of approaches (see Chapter 13).

Slowing of LV relaxation occurs in myocardial dysfunction regardless of etiology and causes a

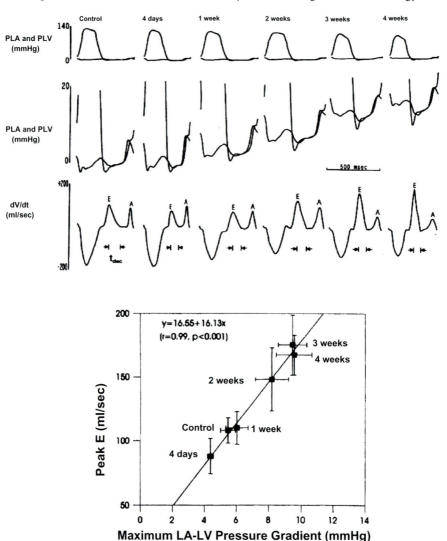

FIGURE 6.12. Changes in transmitral flow pattern and relationship to transmitral pressure gradient during development of congestive heart failure in a dog model. **(Top)** Analog recordings of left atrial and left ventricular pressures (PLA, PLV) along with the time derivative of left ventricular (LV) volume (dV/dt). In diastole, the latter measures transmitral filling rates. Peak early (E) and atrial-induced (A) filling are indicated. During the early phase of heart failure there is a drop in E. With more advanced heart failure, when there is a marked increase in PLA, there is tall E and small A. **(Bottom)** Changes in peak E correlate strongly with peak transmitral pressure gradient. (From Ohno et al.,[28])

FIGURE 6.13. Deceleration time of early filling (t_{dec}) reflects left ventricular stiffness (KLV). (From Ohno et al.,[28])

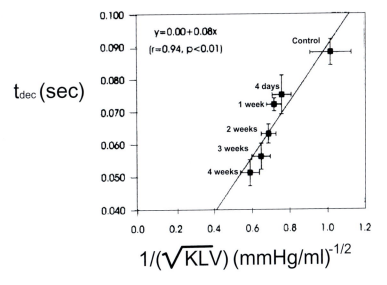

decrease in peak E velocity, with a compensatory increase in peak A velocity. This shift in filling from early to late diastole, measured as a decrease in the E/A ratio, is described clinically as a pattern of *impaired relaxation* (see Chapter 10).

As heart failure progresses and left atrial pressure becomes elevated, there is typically an increase in the early diastolic transmitral pressure gradient, which increases peak E velocity, and the E/A ratio may become normal (Figure 6.12). Clinically this is described as a *pseudonormalized* filling pattern.

When heart failure progresses further, left atrial pressure may become markedly elevated and the early diastolic transmitral pressure gradient increases, leading to supernormal peak E velocity. Because elevation of LV diastolic pressure causes the ventricle to operate on a steeper portion of its PV curve, indicating reduced chamber compliance, there is little further increase in LV volume during atrial contraction. This is measured as a small and abbreviated transmitral A velocity. Furthermore, because of reduced LV chamber compliance, the early filling velocity decelerates rapidly.[31,32] This filling pattern with increased E/A ratio and short E deceleration time is described as *restrictive physiology*. An additional feature of this filling pattern is abbreviated IVRT due to premature opening of the mitral valve caused by the elevated left atrial pressure. As demonstrated in Figure 6.13, E deceleration time is directly related to LV stiffness.

Atrial contraction causes the late diastolic transmitral filling wave (A wave). The A wave is determined by left atrial systolic function, by the LV diastolic PV curve, and by intracavitary LV pressure. Figure 6.11 demonstrates the relationship between the E/A ratio and LV chamber compliance.[33]

Intraventricular Filling

Similar to transmitral filling, intraventricular filling has an early and an atrial-induced filling phase. This is illustrated in Figure 6.14, which shows transmitral and intraventricular filling in a normal individual. In cardiac disease intraventricular filling may be disturbed, and the abnormal filling patterns have been introduced as markers of LV function and dysfunction. However, assessing intraventricular filling is more complex than measuring flow velocities in blood vessels and across heart valves because of the multitude of variables that determine intraventricular flow. Not only driving pressure, inertial forces, and viscous friction but also geometry, regional differences in function, and asynchronies in contraction play major roles as well. Furthermore, flow occurs in multiple and rapidly changing

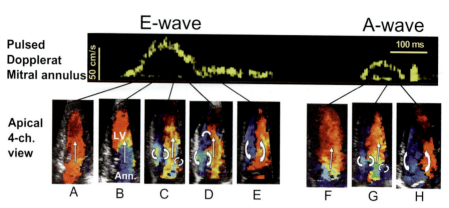

FIGURE 6.14. Left ventricular two-dimensional color flow and transmitral flow velocities in a middle-aged healthy person. Images are four-chamber apical views. Blood moving toward the transducer is depicted in shades of red and yellow, whereas blood moving away from the transducer is in shades of blue and yellow. With the use of low pulse repetition frequency, a multicolored pattern secondary to aliasing occurs at relatively low velocities. Arrows schematically indicate flow patterns interpreted from the velocity signals. Letters indicate sequential recordings, and their timing in relation to transmitral flow is indicated. (Modified from Rodevand O, Bjornerheim R, Edvardsen T, Smiseth OA, Ihlen H. Diastolic flow pattern in the normal left ventricle. J Am Soc Echocardiogr 1999;12(6):500–507.)

directions, forming complex vortex patterns.[34,35] It is therefore difficult to relate measures of intraventricular flow to LV function. There is, however, a well-defined intraventricular flow disturbance that has proven to be a marker of LV dysfunction, that is, mitral-to-apical flow propagation or timing of early diastolic apical filling. The mechanisms of mitral-to-apical flow propagation and how this variable may be related to diastolic function are discussed.

Intraventricular Pressure Gradients and Apical Suction

Similar to transmitral filling, normal LV intracavitary filling is dominated by an early wave and an atrial-induced wave. Most of the attention has been toward the early diastolic filling wave as it has proven to change markedly during myocardial ischemia and LV failure.[36,37] In the normal ventricle the early filling wave propagates rapidly toward the apex and is driven by a pressure gradient between LV base and apex.[38–40] In LV dysfunction there is reduction of the gradient and therefore slowing of mitral-to-apical flow propagation.[41] Nikolic et al.[42] demonstrated that the LV base-to-apex diastolic pressure gradient was related to the magnitude of LV restoring forces. Figure 6.15 illustrates intraventricular pressure gradients in a patient.

Because restoring forces are assumed to be the mechanism of diastolic suction, it is possible that mitral-to-apical early diastolic pressure gradient can be a marker of diastolic suction. The idea is that blood is sucked toward the apex in early diastole because of the pressure gradient caused by restoring forces. Doppler echocardiography represents a means to estimate the mitral-to-apical pressure gradient in patients and has the potential to become a diagnostic tool to quantify diastolic suction.[40,43,44] The analysis needed to calculate intraventricular gradient by Doppler, however, is complicated. An alternative method for assessing apical suction is measurement of mitral-to-apical flow propagation. The normal rapid apical filling may be a marker of apical suction, and retardation of apical filling in LV dysfunction may indicate loss of apical suction.[41] Figure 6.16 shows slowing of flow propagation during acute myocardial ischemia.

6. Filling Velocities

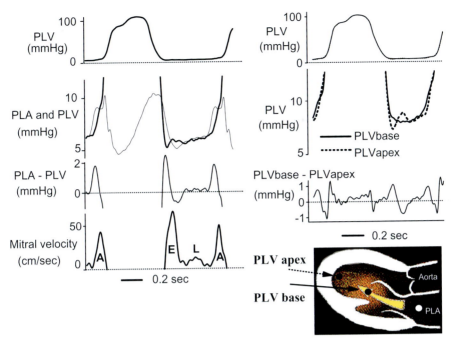

FIGURE 6.15. Left atrial and intraventricular pressures recorded intraoperatively prior to coronary surgery. Recordings were obtained via a catheter with three micromanometers and an electromagnetic fluid velocity sensor (model SSD-827, Millar Instruments, Houston, TX). The catheter was inserted via a pulmonary vein and was first advanced toward the left ventricular apex, and pressures were recorded 4 cm apart **(right)**. Then it was withdrawn such that the velocity sensor was near the mitral leaflet tips, and pressures were recorded 7 cm apart across the mitral valve **(left)**. Across the mitral valve and inside the ventricle there is first a positive diastolic gradient, which accounts for the early filling wave, and subsequently the gradient reverses and causes deceleration of flow. PLA, left atrial pressure; PLV, left ventricular pressure. (Reprinted with permission from Smiseth OA, Thompson CR. Atrioventricular filling dynamics, diastolic function and dysfunction. Heart Fail Rev 2000;5:291–299.)

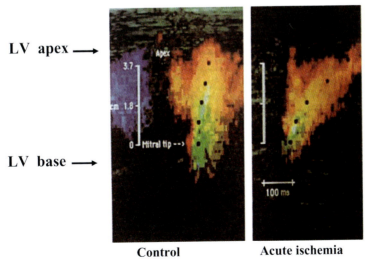

FIGURE 6.16. Effect of acute myocardial ischemia on early diastolic mitral-to-apical flow propagation. Color M-mode Doppler recording of early diastolic inflow in a patient before balloon angioplasty, during balloon inflation, and 5 minutes after balloon deflation. The black dots indicate peak velocities. Before balloon occlusion flow propagates rapidly toward the apex. During ischemia, however, there is a change in the flow image with apparent slowing of flow propagation. LV, left ventricle. (Modified from Stugaard et al.[37])

Left Ventricular Intracavitary Filling in Heart Failure — Role of Vortices

Experimental and model studies suggest that mitral-to-apical flow propagation is caused by two different mechanisms. In the normal ventricle blood propagates rapidly from the mitral tips toward the apex as if an entire column of blood moves toward the apex, attributed in part to apical suction. This type of filling has been denoted *column motion*.[45] Thereafter, there is a phase of protracted filling that appears to represent smoke ring vortices that move slowly toward the apex.[45-47] In the normal ventricle the early rapid column motion dominates. In the failing and in the ischemic ventricle the rapid column motion is reduced or lost and mitral-to-apical flow is attributed mainly to smoke ring vortices that move slowly toward the apex. Figure 6.17 illustrates schematically the smoke ring vortices, and Figure 6.16 illustrates the two phases of filling, with a dominance of rapid early filling during baseline and a dominance of protracted filling during ischemia. Therefore, when color M-mode Doppler is used to estimate mitral-to-apical flow propagation, two different phenomena are quantified.

The slow mitral-to-apical flow propagation in the failing ventricle is attributed to ring vortices that move slowly toward the apex, and the propagation velocity observed by color M-mode Doppler reflects how fast the vortex is moving toward the apex.[45,48] Not only rate of LV relaxation but also ventricular geometry and the ratio between mitral orifice size and LV cavity size influence vortex formation and mitral-to-apical flow propagation velocity.[45,49] A relative reduction in the size of the mitral orifice enhances vortex formation and causes slowing of mitral-to-apical flow propagation in the diseased ventricle.

Therefore, it is not a straightforward relationship between mitral-to-apical flow propagation velocity and LV diastolic function. This complicates the interpretation of intraventricular flow patterns and the use of intraventricular flow as a marker of dysfunction. Marked slowing of mitral-to-apical flow propagation is definitely a sign of LV disease, but the magnitude of flow propagation is determined by a number of factors other than diastolic function. The complexity of intraventricular flow and the limitations of current imaging techniques make it difficult to relate intraventricular flow patterns to LV wall function in a quantitative manner. This complexity limits the utility of assessing mitral-to-apical filling. Furthermore, in most patients with grossly abnormal intraventricular flow there are a number of other hemodynamic signs of impaired LV function, and assessment of intraventricular flow often becomes redundant as a means to identify dysfunction. However, as outlined in Chapter 13, it

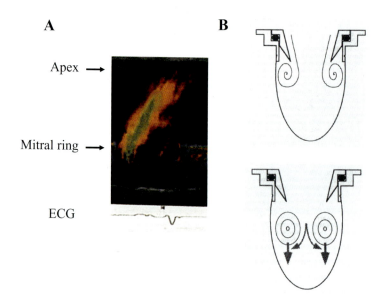

FIGURE 6.17. Retarded left ventricular apical filling and smoke ring vortices. **(A)** Intraventricular filling by color M-mode Doppler in a patient with reduced left ventricular ejection fraction. Note that apical filling is markedly delayed relative to transmitral flow. (From Stugaard M, Steen T, Lundervold A, Smiseth OA, Ihlen H. Visual assessment of intraventricular filling from colour M-mode Doppler images. Int J Card Imaging 1994;10:279–287.) **(B)** Illustration of smoke ring vortices that propagate toward the apex. It seems that retarded apical filling in heart failure reflects slow propagation of vortices toward the apex. (From Steen and Steen.[45])

has proven to be of some value in the noninvasive assessment of LV diastolic pressure.

References

1. Nishimura RA, Abel MD, Hatle LK, Tajik AJ. Relation of pulmonary vein to mitral flow velocity by transesophageal Doppler echocardiography. Effect of different loading conditions. Circulation 1990; 81:1488–1497.
2. Rossvoll O, Hatle LK. Pulmonary venous flow velocities recorded by transthoracic Doppler ultrasound: relation to left ventricular diastolic pressures. J Am Coll Cardiol 1993;21:1687–1696.
3. Appleton CP, Galloway JM, Gonzalez MS, Gaballa M, Basnight MA. Estimation of left ventricular filling pressures using two-dimensional and Doppler echocardiography in adult patients with cardiac disease. Additional value of analyzing left atrial size, left atrial ejection fraction and the difference in duration of pulmonary venous and mitral flow velocity at atrial contraction. J Am Coll Cardiol 1993;22:1972–1982.
4. Myreng Y, Smiseth OA, Risøe C. Left ventricular filling at elevated diastolic pressures. Relationship between transmitral Doppler flow velocities and atrial contribution. Am Heart J 1990;119:620–626.
5. Steen T, Voss BMR, Smiseth OA. Influence of heart rate and left atrial pressure on pulmonary venous flow pattern in the dog. Am J Physiol 1994;266: H2296–H2302.
6. Guntheroth WG, Gould R, Butler J, Kinnen E. Pulsatile flow in pulmonary artery, capillary, and vein in the dog. Cardiovasc Res 1974;8:330–337.
7. Morkin E, Collins JA, Goldman HS, Fishman AP. Pattern of blood flow in the pulmonary veins of dog. J Appl Physiol 1965;20:1118–1128.
8. Pinkerson AL. Pulse-wave propagation through the pulmonary vascular bed of dogs. Am J Physiol 1967;21:450–454.
9. Szidon JP, Ingram RH, Fishman AP. Origins of the pulmonary venous flow pulse. Am J Physiol 1968; 214:10–14.
10. Morgan BC, Abel FL, Mullins GL, Guntheroth WG. Flow patterns in cavae, pulmonary artery, pulmonary vein and aorta in intact dogs. Am J Physiol 1996;210:903–909.
11. Rajagopalan B, Friend JA, Stallard T, Lee de J. Blood flow in pulmonary veins. I. Studies in dog and man. Cardiovasc Res 1979;13:667–676.
12. Rajagopalan B, Friend J A, Stallard T, Lee de J. Blood flow in pulmonary veins. II. The influence of events transmitted from the right and left sides of the heart. Cardiovasc Res 1979;13:677–683.
13. Keren G, Sherez J, Megidish R, Levitt B, Lanaido S. Pulmonary venous flow pattern — its relationship to cardiac dynamics. A pulsed Doppler echocardiographic study. Circulation 1985;71:1105–1112.
14. Barbier P, Solomon S, Schiller NB, Glantz SA. Determinants of forward pulmonary vein flow: an open pericardium pig model. J Am Coll Cardiol 2000;35:1947–1959.
15. Parker KH, Jones CHJ. Forward and backward running waves in the arteries: analysis using the method of characteristics. ASME J Biomech Eng 1990;112:322–326.
16. Smiseth OA, Thompson CR, Lo K, Ling H, Abel JG, Miyagishima RT, Lichtenstein S, Bowering J. The pulmonary venous systolic flow pulse — its origin and relationship to left atrial pressure. J Am Coll Cardiol 1999;34:802–809.
17. Hellevik LR, Segers P, Stergiopulos N, Irgens F, Verdonck P, Thompson CR, Lo K, Miyagishima RT, Smiseth OA. Mechanism of pulmonary venous pressure and flow waves. Heart Vessels 1999;14: 67–71.
18. Kuecherer HF, Muhuidenn IA, Kusumoto F, Lee E, Moulinier LE, Cahalan MK, Schiller NB. Estimation of mean left atrial pressure from transesophageal pulsed Doppler echocardiography of pulmonary venous flow. Circulation 1990;82:1127–1139.
19. Hofmannn T, Keck A, Ingen G van, Ostermeyer J, Meinertz T. Simultaneous measurement of pulmonary venous flow by intravascular catheter Doppler velocimetry and transesophageal Doppler echocardiography: relation to left atrial and left ventricular function. JAAC 1995;26:239–249.
20. Hunderi JO, Thompson CR, Smiseth OA. Deceleration time of systolic pulmonary venous flow: a new clinical marker of left atrial pressure and compliance. J Appl Physiol 2006;100:685–689.
21. Kinnaird TD, Thompson CR, Munt BI. The deceleration time of pulmonary venous diastolic flow is more accurate than the pulmonary artery occlusion pressure in predicting left atrial pressure. J Am Coll Cardiol 2001;38(2):586.
22. Myreng Y, Smiseth OA. Assessment of left ventricular relaxation by Doppler echocardiography. Comparison of isovolumic relaxation time and transmitral flow velocities with time constant of isovolumic relaxation. Circulation 1990;81(1):260–266.
23. Holen J, Aaslid R, Landmark K, Simonsen S. Determination of pressure gradient in mitral stenosis with a non-invasive ultrasound Doppler technique. Acta Med Scand 1976;199(6):455–460.

24. Yellin EL, Nikolic S, Frater RW. Left ventricular filling dynamics and diastolic function. Prog Cardiovasc Dis 1990;32(4):247–271.

25. Thomas JD, Weyman AE. Fluid dynamics model of mitral valve flow: description with in vitro validation. J Am Coll Cardiol 1989;13(1):221–233.

26. Nakatani S, Firstenberg MS, Greenberg NL, Vandervoort PM, Smedira NG, McCarthy PM, Thomas JD. Mitral inertance in humans: critical factor in Doppler estimation of transvalvular pressure gradients. Am J Physiol Heart Circ Physiol 2001;280(3): H1340–H1345.

27. Ishida Y, Meisner JS, Tsujioka K, Gallo JI, Yoran C, Frater RWM, Yellin EL. Left ventricular filling dynamics: influence of left ventricular relaxation and left atrial pressure. Circulation 1986;74:187–196.

28. Ohno M, Cheng C-P, Little WC. Mechanism of altered patterns of left ventricular filling during the development of congestive heart failure. Circulation 1994;89:2241–2250.

29. Greenberg NL, Vandervoort PM, Thomas JD. Instantaneous diastolic transmitral pressure differences from color M mode echocardiography. Am J Physiol 1996;271:H1267–H1276.

30. Gibbons Kroeker CA, Tyberg JV, Beyar R. Effects of load manipulations, heart rate, and contractility on left ventricular apical rotation. An experimental study in anesthetized dogs. Circulation 1995;92(1):130–141.

31. Flachskampf FA, Weyman AE, Guerrero JL, Thomas JD. Calculation of atrioventricular compliance from the mitral flow profile: analytic and in vitro study. J Am Coll Cardiol 1992;19:998–1004.

32. Little WC, Ohno M, Kitzman DW, Thomas JD, Cheng C-P. Determination of left ventricular chamber stiffness from the time for deceleration of early left ventricular filling. Circulation 1995;92:1933–1939.

33. Myreng Y, Smiseth OA, Risøe C. Left ventricular filling at elevated diastolic pressures: relationship between transmitral Doppler flow velocities and atrial contribution. Am Heart J 1990;119:620–626.

34. Yellin EL, Peskin CS, Yoran C, Koenigsberg M, Matsumoto M, Laniado S, McQueen D, Shore D, Frater RWM. Mechanism of mitral valve motion during diastole. Am J Physiol 1981;241:389–H400.

35. Meisner JS, McQueen DM, Ishida Y, Vetter HO, Bortoloffi U, Strom JA, Frater RWM, Peskin CS, Yellin EL. Effects of timing of atrial systole on LV filling and mitral valve closure: computer and dog studies. Am J Physiol 1985;249:H604–H619.

36. Brun P, Tribouilloy C, Duval AM, Iserin L, Meguira A, Pelle G, Dubois-Rande JL. Left ventricular flow propagation during early filling is related to wall relaxation: a color M-mode Doppler analysis. J Am Coll Cardiol 1992;20:420–432.

37. Stugaard M, Smiseth OA, Risoe C, Ihlen H. Intraventricular early diastolic filling during acute myocardial ischemia. Assessment by multigated color M-mode Doppler echocardiography. Circulation 1993;88:2705–2713.

38. Ling D, Rankin JS, Edwards CH 2d, McHale PA, Anderson RW. Regional diastolic mechanics of the left ventricle in the conscious dog. Am J Physiol 1979;236:H323–H330.

39. Courtois M, Kovacs SJ Jr, Ludbrook PA. Physiological early diastolic intraventricular pressure gradient is lost during acute myocardial ischemia. Circulation 1990;81:1688–1696.

40. Firstenberg MS, Smedira NG, Greenberg NL, Prior DL, McCarthy PM, Garcia MJ, Thomas JD. Relationship between early diastolic intraventricular pressure gradients, an index of elastic recoil, and improvements in systolic and diastolic function. Circulation 2001;104(12 Suppl 1):I330-I335.

41. Steine K, Stugaard M, Smiseth OA. Mechanisms of retarded apical filling in acute ischemic left ventricular failure. Circulation 1999;99:2048–2054.

42. Nikolic SD, Feneley MP, Pajaro OE, Rankin JS, Yellin EL. Origin of regional pressure gradients in the left ventricle during early diastole. Am J Physiol 1995;268:H550–H557.

43. Greenberg NL, Vandervoort PM, Firstenberg MS, Garcia MJ, Thomas JD. Estimation of diastolic intraventricular pressure gradients by Doppler M-mode echocardiography. Am J Physiol Heart Circ Physiol 2001;280(6):H2507–H2515.

44. Yotti R, Bermejo J, Antoranz JC, Desco MM, Cortina C, Rojo-Alvarez JL, Allue C, Martin L, Moreno M, Serrano JA, Munoz R, Garcia-Fernandez MA. A noninvasive method for assessing impaired diastolic suction in patients with dilated cardiomyopathy. Circulation 2005;112(19):2921–2929.

45. Steen T, Steen S. Filling of a model left ventricle studied by colour M mode Doppler. Cardiovasc Res 1994;28:1821–1827.

46. Beppu S, Izumi S, Miyatake K, Nagata S, Park Y-D, Sakakibara H, Nimura Y. Abnormal blood pathways in left ventricular cavity in acute myocardial infarction. Experimental observations with special reference to regional wall motion abnormality and hemostasis. Circulation 1988;78:157–164.

47. Delemarre BJ, Bot H, Visser CA, Dunning AJ. Pulsed Doppler echocardiographic description of a circular flow pattern in spontaneous left ventricular contrast. J Am Soc Echo 1988;1:114–118.

6. Filling Velocities

48. Vierendeels JA, Dick E, Verdonck PR. Hydrodynamics of color M-mode Doppler flow wave propagation velocity V(p): a computer study. J Am Soc Echocardiogr 2002;15(3):219–224.

49. Hasegawa H, Little WC, Ohno M, Brucks S, Morimoto A, Cheng HJ, Cheng CP. Diastolic mitral annular velocity during the development of heart failure. J Am Coll Cardiol 2003;41(9):1590–1597.

Further Reading

Helle-Valle T, Crosby J, Edvardsen T, Lyseggen E, Amundsen BH, Smith HJ, Rosen BD, Lima JA, Torp H, Ihlen H, Smiseth OA. New noninvasive method for assessment of left ventricular rotation: speckle tracking echocardiography. Circulation 2005;112(20):3149–3156.

Rodevand O, Bjornerheim R, Edvardsen T, Smiseth OA, Ihlen H. Diastolic flow pattern in the normal left ventricle. J Am Soc Echocardiogr 1999;12(6):500–507.

Smiseth OA, Thompson CR. Atrioventricular filling dynamics, diastolic function and dysfunction. Heart Fail Rev 2000;5:291–299.

Stugaard M, Risøe C, Ihlen H, Smiseth OA. Intracavitary filling pattern in the failing left ventricle assessed by color M-mode Doppler echocardiography. J Am Coll Cardiol 1994;24:663–670.

Stugaard M, Steen T, Lundervold A, Smiseth OA, Ihlen H. Visual assessment of intraventricular filling from colour M-mode Doppler images. Int J Card Imaging 1994;10:279–287.

velocity is determined by cardiac translational motion. The motion of the mitral annulus reflects integrated longitudinal shortening and lengthening of myocardium located between the apex and the measurement site. For example, in the setting of apical infarction, velocities in the basal portion of the ventricle will also be diminished, which may lead to misdiagnosis of dysfunction in these segments. On the other hand, the contraction of normal regions causes passive motion registered in neighboring nonviable myocardium. Recently introduced techniques based on TDE — strain and strain rate imaging — may overcome these limitations (Figure 7.4).[6,7]

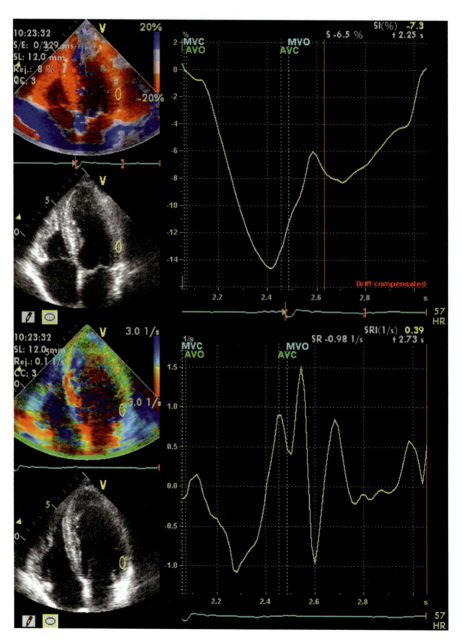

FIGURE 7.4. Normal left ventricular strain **(top)** and strain rate **(bottom)** curves recalculated from tissue Doppler velocities. Examples of the strain curves are from the basal lateral segment of the left ventricle. Cardiac cycle markers are shown on the graph. AVO, aortic valve opening; AVC, aortic valve closure; MVO, mitral valve opening; MVC, mitral valve closure.

Strain is a measure of deformation, occurring whenever myocardium contracts or relaxes. During the contraction of the ventricle, myocardium shortens longitudinally and circumferentially (negative strain) and thickens radially (positive strain). Diastole is characterized by reverse values of strain.

Strain rate describes how fast myocardial shortening or lengthening occurs. It is calculated from myocardial Doppler velocities (V1 and V2) measured at two locations separated by a distance (L). During contraction, when myocardial shortening occurs, these two locations are getting closer, and, when the two locations are moving apart, lengthening takes place. Strain rate is defined as the instantaneous spatial velocity gradient[8,9] with the unit of s^{-1}:

$$\text{Strain rate SR } (s^{-1}) = (V2 - V1)/L$$

Strain (or myocardial deformation, ε) represents the fractional or percentage change in dimension and is calculated as change in length $(L - L_0)$ divided by original length (L_0).[10] The reference noninvasive method that provides quantitative data about myocardial deformation in multiple planes is tagged MRI. In 1998, Heimdal et al.[11] introduced a clinical method to calculate strain rate from regional Doppler velocity gradients. Later, Urheim et al.[12] reported noninvasive measurements of strain by TDE, calculated as the time integral of strain rate. Clinically, strain can be calculated by several different formulas, but it is most often reported as Lagrangian strain (defined as current length divided by original length, or percent change in length). Regional diastolic longitudinal strain may be interpreted as regional lengthening fraction and radial strain as regional thinning fraction. Comparing the two parameters, strain rate is less load dependent and appears to be a better measure of local contractility than strain,[13] closely related to dP/dt_{max}. On the other hand, strain rate imaging is more angle dependent than other Doppler techniques. Because of its load dependency,[14] strain (similar to ejection fraction) is still not a perfect measure of contractility or efficacy of diastole, but its local assessment provides valuable insight into timing and amplitude of systolic and diastolic events. Another related modality derived from TDE myocardial velocity data is tissue tracking.[15] Using tissue tracking, tissue displacement is recalculated as the time integral of local velocities and color coded in consecutive phases of cardiac motion; however, there is little experience regarding the assessment of diastole.

Tissue Doppler echocardiography data can also be converted into color-coded maps of cardiac cycle intervals (e.g., tissue synchronicity imaging[16]) that can be applied to detect diastolic phase abnormalities. The current echocardiographic modalities used in humans for the study of local myocardial function are summarized in Table 7.1.

Two-Dimensional Echocardiographic Velocity and Strain Measurements — Speckle Tracking Echocardiography

The Doppler technique has significant limitations mainly related to the ability to detect only the velocity component parallel to the ultrasound beam. Therefore, alternative strain measurement techniques are being sought. Recent progress in computing allows calculation of myocardial velocities and strain based on the detection of motion of a recognizable image pattern between consecutive image frames. This approach has no angle dependency and thus offers the potential to monitor myocardial strain in two dimensions. Human studies were performed using the comparison of adjacent radiofrequency signals[17] and speckle tracking techniques.[18] These studies confirm that myocardial speckles are highly reproducible tissue ultrasound reflectors that can be analyzed similar to magnetic resonance tags. Various software implementations of the technique are currently available, for example, under the trade names 2-Dimensional Strain (Figure 7.5) and Velocity Vector Imaging (Figure 7.6).[19] It has been shown that the method also allows the calculation of novel indexes potentially useful for the assessment of diastolic physiology, such as ventricular torsion.[20,21]

Currently the technique is undergoing human validation, and signal to noise ratio versus frame rate tradeoff appears to be the main issue. In the future, the tracking algorithms may be applied to obtain three-dimensional velocity and deformation estimates.[22]

TABLE 7.1. Echocardiographic modalities used to study myocardial motion.

Modality	Parameters	Comments
Myocardial velocities by pulsed wave TDE*	Myocardial velocities measured in individual segments	Assesses local myocardial function; possible detection of early changes (e.g., ischemic dysfunction during stress echocardiography)
Mitral annulus velocities by pulsed wave TDE*	Peak diastolic annulus velocities and early to late diastolic velocity ratio	Stratifies diastolic dysfunction and diagnoses pseudonormalization. Reflects total longitudinal function of the selected ventricular wall and diastolic asynchrony of the left ventricle.
	Ratio of peak early diastolic mitral inflow velocity to peak early diastolic mitral annulus velocity (E/E′)	Thoroughly validated for noninvasive estimation of left ventricular filling pressure and prognostic stratification
Myocardial strain by TDE	Color-coded two-dimensional or curved M-mode) display of myocardial deformation (shortening and lengthening)	Measures deformation present in actively contraction or elongating myocardium. Detects abnormalities in amplitude and timing of regional myocardial function independent of passive heart motion. Attempts to assess atrial function
Myocardial strain rate by TDE	Color-coded (two-dimensional or curved M-mode) display of rate of myocardial shortening or lengthening (instantaneous spatial velocity gradient)	Less load-dependent measure of contractility than strain. Reproducibility problems, high sensitivity to noise
Myocardial displacement by TDE (e.g., tissue tracking)	Color-coded (two-dimensional or curved M-mode) display of temporal sequence of myocardial displacement in systole or diastole	Detects abnormalities in amplitude and timing of regional myocardial function
Myocardial strain and velocity by speckle tracking echocardiography (STE)	Non-Doppler myocardial motion detection by computerized tracking of speckle patterns in B-mode images	Detects motion regardless of its direction and allows calculation of strain components in orthogonal directions (two-dimensional strain). Recently validated; good correlation between STE and sonomicrometry or magnetic resonance imaging tagging for systolic strain
Myocardial velocity vector imaging	Non-Doppler myocardial velocity detection by computerized tracking of speckle patterns in B-mode image, displayed by arrows corresponding to instantaneous velocity vectors	Composite method incorporating the principle of speckle tracking echocardiography; calculation of instantaneous velocity vectors relative to an operator-selected reference point
Left ventricular torsion by speckle tracking echocardiography	Local left ventricular rotation can be measured by myocardial speckle tracking. Twist (torsion) is calculated as difference between rotation of apex and base	Potential tool for measuring systolic twist and diastolic untwist of the left ventricle

*Comparable data can be reconstructed from high temporal resolution acquisitions of a cardiac cycle using color mode tissue Doppler echocardiography (TDE). Color mode provides mean velocities, whereas pulsed mode provides peak velocities.

Magnetic Resonance Imaging

An alternative method for measuring local myocardial velocities is MRI. Phase-contrast MRI has been used to measure transmitral and pulmonary vein flow. Phase-contrast MRI allows velocity encoding of moving structures in any direction at 14–18 ms temporal resolution and thus obtaining myocardial velocity estimates. Preliminary experience with a retrospective electrocardiographically triggered Flash phase-contrast MRI technique with a velocity coding of 30 cm/s has been reported.[23,24] However, the values obtained at lower frame rates available with current MRI technology are only moderately correlated with TDE data, and thus their clinical relevance remains yet unsettled.

More data are available regarding the three-dimensional evaluation of myocardial deformation using myocardial tagging by MRI.[25] The data are usually obtained using electrocardiographically gated, segmented k-space, fast gradient-echo pulse sequences with spatial modulation of magnetization to generate a grid tag pattern that can be followed to analyze deformation[26] and

7. Myocardial Velocities

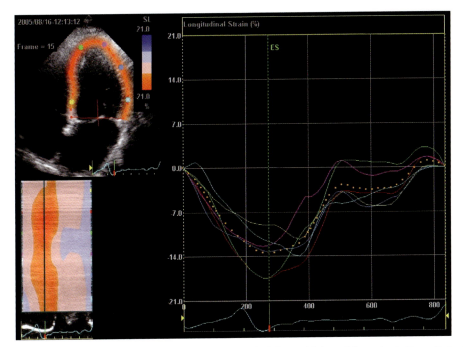

FIGURE 7.5. Quantitative analysis of left ventricular longitudinal strain recorded using the speckle tracking technique (two-dimensional strain) from an apical four-chamber view. Individual strain curves are calculated from six individual locations selected within the apical four-chamber view. At bottom left, the color strain data are reformatted into curvilinear M-Mode (the contour of the left ventricle is straightened onto the vertical axis, and the horizontal axis, time, corresponds to the single cardiac cycle duration). Diastolic strain shows early diastolic increase due to early filling and a smaller degree of late diastolic increase after left atrial contraction. SL, longitudinal strain; ES, end-systole.

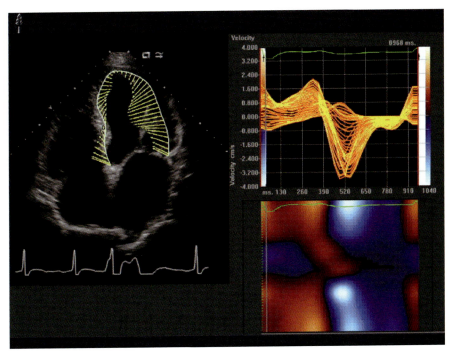

FIGURE 7.6. Vector velocity imaging of myocardial velocities in a patient with cardiomyopathy. Vectors represent instantaneous velocities and direction (**left panel**, vector length is proportional to instantaneous velocity) and can be displayed as a velocity graph in the time domain (**top right panel**) or as a curved color M-Mode graph (**bottom right panel**). (Courtesy of Siemens.)

calculate local strain. Another MRI option offering similar features is displacement encoding with stimulated echoes (DENSE).[27] However, application of these techniques to the assessment of diastolic dysfunction is limited to preclinical studies,[28] including specific aspects of diastolic physiology such as LV untwisting.[29]

Clinical Interpretation of Myocardial Velocities

Easily available noninvasive measurements of local myocardial velocities were rapidly incorporated into diagnostic strategies for many cardiac pathologies. Normal LV myocardium presents with a distinct sequence of myocardial velocities depicted by pulsed wave or reconstructed color-coded tissue Doppler (see Figures 7.1 and 7.3). The main velocity components are the systolic wave (S′ or Sm) corresponding to ventricular ejection, early diastolic wave (E′ or Em) corresponding to early ventricular filling, and late diastolic wave (A′ or Am) during atrial contraction, corresponding to the late phase of ventricular filling. Additionally, brief velocities can be recorded during isovolumic contraction immediately before S′ (usually predominantly directed toward the apex) and during isovolumic relaxation immediately before E′ (usually predominantly away from the apex). The appearance and direction of the isovolumic phase velocities is quite variable, their significance is unclear, and diagnostic utility is controversial. Peak acceleration during isovolumic relaxation was proposed as a load-independent measure of diastolic function. Peak septal acceleration during isovolumic relaxation correlated better than peak lateral wall acceleration with both pressure-derived peak negative dP/dt (r = −0.80) and *tau* (*tau* is the time constant for LV isovolumic pressure fall (r = −0.87) but not with left atrial pressure.[30] However, peak acceleration during the diastolic filling period did correlate (r = −0.81) with mean left atrial pressure.[31]

There is a myocardial velocity gradient between the LV base and apex for both the systolic S′ and the diastolic E′ and A′ velocity waves. Both S′ and E′ wave velocities decrease with age, whereas the A wave velocity increases. Perez-David et al.[32] studied age-related changes in myocardial veloci-

ties in subendocardial, mesocardial, and subepicardial layers of myocardium. The decrease in early diastolic peak velocity was the most pronounced aging-related change. Color M-mode tissue Doppler imaging multilayer analysis showed also that subendocardium is more susceptible to age-related changes involving diastolic function. Yamada et al.[33] evaluated the effect of aging on diastolic LV wall motion velocity in 80 healthy persons with pulsed tissue Doppler imaging. In both posterior wall and ventricular septum, peak E′ diastolic wall motion velocities correlated inversely with age, and the peak atrial A′ wall motion velocities correlated directly with age.

Mitral annular velocities, reflecting the dynamics of the longitudinal axis of the heart, appear to be less dependent on loading conditions than mitral inflow velocities, which makes them potentially useful as markers of diastolic physiology. In an experimental study, Hasegawa et al.[34] examined the effect of progressive diastolic dysfunction produced by rapid pacing on the dynamics of LV filling and the mitral annulus motion. Velocity of the early wave of mitral inflow decreased with mild diastolic dysfunction but progressively increased in response to elevations in left atrial pressure. In contrast, E′ progressively declined with worsening of heart failure, despite the increases in left atrial pressure and the left atrial to LV pressure gradient, accurately reflecting the progressive slowing of LV relaxation as heart failure developed. Consistent with the experimental findings of Firstenberg et al.[35] Hasegawa et al. found that in the presence of normal LV relaxation, E′ is sensitive to changes in the left atrial to LV pressure gradient, but, with slowed relaxation, the dependence of E′ on the pressure gradient is greatly reduced. When LV relaxation is slowed, E′ occurs after LV pressure equals or later in diastole when LV pressure again exceeds left atrial pressure, and it is much less dependent on the pressure gradient.

Numerous studies have assessed the impact of preload on myocardial diastolic velocities. The simplest parameter that can be derived from pulsed tissue Doppler recording is E′ diastolic mitral annular velocity, which at first was reported as a load-independent index of LV diastolic function. According to later studies, acute reduction of preload (usually hemodialysis model) was observed to affect not only mitral inflow parameters but also tissue E' wave velocity and mitral-to-apical flow propagation velocity.[36–38] Effects of the reduction of preload on left and right ventricular myocardial velocities in healthy subjects was assessed by Pela et al.[39] Lower body negative pressure caused progressive preload reduction that resulted in a significant decrease of E' and A' myocardial velocities at the mitral and tricuspid annulus but without changing the E'/A' ratio. On the other hand, during physiologic preload-altering maneuvers, which included Trendelenburg, reverse Trendelenburg, and amyl nitrate inhalation, Doppler tissue early diastolic velocities were not significantly affected, in contrast to standard transmitral Doppler filling indices. This suggests, within certain limits, a degree of load independence that is advantageous for a practical index of diastolic dysfunction.[40]

Bruch et al.[41] documented an impact of increased stroke volume on mitral annulus motion measured by TDE. Systolic and early diastolic mitral annular velocities were elevated in the increased stroke volume group (due to mitral disease) compared with the controls and were significantly reduced in the group with reduced stroke volume (after myocardial infarction, dilated cardiomyopathy, or hypertensive heart disease).

The advantages of TDE for the assessment of local diastolic function have been most widely applied in the following fields:

- Improved grading of diastolic dysfunction
- Identification of elevated filling pressures
- High sensitivity detection of early stage myocardial disease
- Evaluation of regional diastolic asynchrony
- Differentiation between restrictive and constrictive physiology of diastolic dysfunction
- Prognostic stratification

The interest in the significance of local myocardial velocities led to a series of clinically oriented studies, especially in coronary artery disease — by definition a regional entity. Even though not routinely used for the detection of ischemia, change in diastolic velocity parameters, including decrease of peak early diastolic velocity and decrease of tissue E'/A' ratio, have been documented in segments supplied by stenotic arteries. In contrast, no differences in myocardial function were observed between well-perfused segments in patients with coronary artery disease and controls.[42] The number of abnormally relaxing segments was shown to determine the global mitral inflow profile. The subjects with coronary artery disease and normal mitral inflow had on average 3.7 ± 2.7 segments with impaired regional diastolic function, and patients with delayed relaxation profile had 10.3 ± 3 segments, which gave distinct statistical significance ($p < 0.001$).[42]

In the study by Moreno et al.,[43] pulsed tissue Doppler was useful in differentiating between viable and nonviable segments in patients with three-vessel coronary artery disease. In another study, viable segments presented higher early diastolic velocities than nonviable segments and a lower prevalence of E/A ratio <1. The assessment of regional myocardial early diastolic velocities was also performed during dobutamine infusion. Greater than 2 cm/s decrease of early diastolic velocity for the examined segment had a higher diagnostic accuracy for ischemia (84% sensitivity and 93% specificity) than two-dimensional echocardiography (78% sensitivity and 71% specificity) or even radionuclide scintigraphy (61% sensitivity and 86% specificity).[44] Tissue Doppler echocardiography was also used for intraoperative monitoring of LV function during coronary grafting with left internal mammary artery using transesophageal echocardiography.[45] Immediately after mammary artery grafting, the peak systolic and late diastolic anterior wall velocities increased, indicating improvement in the systolic but concomitant impairment in the diastolic function of the grafted anterior wall.

Myocardial Velocities and Grading of Diastolic Dysfunction

The left ventricle fills in diastole in response to the pressure gradient from the left atrium to the left ventricle early in diastole after mitral valve opening and late in diastole during atrial systole. With mild diastolic dysfunction, transmitral E is reduced due to a slowing of the rate of LV relaxation. In more advanced levels of diastolic dysfunction, E returns to its normal values (pseudonormalization) due to the effect of increasing left atrial pressure, which increases the early diastolic transmitral pressure gradient. With even more severe dysfunction, the peak E rate may be higher than normal.[46,47] Transmitral flow is determined by multiple parameters such as filling pressure, LV elastic recoil and myocardial relaxation, atrial function, and the compliance of receiving chambers. In addition, flow can be modified by mitral valve abnormalities or pericardial constraint. Thus, many additional parameters, including early diastolic ventricular filling propagation velocity, pulmonary venous flow velocities and duration, responses to preload modifications by Valsalva maneuver, nitroprusside administration, and leg elevation, have been proposed to improve the definition of diastolic physiology. The ability of TDE to record myocardial velocities in vivo has been well validated for this application.

In the setting of normal LV relaxation, peak early mitral annular velocity (E′) precedes peak early transmitral flow (E) recorded by pulsed wave Doppler. In impaired relaxation E′ follows E.[48] Rodriguez et al.[49] suggested that in patients with diastolic dysfunction elastic recoil related to mitral annular motion is lost. Hemodynamic reflection of the elastic recoil, the minimal pressure recorded in the left ventricle, tends to be low in subjects with normal recoil.[50] Nagueh et al.[51] aimed to identify the hemodynamic determinants of the mitral annulus diastolic velocities measured by tissue Doppler in an experimental study in dogs. The authors observed a positive relation between E′ and the transmitral pressure gradient ($r = 0.57$, $p = 0.04$) and strong correlations with the time constant (tau) for LV isovolumic pressure fall ($r = -0.83$, $p < 0.001$), peak LV $-dP/dt$ ($r = 0.8$, $p < 0.001$) and minimal LV pressure ($r = -0.76$, $p < 0.01$). The relation between E′ and the transmitral pressure gradient was abolished in the settings when *tau* was longer than 50 ms. The late diastolic velocity of the mitral annulus also had significant positive relations with left atrial dP/dt, left atrial relaxation, and inverse correlation with LV end-diastolic pressure.

Also in patients, in contrast to the curvilinear relationship of traditional Doppler indices with the severity of myocardial disease as they progress from normal to restrictive physiology, tissue Doppler parameters show a uniphasic decline in velocities (Figure 7.2): the peak velocity of the mitral annulus during early diastole is reduced in patients with impaired relaxation. The E′ declines with age and in LV hypertrophy and is perceived as a useful index of LV relaxation, inversely related to the time constant of relaxation.[52] Patients with diastolic dysfunction often have increased endocardial and perivascular fibrosis, which alter E′ velocity.[53] Contrary to E, E′ remains reduced in patients with pseudonormalized or restrictive filling patterns, despite elevated left atrial pressure. This has been demonstrated in a classic study by Sohn et al.,[54] which opened way to everyday clinical use of myocardial diastolic velocities and was confirmed in various patient populations.[55–57] Chapter 13 provides a comprehensive review of how to estimate LV filling pressure by TDE and other echocardiographic modalities.

Abnormal Diastolic Velocities as Early Markers of Subclinical Myocardial Disease

Diastolic velocities were proposed in many pathologies as early markers of disease affecting myocardial function. In young, obese, otherwise healthy women, concentric LV remodeling was found to be related with decreased systolic and diastolic functions. Obese women (body mass index >30 kg/m^2) had lower systolic and diastolic myocardial velocities than nonobese, and both parameters were negatively correlated with body mass index. In multivariate analysis, body mass index was the only independent predictor of systolic and diastolic myocardial velocities.[58]

Regional changes in myocardial systolic and diastolic velocities can be detected by TDE in patients with hypertrophic cardiomyopathy. A significantly decreased myocardial function in basal septum was observed in hypertrophic cardiomyopathy patients compared with hypertensives.[59] Although regional function is most abnormal in markedly hypertrophied walls, the impairment is also seen in segments not affected by hypertrophy and in patients with a mutation for hypertrophic cardiomyopathy but without clear phenotypic changes.[60]

Impairment of diastolic function measured by tissue Doppler was seen also in uremic patients without overt cardiac dysfunction who showed a lower E′, a higher A′ velocity, and a reduced E′/A′ ratio of both interventricular septum and lateral wall compared with controls.[61] Moreover, in these patients the E′/A′ ratio of septum and lateral wall were negatively correlated with serum phosphorus and the calcium phosphate product.

Another study characterized LV function in 70 hypertensive patients with type 2 diabetes and normal ejection fraction (>55%) and without any cardiac symptoms.[62] The control group consisted of 35 nondiabetic subjects. Left ventricular longitudinal function was examined by tissue Doppler–derived myocardial strain rate and peak systolic velocities. Diastolic dysfunction was related to increased diastolic blood pressure, nondipping blood pressure profile, and increased urinary albumin excretion. Similarly, reduced exercise capacity in patients with type 2 diabetes is associated with depressed early diastolic velocity, diabetes control, and impaired heart rate recovery (measured as the heart rate difference between peak and 1 minute after exercise).[63] The authors searched for determinants of exercise capacity in 170 patients with type 2 diabetes with negative exercise echocardiograms and in 56 control subjects. Exercise capacity, measured as metabolic equivalents, strain rate, peak early diastolic velocity in basal segments of each wall (E′), and heart rate recovery were significantly reduced in type 2 diabetes. The strongest correlate of exercise capacity was E′ (r = 0.43). In the same study E′, age, male sex, body mass index, heart rate recovery, and HbA$_1$C were independent predictors of exercise capacity — thus reduced exercise capacity in patients with type 2 diabetes is associated with subclinical LV dysfunction detectable with diastolic velocity measurements.

In the study of Skaluba and Litwin,[64] the ratio of early mitral flow velocity (E) to early diastolic mitral annular velocity E′ was the best echocardiographic correlate of heart rate recovery after exercise (r = −0.781, $p < 0.001$), a strong predictor of increased long-term mortality. Patients whose E/E′ was <10 had a faster 1-minute heart rate recovery and a greater chronotropic response during exercise than those with E/E′ ≥10. An E/E′ ratio ≥10.3 predicted 1-minute heart rate recovery of ≤18 beats/min, with 83% sensitivity and 100% specificity. Neither LV ejection fraction nor the presence of a "slow relaxation" mitral inflow pattern (E/A <1.0) was predictive of impaired heart rate recovery.[64]

Lee et al.[65] showed that in coronary artery disease patients abnormal diastolic physiology assessed by TDE was closely associated with increased platelet activation and endothelial dysfunction independent of systolic function. Patients with coronary artery disease had significantly lower systolic and early diastolic velocities of mitral annulus and a higher ratio of early transmitral flow E/E′ compared with controls (all $p < 0.05$). On multivariate analysis, the differences in the group means of von Willebrand factor (a marker of endothelial dysfunction), soluble P-selectin (reflecting platelet activation), and fibrinogen remained significantly different between the low and high values of TDE indexes.

Tissue Doppler echocardiography can also be used to confirm the improvement of diastolic function measured at rest and under stress using peak early mitral annulus velocity in patients after coronary artery bypass graft.[66] Similar results concerning improvement of tissue Doppler indices of the mitral annulus reflecting both the diastolic and systolic functions were reported early after successful percutaneous transluminal coronary angioplasty. In a study of 48 young patients after heart transplantation, E/propagation velocity and E/E′ ratios were predictive for graft rejection in addition to pulmonary capillary wedge pressure and intraventricular flow propagation velocity.[67]

Asynchrony of Local Diastolic Function

The ability of detecting asynchrony of local events throughout the cardiac cycle has contributed to a better understanding of the pathophysiology of heart failure and led to development of novel efficient modes of treatment, including cardiac resynchronization therapy. However, the majority of publications deal with the asynchrony of systole. The concept that diastolic events may also be asynchronous (see Figure 7.3) is not new.[68] The asynchrony during the isovolumic relaxation period has been initially reported to be a marker of significant coronary stenosis. Significant significantly lower in obese patients than in controls at both the septum and lateral wall levels. These strain and strain rate abnormalities were significantly related to body mass index. In addition, the early diastolic strain rate was compromised in obese patients ($p < 0.001$). Another finding of the study was that myocardial deformation (systolic strain) showed a correlation with insulin resistance level defined as homeostasis model assessment insulin resistance index.[83] In the recent study of Izawa et al.,[84] 12 months of treatment with spironolactone in mildly symptomatic patients with idiopathic dilated cardiomyopathy (New York Heart Association classes I and II) ameliorated LV diastolic dysfunction and reduced chamber stiffness in association with regression of myocardial fibrosis as shown by measurements of early diastolic strain rate. These effects appeared limited, however, to patients with increased myocardial collagen accumulation.

Recently several papers reported the potential of strain and strain rate measurements during stress echocardiography. In an animal model of healing canine infarctions, among several indexes diastolic strain rate during dobutamine infusion readily identified segments with >20% transmural infarction and related best to the extent of interstitial fibrosis ($r = -0.86$, $p < 0.01$), appearing to be a promising novel index of myocardial viability.[85]

After improvement in wall motion, low-dose strain/strain rate dobutamine stress echocardiography was performed to determine the underlying ischemic substrate in takotsubo cardiomyopathy. This illness is characterized by an atypical distribution of LV dyssynergy with apical ballooning and compensatory basal hyperkinesis in the presence of normal coronary angiography. Although the pathophysiology of takotsubo cardiomyopathy is poorly understood, high catecholamine levels (due to physical or emotional stress), multivessel epicardial coronary spasm, and diffuse microvascular spasm are postulated as underlying factors. Regional deformation changes during dobutamine stress echocardiography showed the affected myocardium to have the typical response diagnostic of regional stunning.[86]

In summary, strain and strain rate imaging offer interesting opportunities to improve the sensitivity of stress echocardiography, assess myocardial function after resynchronization therapy, and refine estimation of regional ventricular function, including separate analysis of myocardial layers (subendocardial vs. subepicardial).[87–91] The method is still new, and more extensive clinical validation is needed also in terms of comparison of Doppler and speckle tracing–based values (see Figure 7.4) of myocardial deformation.

References

1. Torrent-Guasp F, Kocica MJ, Corno A, Komeda M, Cox J, Flotats A, Ballester-Rodes M, Carreras-Costa F. Systolic ventricular filling. Eur J Cardiothorac Surg 2004;25:376–386.
2. Notomi Y, Setser RM, Shiota T, Martin-Miklovic MG, Weaver JA, Popovic ZB, Yamada H, Greenberg NL, White RD, Thomas JD. Assessment of left ventricular torsional deformation by Doppler tissue imaging: validation study with tagged magnetic resonance imaging. Circulation 2005;111:1141–1147.
3. McDicken WN, Sutherland GR, Moran CM, Gordon LN. Colour Doppler velocity imaging of the myocardium. Ultrasound Med Biol 1992;18:651–654.
4. Donovan CL, Armstrong WF, Bach DS. Quantitative Doppler tissue imaging of the left ventricular myocardium: validation in normal subjects. Am Heart J 1995;130:100–104.
5. Smiseth OA, Ihlen H. Strain rate imaging: why do we need it? J Am Coll Cardiol 2003;9:1584–1586.
6. Kowalski M, Kukulski T, Jamal F, D'Hooge J, Weidemann, F, Rademakers F, Bijnens B, Hatle L, Sutherland GR. Can natural strain and strain rate quantify regional myocardial deformation? A study in healthy subjects. Ultrasound Med Biol 2001;27:1087–1097.
7. Marwick, TH. Measurement of strain and strain rate by echocardiography — ready for prime time? J Am Coll Cardiol 2006;47:1313–1327.
8. Uematsu M, Miyatake K, Tanaka N, Matsuda H, Sano A, Yamazaki N, Hirama M, Yamagishi M. Myocardial velocity gradient as a new indicator of regional left ventricular contraction: detection by a two-dimensional tissue Doppler imaging technique. J Am Coll Cardiol 1995;26:217–223.
9. Derumeaux G, Ovize M, Loufoua J, Pontier G, Andre-Fouet X, Cribier A. Assessment of nonuniformity of transmural myocardial velocities by color-coded tissue Doppler imaging. Circulation 2000;101:1390–1395.

10. Mirsky I, Pamley WW. Assessment of passive elastic stiffness for isolated heart muscle and the intact heart. Circ Res 1973;33:233–243.

11. Heimdal A, Steylen A., Torp H, Skjaerpe T. Real-time strain rate imaging of the left ventricle by ultrasound. J Am Soc Echocardiogr 1998;11:1013–1019.

12. Urheim S, Edvardsen T, Torp H, Angelsen B, Smiseth OA. Myocardial strain by Doppler echocardiography. Validation of a new method to quantify regional myocardial function. Circulation 2000; 102:1158–1164.

13. Greenberg NL, Firstenberg MS, Castro PL, Main M, Travaglini A, Odabashian JA, Drinko JK, Rodriguez LL, Thomas JD, Garcia MJ. Doppler-derived myocardial systolic strain rate is a strong index of left ventricular contractility. Circulation 2002;105:99–105.

14. Weidemann F, Jamal F, Sutherland GR, Claus P, Kowalski M, Hatle L, De Scheerder I, Bijnens B, Rademakers FE. Myocardial function defined by strain rate and strain during alterations in inotropic states and heart rate. Am J Physiol Heart Circ Physiol 2002;283:H792–H799.

15. Borges AC, Kivelitz D, Walde T, Reibis RK, Grohmann A, Panda A, Wernecke KD, Rutsch W, Hamm B, Baumann G. Apical tissue tracking echocardiography for characterization of regional left ventricular function: comparison with magnetic resonance imaging in patients after myocardial infarction. J Am Soc Echocardiogr. 2003;16:254–262.

16. Yu CM, Zhang Q, Fung JW, Chan HC, Chan YS, Yip GW, Kong SL, Lin H, Zhang Y, Sanderson JE. A novel tool to assess systolic asynchrony and identify responders of cardiac resynchronization therapy by tissue synchronization imaging. J Am Coll Cardiol 2005;45:677–684.

17. D'hooge J, Konofagou E, Jamal F, Heimdal A, Barrios L, Bijnens B, Thoen J, Van de Werf F, Sutherland G, Suetens P. Two-dimensional ultrasonic strain rate measurement of the human heart in vivo. IEEE Trans Ultrason Ferroelectr Freq Control 2002;49:281–286.

18. Leitman M, Lysyansky P, Sidenko S, Shir V, Peleg E, Binenbaum M, Kaluski E, Krakover R, Vered Z. Two-dimensional strain — a novel software for real-time quantitative echocardiographic assessment of myocardial function J Am Soc Echocardiogr 2004;17:1021–1029.

19. Vannan MA, Pedrizzetti G, Li P, Gurudevan S, Houle H, Main J, Jackson J, Nanda NC. Effect of cardiac resynchronization therapy on longitudinal and circumferential left ventricular mechanics by velocity vector imaging: description and initial clinical application of a novel method using high-frame rate B-mode echocardiographic images. Echocardiography 2005;22:826–830.

20. Notomi Y, Lysyansky P, Setser RM, Shiota T, Popovic ZB, Martin-Miklovic MG, Weaver JA, Oryszak SJ, Greenberg N, White RD, Thomas JD. Measurement of ventricular torsion by two-dimensional ultrasound speckle tracking imaging. J Am Coll Cardiol 2005;45;2034–2041.

21. Helle-Valle T, Crosby J, Edvardsen T, Lyseggen E, Amundsen BH, Smith HJ, Rosen BD, Lima JA, Torp H, Ihlen H, Smiseth OA. New noninvasive method for assessment of left ventricular rotation: speckle tracking echocardiography. Circulation 2005;112: 3149–3156.

22. Chen X, Xie H, Erkamp R, Kim K, Jia C, Rubin JM, O'Donnell M. 3-D correlation-based speckle tracking. Ultrason Imaging 2005;27:21–36.

23. Paelinck BP, de Roos A, Bax JJ, Bosmans JM, van Der Geest RJ, Dhondt D, Parizel PM, Vrints CJ, Lamb HJ. Feasibility of tissue magnetic resonance imaging: a pilot study in comparison with tissue Doppler imaging and invasive measurement. J Am Coll Cardiol 2005;45:1109–1116.

24. Jung B, Markl M, Foll D, Hennig J. Investigating myocardial motion by MRI using tissue phase mapping. Eur J Cardiothorac Surg 2006;29(Suppl 1):S158–S164.

25. Paelinck BP, Lamb HJ, Bax JJ, Van der Wall EE, de Roos A. Assessment of diastolic function by cardiovascular magnetic resonance. Am Heart J 2002;144: 198–205.

26. Axel L, Dougherty L. Heart wall motion: improved method of spatial modulation of magnetization for MR imaging. Radiology 1989;172:349–350.

27. Kim D, Gilson WD, Kramer CM, Epstein FH. Myocardial tissue tracking with two-dimensional cine displacement-encoded MR imaging: development and initial evaluation. Radiology 2004;230:862–871.

28. Azevedo CF, Amado LC, Kraitchman DL, Gerber BL, Osman NF, Rochitte CE, Edvardsen T, Lima JA. Persistent diastolic dysfunction despite complete systolic functional recovery after reperfused acute myocardial infarction demonstrated by tagged magnetic resonance imaging. Eur Heart J 2004;25:1419–1427.

29. Rademakers FE, Buchalter MB, Rogers WJ, Zerhouni EA, Weisfeldt ML, Weiss JL, Shapiro EP. Dissociation between left ventricular untwisting and filling. Accentuation by catecholamines. Circulation 1992;85:1572–1581.

30. Hashimoto I, Li XK, Bhat AH, Jones M, Sahn DJ. Quantitative assessment of regional peak myocardial acceleration during isovolumic contraction

and relaxation times by tissue Doppler imaging. Heart 2005;91:811–816.

31. Hashimoto I, Bhat AH, Li X, Jones M, Davies CH, Swanson JC, Schindera ST, Sahn DJ. Tissue Doppler–derived myocardial acceleration for evaluation of left ventricular diastolic function. J Am Coll Cardiol 2004;44:1459–1466.

32. Perez-David E, Garcia-Fernandez MA, Ledesma MJ, Malpica N, Lopez Fernandez T, Santos A, Moreno M, Antoranz JC, Bermejo J, Desco M. Age-related intramyocardial patterns in healthy subjects evaluated with Doppler tissue imaging. Eur J Echocardiogr 2005;6:175–185.

33. Yamada H, Oki T, Mishiro Y, Tabata T, Abe M, Onose Y, Wakatsuki T, Ito S. Effect of aging on diastolic left ventricular myocardial velocities measured by pulsed tissue Doppler imaging in healthy subjects. J Am Soc Echocardiogr 1999;12:574–581.

34. Hasegawa H, Little WC, Ohno M, Brucks S, Morimoto A, Cheng HJ, Cheng CP. Diastolic mitral annular velocity during the development of heart failure. J Am Coll Cardiol 2003;41:1590–1597.

35. Firstenberg MS, Greenberg NL, Main ML, Drinko JK, Odabashian JA, Thomas JD, Garcia MJ. Determinants of diastolic myocardial tissue Doppler velocities: influences of relaxation and preload. J Appl Physiol 2001;90:299–307.

36. Ie EH, Vletter WB, ten Cate FJ, Nette RW, Weimar W, Roelandt JR, Zietse R. Preload dependence of new Doppler techniques limits their utility for left ventricular diastolic function assessment in hemodialysis patients. J Am Soc Nephrol 2003;14:1858–1862.

37. Dincer I, Kumbasar D, Nergisoglu G, Atmaca Y, Kutlay S, Akyurek O, Sayin T, Erol C, Oral D. Assessment of left ventricular diastolic function with Doppler tissue imaging: effects of preload and place of measurements. Int J Cardiovasc Imaging 2002;18:155–160.

38. Hung KC, Huang HL, Chu CM, Chen CC, Hsieh IC, Chang ST, Fang JT, Wen MS. Evaluating preload dependence of a novel Doppler application in assessment of left ventricular diastolic function during hemodialysis. Am J Kidney Dis 2004;43:1040–1046.

39. Pela G, Regolisti G, Coghi P, Cabassi A, Basile A, Cavatorta A, Manca C, Borghetti A. Effects of the reduction of preload on left and right ventricular myocardial velocities analyzed by Doppler tissue echocardiography in healthy subjects. Eur J Echocardiogr 2004;5:262–271.

40. Yalcin F, Kaftan A, Muderrisoglu H, Korkmaz ME, Flachskampf F, Garcia M, Thomas JD. Is Doppler tissue velocity during early left ventricular filling preload independent? Heart 2002;87:336–339.

41. Bruch C, Stypmann J, Gradaus R, Breithardt G, Wichter T. Stroke volume and mitral annular velocities. Insights from tissue Doppler imaging. Z Kardiol 2004;93:799–806.

42. Garcia-Fernandez MA, Azevedo J, Moreno M, Bermejo J, Perez-Castellano N, Puerta P, Desco M, Antoranz C, Serrano JA, Garcia E, Delcan JL. Regional diastolic function in ischaemic heart disease using pulsed wave Doppler tissue imaging. Eur Heart J 1999;20:496–505.

43. Moreno R, Garcia-Fernandez MA, Zamorano LJ, Moreno M, De Isla PL, Ortega A, Puerta P, Bermejo J, Allue C, Lopez-Sendon J. Regional diastolic function is more preserved in viable than non-viable myocardium. Demonstration by pulsed-wave Doppler tissue imaging in basal conditions. Rev Esp Cardiol 2001;54:592–596.

44. Bibra H, Tuchnitz A, Klein A, Schneider-Ecke J, Schoming A, Schweiger M. Regional diastolic function by pulsed Doppler myocardial mapping for the detection of left ventricular ischemia during pharmacologic stress testing. A comparison with stress echocardiography and perfusion scintigraphy. J Am Coll Cardiol 2000;36:444–452.

45. Skarvan K, Filipovic M, Wang J, Brett W, Seeberger M. Use of myocardial tissue Doppler imaging for intraoperative monitoring of left ventricular function. Br J Anaesth 2003;91(4):473–480.

46. Ohno M, Cheng CP, Little WC. Mechanism of altered patterns of left ventricular filling during the development of congestive heart failure. Circulation 1994;89:2241–2250.

47. Appleton CP. Doppler assessment of left ventricular diastolic function: the refinements continue. J Am Coll Cardiol 1993;21:1697–1700.

48. Nagueh SF, Sun H, Kopelen HA, Middleton KJ, Khoury DS. Haemodynamic determinants of the mitral annulus diastolic velocities by tissue Doppler. J Am Coll Cardiol 2001,37:278–285.

49. Rodriguez L, Garcia M, Ares M, Griffin BP, Nakatani S, Thomas JD. Assessment of mitral annulus dynamics during diastole by Doppler tissue imaging: comparison with mitral Doppler inflow in subjects without heart disease and in patients with left ventricular hypertrophy. Am Heart J 1996;131:982–987.

50. Ohte N, Narita H, Hashimoto T, Akita S, Kurokawa K, Fujinami T. Evaluation of left ventricular early diastolic performance by tissue Doppler imaging of the mitral annulus. Am J Cardiol 1998,82:1414–1417.

51. Nagueh SF, Sun H, Kopelen HA, Middleton KJ, Khoury DS. Hemodynamic determinants of the

mitral annulus diastolic velocities by tissue Doppler. J Am Coll Cardiol 2001;37:278–285.

52. Nagueh SF, Middleton KJ, Kopelen HA, Zoghbi WA, Quinones MA. Doppler tissue imaging: a non-invasive technique for evaluation of left ventricular relaxation and estimation of filling pressures. J Am Coll Cardiol 1997;30:1527–1533.

53. Shan K, Bick RJ, Poindexter BJ, Shimoni S, Letsou GV, Reardon MJ, Howell JF, Zoghbi WA, Nagueh SF. Relation of tissue Doppler derived myocardial velocities to myocardial structure and beta-adrenergic receptor density in humans. J Am Coll Cardiol 2000;36:891–896.

54. Sohn DW, Chai IH, Lee DJ, Kim HC, Kim HS, Oh BH, Lee MM, Park YB, Choi YS, Seo JD, Lee YW. Assessment of mitral annulus velocity by Doppler tissue imaging in the evaluation of left ventricular diastolic function. J Am Coll Cardiol 1997;30:474–480.

55. Nagueh SF, Middleton KJ, Kopelen HA, Zoghbi WA, Quinones MA. Doppler tissue imaging: a non-invasive technique for evaluation of left ventricular relaxation and estimation of filling pressures. J Am Coll Cardiol 1997;30:1527–1533.

56. Nagueh SF, Lakkis NM, Middleton KJ, Spencer WH III, Zoghbi WA, Quinones MA. Doppler estimation of left ventricular filling pressures in patients with hypertrophic cardiomyopathy. Circulation 1999;99: 254–261.

57. Wierzbowska-Drabik K, Drozdz J, Plewka M, Trzos E, Krzeminska-Pakula M, Kasprzak JD. The utility of pulsed tissue Doppler parameters for the diagnosis of advanced left ventricular diastolic dysfunction. Echocardiography 2006;23:189–196.

58. Peterson LR, Waggoner AD, Schechtman KB, Meyer T, Gropler RJ, Barzilai B, Davila-Roman VG. Alterations in left ventricular structure and function in young healthy obese women. J Am Coll Cardiol 2004;43:1399–1404.

59. Nunez J, Zamorano JL, Perez De Isla L, Palomeque C, Almeria C, Rodrigo JL, Corteza J, Banchs J, Macaya C. Differences in regional systolic and diastolic function by Doppler tissue imaging in patients with hypertrophic cardiomyopathy and hypertrophy caused by hypertension. J Am Soc Echocardiogr 2004;17:717–722.

60. Rajiv C, Vinereanu D, Fraser AG Tissue Doppler imaging for the evaluation of patients with hypertrophic cardiomyopathy. Curr Opin Cardiol 2004;19:430–436.

61. Galetta F, Cupisti A, Franzoni F, Femia FR, Rossi M, Barsotti G, Santoro G. Left ventricular function and calcium phosphate plasma levels in uraemic patients. J Intern Med 2005;258:378–384.

62. Andersen NH, Poulsen SH, Poulsen PL, Knudsen ST, Helleberg K, Hansen KW, Berg TJ, Flyvbjerg A, Mogensen CE. Left ventricular dysfunction in hypertensive patients with type 2 diabetes mellitus. Diabet Med 2005;22:1218–1225.

63. Fang ZY, Sharman J, Prins JB, Marwick TH. Determinants of exercise capacity in patients with type 2 diabetes. Diabetes Care 2005;28:1643–1648.

64. Skaluba SJ, Litwin SE. Doppler-derived left ventricular filling pressures and the regulation of heart rate recovery after exercise in patients with suspected coronary artery disease. Am J Cardiol 2005;95:832–837.

65. Lee KW, Blann AD, Lip GY. Impaired tissue Doppler diastolic function in patients with coronary artery disease: relationship to endothelial damage/dysfunction and platelet activation. Am Heart J 2005;150:756–766.

66. Hedman A, Samad BA, Larsson T, Zuber E, Nordlander R, Alam M. Improvement in diastolic left ventricular function after coronary artery bypass grafting as assessed by recordings of mitral annular velocity using Doppler tissue imaging. Eur J Echocardiogr 2005;6:202–209.

67. Eun LY, Gajarski RJ, Graziano JN, Ensing GJ. Relation of left ventricular diastolic function as measured by echocardiography and pulmonary capillary wedge pressure to rejection in young patients (≤31 years) after heart transplantation. Am J Cardiol 2005;96:857–860.

68. Bruch C, Schmermund A, Bartel T, Schaar J, Erbel R. Tissue Doppler imaging (TDI) for on-line detection of regional early diastolic ventricular asynchrony in patients with coronary artery disease. Int J Card Imaging 1999;15:379–390.

69. Pai RG, Gill KS. Amplitudes, durations, and timings of apically directed left ventricular myocardial velocities: II. Systolic and diastolic asynchrony in patients with left ventricular hypertrophy. J Am Soc Echocardiogr 1998;11:112–118.

70. Schuster I, Habib G, Jego C, Thuny F, Avierinos JF, Derumeaux G, Beck L, Medail C, Franceschi F, Renard S, Ferracci A, Lefevre J, Luccioni R, Deharo JC, Djiane P. Diastolic asynchrony is more frequent than systolic asynchrony in dilated cardiomyopathy and is less improved by cardiac resynchronization therapy. J Am Coll Cardiol 2005;46:2250–2257.

71. Waggoner AD, Rovner A, de las Fuentes L, Faddis MN, Gleva MJ, Sawhney N, Davila-Roman VG. Clinical outcomes after cardiac resynchronization therapy: importance of left ventricular diastolic function and origin of heart failure. J Am Soc Echocardiogr 2006;19:307–313.

72. Waggoner AD, Faddis MN, Gleva MJ, de las Fuentes L, Davila-Roman VG. Improvements in left ventricular diastolic function after cardiac resynchronization therapy are coupled to response in systolic performance. J Am Coll Cardiol 2005;46:2244–2249.

73. Dokainish H, Zoghbi WA, Lakkis NM, Ambriz E, Patel R, Quinones MA, Nagueh SF. Incremental predictive power of B-type natriuretic peptide and tissue Doppler echocardiography in the prognosis of patients with congestive heart failure. J Am Coll Cardiol 2005;45:1223–1226.

74. Wang M, Yip G, Yu CM, Zhang Q, Zhang Y, Tse D, Kong SL, Sanderson JE. Independent and incremental prognostic value of early mitral annulus velocity in patients with impaired left ventricular systolic function. J Am Coll Cardiol 2005;45:272–277.

75. Liang HY, Cauduro SA, Pellikka PA, Bailey KR, Grossardt BR, Yang EH, Rihal C, Seward JB, Miller FA, Abraham TP. Comparison of usefulness of echocardiographic Doppler variables to left ventricular end-diastolic pressure in predicting future heart failure events. Am J Cardiol 2006;97:866–871.

76. Yilmaz R, Celik S, Baykan, Kasap H, Kaplan S, Kucukosmanoglu M, Erdol C. Assessment of mitral anular velocities by Doppler tissue imaging in predicting left ventricular thrombus formation after first anterior acute myocardial infarction. J Am Soc Echocardiogr 2005;18:632–637.

77. Troughton RW, Prior DL, Pereira JJ, Martin M, Fogarty A, Morehead A, Yandle TG, Richards AM, Starling RC, Young JB, Thomas JD, Klein AL. Plasma B-type natriuretic peptide levels in systolic heart failure importance of left ventricular diastolic function and right ventricular systolic function. J Am Coll Cardiol 2004;43:416–422.

78. Edvardsen T, Skulstad H, Aakhus S, Urheim S, Ihlen H. Regional myocardial systolic function during acute myocardial ischemia assessed by strain Doppler echocardiography. J Am Coll Cardiol 2001;37:726–730.

79. Park TH, Nagueh SF, Khoury DS, Kopelen HA, Akrivakis S, Nasser K, Ren G, Frangogiannis NG. Impact of myocardial structure and function postinfarction on diastolic strain measurements: implications for assessment of myocardial viability. Am J Physiol Heart Circ Physiol 2006;290:H724–H731.

80. Hoffmann R, Altiok E, Nowak B, Kuhl H, Kaiser HJ, Buell U, Hanrath P. Strain rate analysis allows detection of differences in diastolic function

between viable and nonviable myocardial segments. J Am Soc Echocardiogr 2005;18:330–335.

81. Takemoto Y, Pellikka PA, Wang J, Modesto KM, Cauduro S, Belohlavek M, Seward JB, Thomson HL, Khandheria B, Abraham TP. Analysis of the interaction between segmental relaxation patterns and global diastolic function by strain echocardiography. J Am Soc Echocardiogr 2005;18:901–906.

82. Edvardsen T, Gerber B, Garot J, Bluemke D, Lima J, Smiseth O. Quantitative assessment of intrinsic regional myocardial deformation by Doppler strain rate echocardiography in humans. Validation against three-dimensional tagged magnetic resonance imaging. Circulation 2002;106:50–56.

83. Di Bello V, Santini F, Di Cori A, Pucci A, Palagi C, Delle Donne MG, Giannetti M, Talini E, Nardi C, Pedrizzetti G, Fierabracci P, Vitti P, Pinchera A, Balbarini A. Relationship between preclinical abnormalities of global and regional left ventricular function and insulin resistance in severe obesity: a color Doppler imaging study. Int J Obes (Lond) 2006;30:948–956.

84. Izawa H, Murohara T, Nagata K, Isobe S, Asano H, Amano T, Ichihara S, Kato T, Ohshima S, Murase Y, Iino S, Obata K, Noda A, Okumura K, Yokota M. Mineralocorticoid receptor antagonism ameliorates left ventricular diastolic dysfunction and myocardial fibrosis in mildly symptomatic patients with idiopathic dilated cardiomyopathy: a pilot study. Circulation 2005;112:2940–2945.

85. Park TH, Nagueh SF, Khoury DS, Kopelen HA, Akrivakis S, Nasser K, Ren G, Frangogiannis NG. Impact of myocardial structure and function postinfarction on diastolic strain measurements: implications for assessment of myocardial viability. Am J Physiol Heart Circ Physiol 2006;290: H724–H731.

86. Merli E, Sutcliffe S, Gori M, Sutherland GG. Tako-Tsubo cardiomyopathy: new insights into the possible underlying pathophysiology. Eur J Echocardiogr 2006;7:53–61.

87. Hanekom L, Jenkins C, Jeffries L, Case C, Mundy J, Hawley C, Marwick TH. Incremental value of strain rate analysis as an adjunct to wall-motion scoring for assessment of myocardial viability by dobutamine echocardiography: a follow-up study after revascularization. Circulation 2005;112:3892–3900.

88. Pham PP, Balaji S, Shen I, Ungerleider R, Li X, Sahn DJ. Impact of conventional versus biventricular pacing on hemodynamics and tissue Doppler imaging indexes of resynchronization postoperatively in children with congenital heart disease J Am Coll Cardiol 2005;46:2284–2289.

89. Ashford MW Jr, Liu W, Lin SJ, Abraszewski P, Caruthers SD, Connolly AM, Yu X, Wickline SA. Occult cardiac contractile dysfunction in dystrophin-deficient children revealed by cardiac magnetic resonance strain imaging. Circulation 2005;112:2462–2467.

90. Yip G, Khandheria B, Belohlavek M, Pislaru C, Seward J, Bailey K, Tajik AJ, Pellikka P, Abraham T. Strain echocardiography tracks dobutamine-induced decrease in regional myocardial perfusion in nonocclusive coronary stenosis. J Am Coll Cardiol 2004;44:1664–1671.

91. Hashimoto I, Li X, Bhat AH, Jones M, Zetts AD, Sahn DJ. Myocardial strain rate is a superior method for evaluation of left ventricular subendocardial function compared with tissue Doppler imaging. J Am Coll Cardiol 2003;42:1574–1583.

8
Diastolic Versus Systolic Heart Failure

Hidekatsu Fukuta and William C. Little

Introduction

Heart failure is defined as the pathologic state in which the heart is unable to pump blood at a rate required by the metabolizing tissues or can do so only with an elevated filling pressure. Inability of the heart to pump blood sufficiently to meet the needs of the body's tissues is due to the inability of the left ventricle (LV) to fill (diastolic performance) and eject (systolic performance). Thus, consideration of the systolic and diastolic performance of the LV provides a conceptual basis to classify and understand the pathophysiology of heart failure.

Left Ventricular Systolic and Diastolic Performance

Systolic Performance

Left ventricular systolic performance is the ability of the LV to empty. The ability of the LV to empty can be quantified as the LV ejection fraction (EF; a ratio of stroke volume to end-diastolic volume). Thus, LV systolic dysfunction is defined as a decreased EF. The EF can be obtained by determining the LV volume by use of two-dimensional echocardiography or contrast or radionuclide ventriculography.

The EF has been used as an index of myocardial contractile performance. The EF, however, is influenced not only by myocardial contractility but also by LV afterload.[1] Furthermore, in the presence of a left-sided valvular regurgitation (mitral or aortic regurgitation) or a left-to-right shunt (ventricular septal defect or patent ductus arteriosus), the LV stroke volume may be high, while the forward stroke volume (stroke volume minus regurgitant volume or shunt volume) is lower. Thus, the effective EF is defined as the forward stroke volume divided by end-diastolic volume.[2] The effective EF is a useful means to quantify systolic function for two reasons. First, the effective EF represents the functional emptying of the LV that contributes to cardiac output. Second, the effective EF is relatively independent of LV end-diastolic volume over the clinically relevant range.

An operational definition of systolic dysfunction is an effective EF of <0.50.[2] When defined in this manner, systolic dysfunction results from impaired myocardial function, increased LV afterload, and/or structural abnormalities of the LV.[2]

Diastolic Performance

For the LV to function effectively as a pump, it must be able not only to eject but also to fill (diastolic function). Diastolic function has conventionally been assessed on the basis of the LV end-diastolic pressure volume relation. A shift of the curve upward and to the left has been considered to be the hallmark of diastolic dysfunction (Figure 8.1, curve A). In this situation, each LV end-diastolic volume is associated with a high end-diastolic pressure, and thus the LV is less distensible. Decreased LV distensibility is caused by

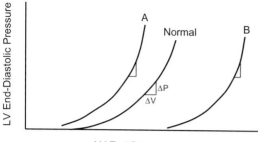

FIGURE 8.1. A shift of the curve to A indicates that a higher left ventricular (LV) pressure will be required to distend the LV to a similar volume, indicating that the ventricle is less distensible. The slope of the LV end-diastolic pressure–volume relation indicates the passive chamber stiffness. Because the relation is exponential in shape, the slope ($\Delta P/\Delta V$) increases as the end-diastolic pressure increases. (From Little,[36] with permission of the American Heart Association.)

aging, systemic hypertension, and hypertrophic or restrictive cardiomyopathy.[2]

Diastolic function has also been assessed based on LV filling patterns by use of Doppler echocardiography.[3] In the absence of mitral stenosis, three patterns of LV filling indicate progressive impairment of diastolic function: (1) reduced early diastolic filling with a compensatory increase in importance of atrial filling (impaired relaxation); (2) most filling early in diastole with normal deceleration of mitral flow (pseudonormalization); and (3) almost all filling of the LV occurring very early in diastole in association with very rapid deceleration of mitral flow (restricted filling) (Figure 8.2).

These LV filling patterns, however, are influenced not only by LV diastolic properties but also by left atrial pressure. In contrast, tissue Doppler measurement of mitral annular velocity and color M-mode measurement of the velocity of propagation of mitral inflow to the apex are much less load sensitive. The peak early diastolic mitral annular velocity provides a relatively load-insensitive measure of LV relaxation in heart failure.[4] Peak early diastolic mitral annular velocity progressively decreases with increasing severity of diastolic dysfunction.[5,6] The color M-mode imaging performed from the apex provides a temporal and

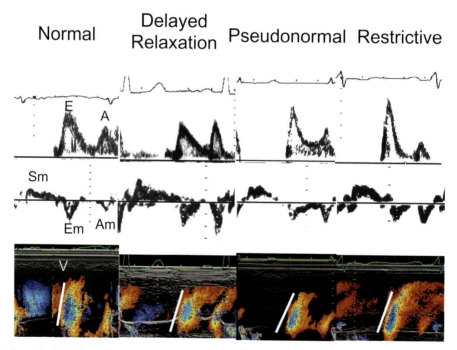

FIGURE 8.2. Transmitral Doppler left ventricular inflow velocity, Doppler tissue velocity, and color M-mode imaging during diastole. A, velocity of LV filling contributed by atrial contraction; Am, myocardial velocity during filling produced by atrial contraction; E, early LV filling velocity; Em, myocardial velocity during early filling; Sm, myocardial velocity during systole; V, velocity of propagation of mitral inflow to the apex.

8. Diastolic Versus Systolic Heart Failure

TABLE 8.1. Stages of diastolic dysfunction.

Parameter	Normal (young)	Normal (adult)	Delayed relaxation	Pseudonormal filling	Restrictive filling
E/A	>1	>1	<1	1–2	>2
DT (ms)	<220	<220	>220	150–200	<150
IVRT (ms)	<100	<100	>100	60–100	<60
S/D	<1	≥1	≥1	<1	<1
AR (cm/s)	<35	<35	<35	≥35	≥25*
Vp (cm/s)	>55	>45	<45	<45	<45
Em (cm/s)	>10	>8	<8	<8	<8

*Unless atrial mechanical failure is present.

Note: AR, pulmonary venous peak atrial contraction reversed velocity; DT, early left ventricular filling deceleration time; E/A, early-to-atrial left ventricular filling ratio; Em, peak early diastolic myocardial velocity; IVRT, isovolumic relaxation time; S/D, systolic-to-diastolic pulmonary venous flow ratio; Vp, color M-mode flow propagation velocity.

Source: Garcia et al.[6] © 1998, with permission of the American College of Cardiology Foundation.

spatial map of the ventricles of blood flow in early diastole along the long axis of the LV. The velocity of propagation of mitral inflow to the apex is reduced in conditions with impaired LV relaxation.[6] A pseudonormalized LV filling pattern can be distinguished from the normal filling pattern by demonstrating reduced peak early diastolic mitral annular velocity or reduced rate of flow propagation into the LV in early diastole. Furthermore, color M-mode imaging provides a noninvasive measurement of diastolic intraventricular pressure gradient between the apex and the base during early diastole.[7] Table 8.1 shows stages of diastolic dysfunction incorporating tissue Doppler and color M-mode indices.[6]

Definition of Systolic and Diastolic Heart Failure

Heart failure is defined as the pathologic state in which the heart is unable to pump blood at a rate required by the metabolizing tissues or can do so only with an elevated filling pressure. When the heart failure results from systolic dysfunction, the pathologic state can be called systolic heart failure (SHF). When the heart failure results from diastolic dysfunction in the absence of a reduced EF, the pathologic state can be called diastolic heart failure (DHF). It is important to recognize that the

heart failure, whether it results from systolic or diastolic dysfunction, is a clinical syndrome and that both SHF and DHF are heterogeneous disorders. Patients with SHF have abnormalities of diastolic function, and patients with DHF may have abnormalities of systolic contractile function.

Left Ventricular Structure and Function in Systolic and Diastolic Heart Failure

Table 8.2 compares the LV structural and functional characteristics in SHF and DHF.[8] Systolic heart failure and DHF have several similarities in LV structural and functional characteristics, including increased LV mass and increased LV end-diastolic pressure. The most significant difference between the two forms of heart failure is the difference in LV geometry and LV function; SHF is characterized by eccentric LV hypertrophy and abnormal systolic function, whereas DHF is characterized by concentric LV hypertrophy, normal systolic function, and abnormal diastolic function. Thus, the pathophysiology of SHF is dependent on progressive LV dilatation and abnormal systolic function. On the other hand, the pathophysiology of DHF is dependent on concentric LV hypertrophy and abnormal diastolic function.

TABLE 8.2. Comparison of left ventricular (LV) structural and functional features of systolic heart failure (SHF) and diastolic heart failure (DHF).

Characteristics	SHF	DHF
Remodeling		
LV end-diastolic volume	↑	N
LV end-systolic volume	↑	N
LV mass	↑ Eccentric	↑ Concentric
Relative wall thickness	↓	↑
Cardiomyocyte	↑ Length	↑ Diameter
Extracellular matrix collagen	↓	↑
Diastolic properties		
LV end-diastolic pressure	↑↑	↑↑
Relaxation time constant	↑	↑↑
Filling rate	↓	↓↓
Chamber stiffness	N–↓	↑
Myocardial stiffness	N–↑	↑
Systolic properties		
Performance		
Stroke volume	↓	N–↓
Stroke work	↓	N
Function		
Ejection fraction	↓	N
Ejection rate	↓	N
PRSW	↓	N
Contractility		
Positive dP/dt	↓	N
Ees	↓	N–↑
FS vs. stress	↓	N
Preload reserve	Exhausted	Limited
Ea	↓	↑
Arterial–ventricular coupling (Ea/Ees)	↓	N

Note: PRSW, preload-recruitable stroke work; Ees, end-systolic elastance; FS, fractional shortening; Ea, effective arterial elastance. N, no change; N–, no change or.
Source: From Zile et al.[8] © 2005, with permission of Elsevier.

Left Ventricular Structure

Concentric Versus Eccentric Hypertrophy

Left ventricular hypertrophy has traditionally been proposed as a mechanism that compensates for increased wall stress generated by a pressure or volume overload.[9] Pressure overload induces concentric hypertrophy, which is characterized by an absence of increased LV volume and increased LV mass with an increased ratio of wall thickness to LV dimension. On the other hand, volume overload induces eccentric hypertrophy, which is characterized by high LV volume and increased LV mass with a normal or decreased ratio of wall thickness to LV dimension. Figure 8.3 shows the morphologic responses to different stimuli. It is important to recognize that LV hypertrophy can occur in the absence of a pressure or volume overload (see later discussion).

Development of Concentric Hypertrophy

Concentric LV hypertrophy is an adaptive mechanism in response to pressure overload. A pressure overload produces a mechanical signal that is translated into the replication of sarcomeres in parallel, in turn increasing wall thickness. According to the Laplace formula, wall stress is equal to the product of pressure times radius divided by two times the wall thickness. Thus, excessive systolic wall stress generated by increased pressure is offset by increased wall thickness. This compensatory hypertrophy, however, is achieved at the cost of impaired LV relaxation and/or reduced LV distensibility. The most common conditions responsible for concentric hypertrophy include hypertensive heart disease and aortic stenosis.

Concentric hypertrophy also occurs in the absence of pressure overload. In hypertrophic cardiomyopathy, concentric hypertrophy may be induced by the abnormalities of myocardial contractile protein.

Transition from Concentric Hypertrophy to Diastolic Heart Failure

The mechanisms by which concentric hypertrophy transforms into DHF are currently undergoing intense study. Several experimental and clinical studies suggest that increased LV fibrosis may play an important role in the transition.[10–12] Thus, the LV fibrosis may be a therapeutic target to prevent the transition to DHF. Other potential mechanisms that may contribute to DHF include ventricular and aortic stiffening,[13,14] which are accelerated by aging.[15,16]

Development of Eccentric Hypertrophy

Eccentric LV hypertrophy is an adaptive mechanism in response to volume overload. Increased end-diastolic stress generated by volume overload triggers the replication of sarcomeres in series and elongates individual myocytes. The increased cell length causes an increase in total ventricular volume. The increase in volume allows for the generation of greater stroke volume and

8. Diastolic Versus Systolic Heart Failure

FIGURE 8.3. The morphologic response to a hemodynamic overload depends on the nature of the stimulus. When the overload is predominantly due to an increase in pressure (e.g., with systemic hypertension or aortic stenosis), the increase in systolic wall stress leads to the parallel additional sarcomeres and widening of the cardiac myocytes, resulting in concentric hypertrophy of the ventricle. When the overload is predominantly due to an increase in ventricular volume, the increase in diastolic wall stress leads to the series addition of sarcomeres, lengthening of cardiac myocytes, and eccentric chamber hypertrophy. (From Colucci WS, Braunwald E. Pathophysiology of heart failure. In Zipes DP, Libby P, Bonow R, Braunwald E, eds. Heart Disease: A Text Book of Cardiovascular Medicine, 7th ed. Philadelphia: WB Saunders; 2004:509–538. © 2004, with permission of Elsevier.)

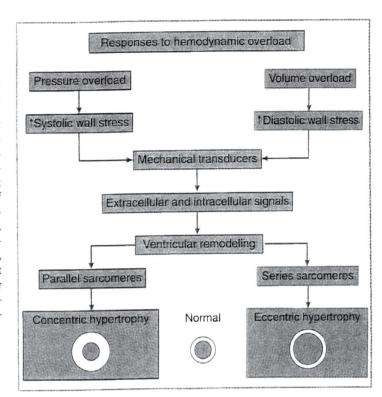

compensates the volume overload. Eccentric hypertrophy develops in patients with regurgitant valvular disease and anemia.

In the absence of volume overload, eccentric hypertrophy frequently occurs as a response to reduced LV wall motion caused by a large anterior myocardial infarction or idiopathic dilated cardiomyopathy to generate a normal stroke volume from a large end-diastolic volume.

Transition from Eccentric Remodeling to Systolic Heart Failure

Regardless of the underlying etiology, as the LV volume increases, wall stress increases not only in diastole but also in systole because of the increased radius of the curvature. Furthermore, the dilated ventricle becomes more spherical. This leads to repositioning of papillary muscles with functional mitral regurgitation, resulting in further LV dilatation. In agreement with the Laplace formula, increased LV volume and sphericity induce excessive wall stress. This leads to impairment of myocardial contractile function and thus overt heart failure.[17–19] In addition, continued activation of the sympathetic nervous and the renin-angiotensin-aldosterone systems, which are initially activated to maintain cardiac output, plays an important role in the progression of LV dilatation and the development of overt heart failure (neurohumoral hypothesis).[20,21] This neurohumoral hypothesis is supported by the success in the treatment of SHF, namely, with angiotensin-converting enzyme inhibitors,[22,23] angiotensin receptor blockers,[24,25] β-blockers,[26–28] and aldosterone inhibitors.[29,30]

Left Ventricular Function

Diastolic Function in Systolic Heart Failure

Although the pathophysiology of SHF is primarily dependent on systolic dysfunction, SHF is accompanied by diastolic dysfunction (Figure 8.4).[2,31] Furthermore, it is increasingly clear that the severity of heart disease and prognosis are related to diastolic dysfunction regardless of the EF.[31–35] This

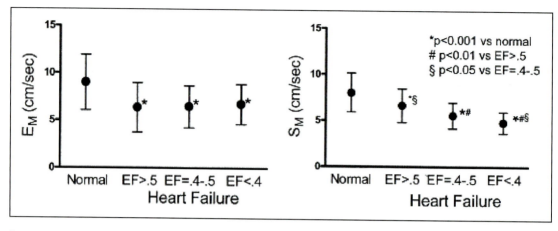

FIGURE 8.4. Peak early diastolic mitral annular velocity (E_M) is similarly decreased in patients who have heart failure regardless of ejection fraction (EF) compared with patients who do not have heart failure. Peak systolic mitral annular velocity (S_M) is progressively decreased in patients who have an EF ≥0.50, 0.40–0.50, and ≤0.40. (From Brucks et al.[31] © 2005, with permission of Excerpta Medica, Inc.)

underscores the importance of understanding the mechanisms of diastolic dysfunction in SHF.

Patients with SHF require a large end-diastolic volume to produce an adequate stroke volume and cardiac output. This is represented as the rightward shift of the LV end-diastolic pressure volume relation (see Figure 8.1, curve B). In this situation, each volume is associated with a lower pressure. This could be interpreted as indicating that the LV is more distensible. Nevertheless, patients with SHF have abnormal LV diastolic filling and markedly elevated left atrial pressure. Although this may merely reflect overfilling of the LV that has displaced the operating point to a portion of the pressure–volume relation at which chamber stiffness (dP/dV) is high, there appear to be other plausible reasons.[36]

First, reduced elastic recoil due to reduced LV contractility contributes to abnormal LV filling in SHF. During LV ejection, energy is stored as myocytes are compressed, and the elastic elements in the myocardial wall are compressed and twisted. Relaxation of myocardial contraction allows this energy to be released as the elastic elements recoil. This causes LV pressure to rapidly fall during isovolumetric relaxation. Furthermore, for the first 30–40 ms after mitral valve opening, the relaxation of LV wall tension is normally rapid enough to cause LV pressure to fall despite an increase in LV volume. This fall in LV pressure produces an early diastolic pressure gradient from the left atrium to the apex. This accelerates blood out of the left atrium and produces rapid early diastolic flow that quickly propagates to the apex. In the hypocontractile LV, however, less energy is stored during systole and released during diastole, which in turn results in a decreased intraventricular pressure gradient.[37] In this situation, the LV filling depends entirely on the elevated left atrial pressure.

Second, LV dilatation itself may contribute to abnormal LV filling in SHF. Yotti et al.[38] investigated the mechanisms of reduced intraventricular diastolic pressure gradient in dilated cardiomyopathy using color M-mode Doppler echocardiography and then applying the Euler equation. The Euler equation relates the pressure gradient to inertial acceleration and convective deceleration.[7] Inertial acceleration is the change in velocity with respect to time, whereas convective deceleration is proportional to the reduction in velocity with respect to distance. Convective deceleration would be expected to be increased in a dilated ventricle because of divergence of the blood flow away from the longitudinal axis of the ventricle, forming vortices (Figure 8.5). Such an increase in convective deceleration would decrease the intraventricular pressure gradient. In fact, Yotti et al.[38] found that the intraventricular diastolic pressure gradient was reduced in dilated

8. Diastolic Versus Systolic Heart Failure

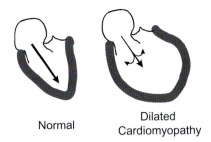

FIGURE 8.5. Diagram of early diastolic left ventricular filling. In the normal heart, recoil of elastic elements produces a progressive pressure gradient from the left atrium to the apex of the left ventricle. This results in acceleration of blood from the left atrium to the left ventricular apex, resulting in rapid diastolic filling. In a patient with a dilated cardiomyopathy there is less elastic recoil. The acceleration of blood to the apex is further reduced by convective deceleration, which is the tendency for blood to diverge from the longitudinal axis forming vortices in the dilated ventricle. (From Little.[36] © 2005 American Heart Association, Inc. All rights reserved. Reprinted with permission.)

cardiomyopathy because of both the impaired inertial acceleration and the enhanced convective deceleration. They also found that the amount of convective deceleration was proportional to the ventricular–annular disproportion; the more dilated the ventricle, the greater the convective deceleration. The reduced inertial acceleration was presumably the result of impaired elastic recoil. Thus, the dilated hypocontractile ventricle produces a lower intraventricular pressure gradient in early diastole as the result of both the reduced elastic recoil and the dilated ventricle itself.

Taken together, eccentric ventricular remodeling impairs not only LV systolic function but also LV diastolic filling. In patients with dilated cardiomyopathy, left atrial pressure is elevated, and LV filling pressure is impaired because of slow relaxation, reduced elastic recoil, displacement onto a stiff portion of the LV end-diastolic pressure volume relation, and impairment of filling from the ventricular dilatation itself. Thus, despite the enhanced passive distensibility, the dilated LV has substantial diastolic dysfunction.

Systolic Function in Diastolic Heart Failure

Because patients with DHF have a normal EF, the systolic function of these patients has implicitly been considered to be normal. However, many patients with DHF have a subtle systolic dysfunction that is not detected by measurement of an EF.

Brucks et al.[31] compared systolic function measured by systolic mitral annular velocity (Sm) in tissue Doppler imaging in patients with heart failure with an EF ≥ 0.50, those with an EF >0.40 and <0.50, those with an EF ≤ 0.40, and age-matched controls. They found that Sm was significantly lower in heart failure patients with an EF ≥ 0.50 than in controls but significantly higher than in heart failure patients with an EF >0.40 and <0.50 and those with an EF ≤ 0.40 (see Figure 8.4). Similarly, Yu et al.[39] showed that Sm was significantly lower in heart failure patients with an EF ≥ 0.50 than in normal controls and in asymptomatic patients with diastolic dysfunction but significantly higher than in heart failure patients with an EF <0.50.

It is possible, however, that Sm may be affected by not only contractility but also coexistent changes in LV loading conditions and geometry. Thus, to determine whether patients with DHF have abnormal systolic function, indices that are independent of loading conditions and geometric changes should be examined. No such indexes, however, have been proposed. Thus, Baicu et al.[40] hypothesized that if multiple indexes were measured and if the results were in general agreement and viewed in aggregate, it should be possible to determine whether patients with DHF have abnormal systolic function. To test the hypothesis, they examined LV systolic properties using echocardiographic and cardiac catheterization data from heart failure patients with an EF >0.50 and normal controls. They found that measurements of systolic performance (stroke volume), function (EF, preload-recruitable stroke work), and contractility (positive dP/dt, stress vs. shortening, end-systolic elastance) were not significantly different in patients with DHF compared with normal controls.

These observations suggest that systolic function assessed by Sm is impaired in DHF compared with normal controls but not as severely impaired in DHF as in SHF and that other LV systolic properties of DHF are similar to those of normal controls. Furthermore, Zile et al.[41] showed that patients with DHF had generally abnormal diastolic properties. Thus, although subtle systolic dysfunction might contribute to DHF to some extent, it appears that the pathophysiology of DHF is predominantly dependent on abnormal LV diastolic properties.

Exercise Intolerance

Limited exercise tolerance due to fatigue and dyspnea is a major symptom and a cause of disability in heart failure. Furthermore, exercise intolerance is often the initial presenting symptom in heart failure patients.

During exercise, the body's oxygen consumption increases. Normally, the increase in oxygen consumption is met by a combination of an increase in cardiac output and a widening of the arteriovenous oxygen difference. In patients with heart failure, however, the ability of the heart to increase cardiac output (central mechanisms) and the ability of the skeletal muscles to utilize oxygen from the delivered blood (peripheral mechanisms) are limited because of the abnormal cardiac function and alterations in the skeletal muscles and vasculature.

It is increasingly clear that exercise capacity is similarly impaired in patients with SHF and those with DHF despite the different pathophysiologies (Figure 8.6).[42] Thus, understanding similar and different mechanisms of exercise intolerance in systolic and DHF may provide a basis for the development of specific therapeutic strategies for exercise intolerance in the two forms of heart failure.

Central Mechanisms

Different Central Hemodynamic Responses to Exercise in Systolic and Diastolic Heart Failure

Both patients with SHF and those with DHF have reduced peak cardiac output and stroke volume, mildly reduced peak heart rate, and slightly reduced peak arteriovenous oxygen difference.[43] The mechanisms of reduced peak stroke volume, however, markedly differ between the two forms. In SHF, the inability of the heart to increase stroke volume is due to impaired enhancement of LV contractility and a blunted ability to increase the LV end-diastolic volume.[44] Furthermore, mitral regurgitation is often present during exercise in SHF because of the dilatation of the mitral annulus; thus, the exercise-induced functional mitral regurgitation reduces forward stroke volume, thereby limiting the increase in cardiac output.[45] In contrast, in DHF, the inability of the heart to increase stroke volume during exercise is due primarily to the limited increase in LV end-diastolic volume despite the normal LV contractility and the increased LV filling pressure (Figure 8.7).[46]

Diastolic Dysfunction as a Cause of Exercise Intolerance

For many years, investigators have focused on the role of systolic dysfunction in abnormal central hemodynamics to explain exercise intolerance in heart failure. Nevertheless, studies have consistently reported that systolic function is not or is

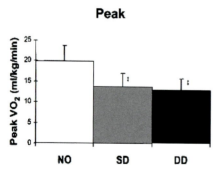 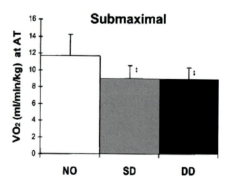

FIGURE 8.6. Exercise oxygen consumption (VO$_2$) during peak exhausted exercise (**left**) and during submaximal exercise at the ventilatory anaerobic threshold (AT; **right**) in age-matched healthy subjects (NO), elderly patients with heart failure due to systolic dysfunction (SD), and elderly patients with heart failure due to diastolic dysfunction (DD). (From Kitzman.[43] © 2005, with permission of Elsevier.)

8. Diastolic Versus Systolic Heart Failure

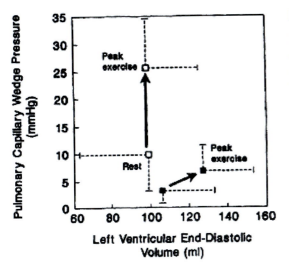

FIGURE 8.7. Plot of pulmonary capillary wedge pressure versus left ventricular end-diastolic volume, indicating the direction change from rest to peak exercise in seven elderly patients with diastolic heart failure (open boxes) versus 10 age-matched normal controls (solid boxes). Note the shift upward and to the left, denoting abnormal diastolic function. (From Kitzman et al.[46] © 1991, with permission of the American College of Cardiology Foundation.)

only weakly related to exercise capacity in heart failure.[44,47] Instead, several lines of evidence suggest that an increase in left atrial pressure may be the most important hemodynamic determinant of exercise capacity in SHF.[48] Thus, diastolic dysfunction may play an important role in the mechanisms of exercise intolerance in both SHF and DHF. In this section, we discuss diastolic dysfunction as a cause of exercise intolerance in heart failure.

Normal Left Ventricular Filling

The LV fills in diastole in response to the pressure gradient from the left atrium to the LV. This occurs at two times during the cardiac cycle: early in diastole after mitral valve opening and late in diastole during atrial systole. Most of LV filling occurs early in diastole, and less than 25% of the LV stroke volume enters the LV during atrial systole. The rate of early LV filling is determined by two factors: the rate of LV relaxation and left atrial pressure at the time of mitral valve opening.

Effect of Exercise on Left Ventricular Filling

During exercise, the LV must increase cardiac output to meet an increase in the body's oxygen consumption. This is accomplished by increased heart rate and maintained or augmented LV stroke volume. An increase in heart rate during exercise, however, decreases the duration of diastole and thus shortens the time for diastolic filling. Thus, LV filling rate must increase to maintain or augment the LV stroke volume. This is accomplished by enhancement of LV relaxation and lower early diastolic LV pressure (Figure 8.8).[49] The mechanisms underlying the enhanced LV relaxation and lower early diastolic LV pressure during exercise are complex and may result from the combined effects of sympathetic stimulation, tachycardia, and/or enhanced elastic recoil due to contraction to lower volume.[49]

Effect of Heart Failure on Response to Exercise

The normal response to exercise is lost during the development of heart failure. In a model of chronic heart failure produced by several weeks of pacing, during exercise after heart failure, the stroke volume, the peak early LV filling rate, and the peak early diastolic pressure gradient increased as during normal exercise.[50] However, the cause of the increased early LV filling during exercise after heart failure was different (Figure 8.9).[50] Instead of the normal response of rapid LV relaxation and lower early diastolic LV pressure, during exercise after heart failure, LV relaxation that was slower at rest was further slowed, and the early diastolic LV pressure increased. Thus, the increased early LV filling rate and mitral valve pressure gradient resulted from an abnormal increase in left atrial pressure during exercise after heart failure. Furthermore, LV relaxation and early diastolic LV pressure that were abnormal at rest were further exacerbated during exercise. Similar observations were reported in patients with dilated cardiomyopathy.[51]

These observations suggest that the enhanced diastolic dysfunction during exercise leads to an increase in left atrial pressure, thereby contributing to the dyspnea that limits exercise tolerance in SHF. Similarly, a left atrial pressure abnormally increases during exercise in DHF (see Figure 8.7).[46] Thus, diastolic dysfunction appears to play

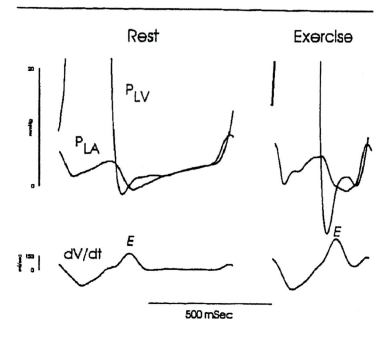

FIGURE 8.8. Recording of left atrial pressure (P_{LA}), left ventricular pressure (P_{LV}), and the rate of change of left ventricular volume (dV/dt) in a conscious animal at rest and during exercise. E, early diastolic left ventricular filling velocity. (From Little WC, Cheng CP. Modulation of diastolic dysfunction in the intact heart. In Lorell BH, Grossmann W, eds. Diastolic Relaxation of the Heart. Boston: Kluwer Academic, 1994:167–146, with permission.)

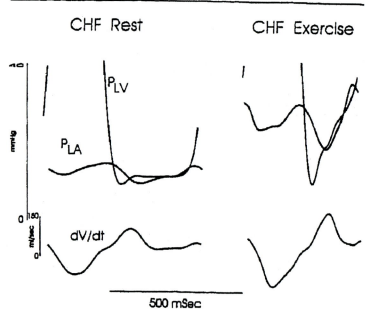

FIGURE 8.9. Recording from the same animal as in Figure 8.8 after the induction of pacing-induced congestive heart failure (CHF). (From Little WC, Cheng CP. Modulation of diastolic dysfunction in the intact heart. In Lorell BH, Grossmann W, eds. Diastolic Relaxation of the Heart. Boston: Kluwer Academic, 1994:167–146, with permission.)

an important role in the mechanisms of exercise intolerance in both SHF and DHF.

Peripheral Mechanisms

The importance of peripheral factors as mechanisms of exercise intolerance in heart failure has been supported by several lines of evidence: (1) exercise capacity and measures of systolic LV function are poorly correlated;[47] and (2) the improvements of central hemodynamics with pharmacologic therapy are rapid, but corresponding improvements in exercise capacity are delayed for weeks or months.[48] Proposed peripheral factors include abnormalities of endothelial function, ergoreflex activation, vasodilatory capacity, and distribution of cardiac output.[44] These factors may contribute to reduced tissue perfusion and/or abnormal oxygen extraction, thereby limiting exercise capacity in heart failure patients. These peripheral factors, however, have been proposed from studies in SHF. The role of peripheral factors in the mechanisms of exercise intolerance in DHF deserves future investigation.

Distinction Between Systolic and Diastolic Heart Failure

A distinction between SHF and DHF is important because these two forms of heart failure have different pathophysiologies and natural histories and thus might potentially require different therapeutic approaches. Nevertheless, clinical symptoms and signs are similar in SHF and DHF (Table 8.3).[52] This may be because SHF is often accompanied by diastolic dysfunction, and thus symptoms and signs related to pulmonary congestion are commonly observed in SHF.[2] Thus, clinical history and physical examination do not provide useful information in discriminating between SHF and DHF.

The most significant differences between SHF and DHF are those in LV volumes, geometries, and functions; SHF is characterized by large volume, eccentric LV remodeling, and a low EF, whereas DHF is characterized by small volume, concentric LV remodeling, and a normal EF (see Table 8.2). Thus, the first requirement for discriminating between SHF and DHF is to assess the

TABLE 8.3. Prevalence of specific symptoms and signs in systolic heart failure (SHF) and diastolic heart failure (DHF).

	SHF	DHF
Symptoms		
Dyspnea on exertion	96	85
Paroxysmal nocturnal dyspnea	50	55
Orthopnea	73	60
Physical examination		
Jugular venous distension	46	35
Rales	70	72
Displaced apical impulse	60	50
S3	65	45
S4	66	45
Hepatomegaly	16	15
Edema	40	30
Chest radiograph		
Cardiomegaly	96	90
Pulmonary venous hypertension	80	75

Note: Values are expressed as percentages.
Source: From Zile and Brutsaert.[52] © 2002 American Heart Association, Inc. All rights reserved. Reprinted with permission.

LV structure and function. For this purpose, echocardiography appears to be the most useful method for several reasons. First, it noninvasively provides information on the LV structure and function. Second, it provides other useful information about regional wall motion abnormalities, valvular disease, and pericardial disease. Thus, echocardiography is useful for not only discriminating between SHF and DHF but also identifying the causes of systolic and diastolic dysfunction.

Is Measurement of Diastolic Function Necessary?

Several criteria have been proposed for the diagnosis of DHF.[53,54] In summary, for the diagnosis of DHF to be made, the following are required: (1) clinical evidence of heart failure, (2) normal or near-normal systolic function (LVEF >0.50), and (3) objective evidence of impaired LV relaxation and/or LV passive stiffness. If strictly applied, the definition of DHF would include patients with acute mitral or aortic regurgitation or mechanical causes of diastolic dysfunction (mitral stenosis or constrictive pericarditis); this could be avoided by additional screening.

Recognizing the difficulties inherent in the clinical assessment of the LV diastolic performance,

Zile et al.[55] tested the hypothesis that measurements of LV relaxation and passive stiffness were not necessary to make the diagnosis of DHF. They studied 63 patients with a history of heart failure, a normal LVEF (>0.50), and an at least mild LV hypertrophy (LV mass ≥125 g/m^2) or concentric LV remodeling (LV chamber dimension <55 mm combined with LV wall thickness ≥11 mm and relative wall thickness ≥0.45). They then assessed LV diastolic function during cardiac catheterization. They found that all the patients had evidence of abnormalities of LV relaxation and passive stiffness.[41,55] Thus, they concluded that objective evidence of abnormalities of LV relaxation or distensibility was not necessary to make the diagnosis of DHF if there was evidence of LV hypertrophy or concentric remodeling.

However, assessment of diastolic dysfunction using Doppler echocardiography provides useful information on the severity of heart failure and the prognosis.[31–35] Specifically, Brucks et al.[31] examined the association of systolic and diastolic function with severity of heart failure assessed by plasma brain natriuretic peptide levels and prognosis in 104 heart failure patients with an EF <0.50 and in 102 heart failure patients with an EF ≥0.50. They found that increasing grade of diastolic dysfunction but not reduced EF was associated with increased plasma brain natriuretic peptide levels. They also found that greater diastolic dysfunction but not reduced EF was associated with a worse 2-year survival rate (Figure 8.10). When analysis was restricted to heart failure patients with an EF <0.50, both reduced EF and the greater diastolic dysfunction was associated with worse survival. Rihal et al.[33] examined the association of systolic and diastolic function with heart failure symptoms and 3-year survival rate in 102 patients with dilated cardiomyopathy and an EF of 0.23 ± 0.08. They found that markers of diastolic dysfunction, including the short deceleration time and the increased peak early diastolic LV inflow velocity, were more strongly associated with symptoms than the reduced EF. They also found that the short (<130 ms) deceleration time had incremental prognostic value to the reduced (<0.25) EF. Similarly, Wang et al.[34] showed that the reduced (<3 cm/s) Em was a powerful predictor for 4-year mortality and provided incremental prognostic value to other clinical risk factors and Doppler echocardiographic variables in 182 heart failure patients with an EF <0.50. These observations suggest that diastolic dysfunction is associated with the severity of heart failure and prognosis independent of the EF. Thus, although measurement of diastolic function may not be necessary for the diagnosis of DHF, it provides useful information for assessment of the severity of heart failure and for risk stratification for all heart failure patients.

Timing of Ejection Fraction Measurement

Vasan and Levy[54] require a normal EF within 72 hours of an episode of pulmonary congestion to make a definite diagnosis of DHF. It is possible,

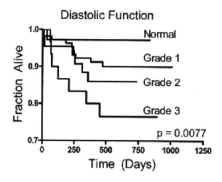 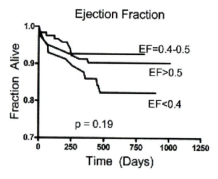

FIGURE 8.10. Kaplan-Meier survival curves for 104 heart failure (HF) patients with an ejection fraction (EF) < 0.50 and 102 HF patients with an EF ≥0.50. Progressively more severe diastolic dysfunction is strongly associated with decreased survival. The EF does not significantly affect survival. For stages of diastolic dysfunction, see Table 8.1. (From Brucks et al.[31] © 2005, with permission from Elsevier.)

however, that the acute pulmonary congestion may be due to transient systolic dysfunction or to acute mitral regurgitation produced by hypertension and/or myocardial ischemia that had resolved by the time the LVEF was measured. To address this issue, Gandhi et al.[56] used Doppler echocardiography to evaluate LVEF, regional wall motion, and mitral regurgitation in 38 patients both during an acute episode of hypertensive pulmonary edema and 24–72 hours later, after treatment and resolution of the hypertension and pulmonary congestion. They found that LVEF and regional wall motion were similar both during the acute episode of hypertensive pulmonary edema and after resolution of the congestion and control of blood pressure. No patient had severe mitral regurgitation during the acute episode. They also found that one-half of the patients had an EF $\geq$0.50 during their presentation with acute pulmonary edema and that 88% of the patients with an EF $\geq$0.50 after treatment had an EF $\geq$0.50 during the acute episode, and all of these patients had an EF of at least 0.43. Thus, they concluded that the EF obtained 1–3 days after the acute presentation of patients with hypertensive pulmonary edema accurately identified patients with a preserved EF during acute presentation. This study suggests that measuring the EF within 72 hours of an acute episode of pulmonary congestion is sufficient to meet the diagnostic criteria proposed by Vasan and Levy.[54]

Current Recommendations

If patients have clinical evidence of heart failure, the EF should be measured within 72 hours of an acute episode of pulmonary congestion. If the EF is <0.50, the diagnosis of SHF can be made. If the EF is >0.50 and there is evidence of LV hypertrophy or concentric remodeling, the diagnosis of DHF can be made. In the absence of LV hypertrophy or concentric remodeling, the diagnosis of DHF may be supported by the presence of left atrial enlargement.[57] When the diagnosis of DHF remains uncertain, Doppler echocardiography or cardiac catheterization provides a definitive diagnosis. Furthermore, assessment of diastolic function using Doppler echocardiography, particularly with tissue Doppler imaging, provides useful information on the severity of heart failure and prognosis regardless of the EF. Thus, it is important to evaluate both systolic and diastolic function not only for differentiating between SHF and DHF but also for assessing the severity of heart failure and identifying high-risk patients.

References

1. Kass DA, Maughan WL. From "Emax" to pressure–volume relations: a broader view. Circulation 1988;77:1203–1212.
2. Little WC, Applegate RJ. Congestive heart failure: systolic and diastolic function. J Cardiothorac Vasc Anesth 1993;7:2–5.
3. Little WC, Warner JG Jr, Rankin KM, et al. Evaluation of left ventricular diastolic function from the pattern of left ventricular filling. Clin Cardiol 1998;21:5–9.
4. Hasegawa H, Little WC, Ohno M, et al. Diastolic mitral annular velocity during the development of heart failure. J Am Coll Cardiol 2003;41:1590–1597.
5. Sohn DW, Chai IH, Lee DJ, et al. Assessment of mitral annulus velocity by Doppler tissue imaging in the evaluation of left ventricular diastolic function. J Am Coll Cardiol 1997;30:474–480.
6. Garcia MJ, Thomas JD, Klein AL. New Doppler echocardiographic applications for the study of diastolic function. J Am Coll Cardiol 1998;32:865–875.
7. Greenberg NL, Vandervoort PM, Firstenberg MS, et al. Estimation of diastolic intraventricular pressure gradients by Doppler M-mode echocardiography. Am J Physiol Heart Circ Physiol 2001;280:H2507–H2515.
8. Zile MR, Baicu CF, Bonnema DD. Diastolic heart failure: definitions and terminology. Prog Cardiovasc Dis 2005;47:307–313.
9. Carabello BA. Concentric versus eccentric remodeling. J Card Fail 2002;8:S258–S263.
10. Masuyama T, Yamamoto K, Sakata Y, et al. Evolving changes in Doppler mitral flow velocity pattern in rats with hypertensive hypertrophy. J Am Coll Cardiol 2000;36:2333–2338.
11. Yamamoto K, Masuyama T, Sakata Y, et al. Myocardial stiffness is determined by ventricular fibrosis, but not by compensatory or excessive hypertrophy in hypertensive heart. Cardiovasc Res 2002;55:76–82.
12. Querejeta R, Lopez B, Gonzalez A, et al. Increased collagen type I synthesis in patients with heart failure of hypertensive origin: relation to myocardial fibrosis. Circulation. 2004;110:1263–1268.
13. Hundley WG, Kitzman DW, Morgan TM, et al. Cardiac cycle–dependent changes in aortic area

and distensibility are reduced in older patients with isolated diastolic heart failure and correlate with exercise intolerance. J Am Coll Cardiol 2001;38:796–802.

14. Kawaguchi M, Hay I, Fetics B, et al. Combined ventricular systolic and arterial stiffening in patients with heart failure and preserved ejection fraction: implications for systolic and diastolic reserve limitations. Circulation 2003;107:714–720.

15. Chen CH, Nakayama M, Nevo E, et al. Coupled systolic-ventricular and vascular stiffening with age: implications for pressure regulation and cardiac reserve in the elderly. J Am Coll Cardiol 1998;32:1221–1227.

16. Redfield MM, Jacobsen SJ, Borlaug BA, et al. Age- and gender-related ventricular–vascular stiffening: a community-based study. Circulation 2005;112:2254–2262.

17. Fedak PW, Verma S, Weisel RD, et al. Cardiac remodeling and failure: from molecules to man (part I). Cardiovasc Pathol 2005;14:1–11.

18. Cohn JN, Ferrari R, Sharpe N. Cardiac remodeling—concepts and clinical implications: a consensus paper from an international forum on cardiac remodeling. On Behalf of an International Forum on Cardiac Remodeling. J Am Coll Cardiol 2000;35:569–582.

19. Mann DL. Mechanisms and models in heart failure: a combinatorial approach. Circulation 1999;100:999–1008.

20. Cohn JN. Structural basis for heart failure. Ventricular remodeling and its pharmacological inhibition. Circulation 1995;91:2504–2507.

21. Francis GS. Pathophysiology of chronic heart failure. Am J Med 2001;110 Suppl 7A:37S–46S.

22. Effects of enalapril on mortality in severe congestive heart failure. Results of the Cooperative North Scandinavian Enalapril Survival Study (CONSENSUS). The CONSENSUS Trial Study Group. N Engl J Med 1987;316:1429–1435.

23. Effect of enalapril on survival in patients with reduced left ventricular ejection fractions and congestive heart failure. The SOLVD Investigators. N Engl J Med 1991;325:293–302.

24. Granger CB, McMurray JJ, Yusuf S, et al. Effects of candesartan in patients with chronic heart failure and reduced left-ventricular systolic function intolerant to angiotensin-converting-enzyme inhibitors: the CHARM-Alternative trial. Lancet 2003;362:772–776.

25. Cohn JN, Tognoni G. A randomized trial of the angiotensin-receptor blocker valsartan in chronic heart failure. N Engl J Med 2001;345:1667–1675.

26. The Cardiac Insufficiency Bisoprolol Study II (CIBIS-II): a randomised trial. Lancet 1999;353:9–13.

27. Packer M, Bristow MR, Cohn JN, et al. The effect of carvedilol on morbidity and mortality in patients with chronic heart failure. U.S. Carvedilol Heart Failure Study Group. N Engl J Med 1996;334:1349–1355.

28. Packer M, Coats AJ, Fowler MB, et al. Effect of carvedilol on survival in severe chronic heart failure. N Engl J Med 2001;344:1651–1658.

29. Pitt B, Zannad F, Remme WJ, et al. The effect of spironolactone on morbidity and mortality in patients with severe heart failure. Randomized Aldactone Evaluation Study Investigators. N Engl J Med 1999;341:709–717.

30. Pitt B, Remme W, Zannad F, et al. Eplerenone, a selective aldosterone blocker, in patients with left ventricular dysfunction after myocardial infarction. N Engl J Med 2003;348:1309–1321.

31. Brucks S, Little WC, Chao T, et al. Contribution of left ventricular diastolic dysfunction to heart failure regardless of ejection fraction. Am J Cardiol 2005;95:603–606.

32. Vanoverschelde JL, Raphael DA, Robert AR, et al. Left ventricular filling in dilated cardiomyopathy: relation to functional class and hemodynamics. J Am Coll Cardiol 1990;15:1288–1295.

33. Rihal CS, Nishimura RA, Hatle LK, et al. Systolic and diastolic dysfunction in patients with clinical diagnosis of dilated cardiomyopathy. Relation to symptoms and prognosis. Circulation 1994;90:2772–2779.

34. Wang M, Yip G, Yu CM, et al. Independent and incremental prognostic value of early mitral annulus velocity in patients with impaired left ventricular systolic function. J Am Coll Cardiol. 2005;45:272–277.

35. Dokainish H, Zoghbi WA, Lakkis NM, et al. Incremental predictive power of B-type natriuretic peptide and tissue Doppler echocardiography in the prognosis of patients with congestive heart failure. J Am Coll Cardiol 2005;45:1223–1226.

36. Little WC. Diastolic dysfunction beyond distensibility: adverse effects of ventricular dilatation. Circulation 2005;112:2888–2890.

37. Firstenberg MS, Smedira NG, Greenberg NL, et al. Relationship between early diastolic intraventricular pressure gradients, an index of elastic recoil, and improvements in systolic and diastolic function. Circulation 2001;104:I330–I335.

38. Yotti R, Bermejo J, Antoranz JC, et al. A noninvasive method for assessing impaired diastolic suction in patients with dilated cardiomyopathy. Circulation 2005;112:2921–2929.

39. Yu CM, Lin H, Yang H, et al. Progression of systolic abnormalities in patients with "isolated" diastolic heart failure and diastolic dysfunction. Circulation 2002;105:1195–1201.
40. Baicu CF, Zile MR, Aurigemma GP, et al. Left ventricular systolic performance, function, and contractility in patients with diastolic heart failure. Circulation 2005;111:2306–2312.
41. Zile MR, Baicu CF, Gaasch WH. Diastolic heart failure—abnormalities in active relaxation and passive stiffness of the left ventricle. N Engl J Med 2004;350:1953–1959.
42. Kitzman DW, Little WC, Brubaker PH, et al. Pathophysiological characterization of isolated diastolic heart failure in comparison to systolic heart failure. JAMA 2002;288:2144–2150.
43. Kitzman DW. Exercise intolerance. Prog Cardiovasc Dis 2005;47:367–379.
44. Pina IL, Apstein CS, Balady GJ, et al. Exercise and heart failure: a statement from the American Heart Association Committee on exercise, rehabilitation, and prevention. Circulation 2003;107:1210–1225.
45. Lapu-Bula R, Robert A, Van CD, et al. Contribution of exercise-induced mitral regurgitation to exercise stroke volume and exercise capacity in patients with left ventricular systolic dysfunction. Circulation 2002;106:1342–1348.
46. Kitzman DW, Higginbotham MB, Cobb FR, et al. Exercise intolerance in patients with heart failure and preserved left ventricular systolic function: failure of the Frank-Starling mechanism. J Am Coll Cardiol 1991;17:1065–1072.
47. Sullivan MJ, Hawthorne MH. Exercise intolerance in patients with chronic heart failure. Prog Cardiovasc Dis 1995;38:1–22.
48. Packer M. Abnormalities of diastolic function as a potential cause of exercise intolerance in chronic heart failure. Circulation. 1990;81:III78–III86.
49. Cheng CP, Igarashi Y, Little WC. Mechanism of augmented rate of left ventricular filling during exercise. Circ Res 1992;70:9–19.
50. Cheng CP, Noda T, Nozawa T, et al. Effect of heart failure on the mechanism of exercise-induced augmentation of mitral valve flow. Circ Res. 1993;72:795–806.
51. Sato H, Hori M, Ozaki H, et al. Exercise-induced upward shift of diastolic left ventricular pressure-volume relation in patients with dilated cardiomyopathy. Effects of beta-adrenoceptor blockade. Circulation 1993;88:2215–2223.
52. Zile MR, Brutsaert DL. New concepts in diastolic dysfunction and diastolic heart failure: Part I: diagnosis, prognosis, and measurements of diastolic function. Circulation 2002;105:1387–1393.
53. How to diagnose diastolic heart failure. European Study Group on Diastolic Heart Failure. Eur Heart J 1998;19:990–1003.
54. Vasan RS, Levy D. Defining diastolic heart failure: a call for standardized diagnostic criteria. Circulation 2000;101:2118–2121.
55. Zile MR, Gaasch WH, Carroll JD, et al. Heart failure with a normal ejection fraction: is measurement of diastolic function necessary to make the diagnosis of diastolic heart failure? Circulation 2001;104:779–782.
56. Gandhi SK, Powers JC, Nomeir AM, et al. The pathogenesis of acute pulmonary edema associated with hypertension. N Engl J Med 2001;344:17–22.
57. Yturralde RF, Gaasch WH. Diagnostic criteria for diastolic heart failure. Prog Cardiovasc Dis 2005;47:314–319.

Section 2
Diagnosis of Diastolic Heart Failure

9
Invasive Evaluation of Diastolic Left Ventricular Dysfunction

Loek van Heerebeek and Walter J. Paulus

Introduction

According to the criteria proposed by the European Study Group on Diastolic Heart Failure, the diagnosis of diastolic heart failure (DHF) is based on the presence of a triad of signs or symptoms of congestive heart failure, a normal left ventricular (LV) ejection fraction, and objective evidence of diastolic LV dysfunction.[1] Objective evidence of diastolic LV dysfunction can be obtained using invasive techniques or noninvasive imaging. Because of questionable sensitivity of noninvasive techniques such as Doppler mitral flow velocity measurements, some investigators proposed restricting the diagnosis of "definite" DHF only to those patients who had invasive evidence of diastolic LV dysfunction.[2] Acquisition of objective evidence of diastolic LV dysfunction by invasive techniques therefore remains important. This objective evidence can consist of an assessment of LV relaxation kinetics or an assessment of LV diastolic distensibility. It requires use of high-fidelity tip-micromanometer catheters to measure LV cavity pressures and LV conductance catheters or LV angiograms to simultaneously measure LV cavity dimensions. If the LV diastolic distensibility assessment is intended to derive myocardial stiffness indices, regional LV stress and strain values need to be determined and the LV pressure and volume measurements therefore need to be implemented with an LV wall thickness measurement usually derived from a simultaneously acquired two-dimensional echocardiogram.[3]

Left Ventricular Relaxation Kinetics

- LV dP/dt_{min} is afterload sensitive.
- The time constant of LV pressure decay (tau) is less afterload sensitive.
- Calculation of tau has to take into consideration the closeness of an exponential fit, the start and end point of the fit, and the asymptote pressure of the fit.

Left ventricular relaxation kinetics can be assessed invasively by LV peak negative dP/dt (LV dP/dt_{min}), that is, the peak rate of LV pressure fall, and by the time constant of LV pressure decay (tau). Diastolic LV dysfunction is said to be present if the absolute value of LV dP/dt_{min} is lower than $1,100 \, mm \, Hg/s^{-1}$ (normal control value: $1,864 \pm 390 \, mm \, Hg/s^{-1}$; mean $\pm$ SD). Low values have been reported in hypertrophic cardiomyopathy ($998 \pm 223 \, mm \, Hg/s^{-1}$) and in congestive cardiomyopathy ($1,060 \pm 334 \, mm \, Hg/s^{-1}$) but not in coronary artery disease or hypertensive heart disease.[4] A valid measurement of this index requires a high-fidelity tip-micromanometer LV pressure signal and adequate signal processing (high-cut filter >100 Hz). The major drawback of LV dP/dt_{min} is its sensitivity to LV end-systolic pressure and the LV afterload profile of the foregoing systole.[5,6] The dependence of LV dP/dt_{min} on LV end-systolic pressure is especially evident on an LV dP/dt versus LV pressure plot (a phase-plane plot of LV pressure) as shown in Figure 9.1, which displays four phase-plane plots of LV

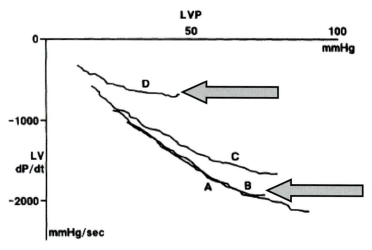

FIGURE 9.1. Dependence of LV dP/dt$_{min}$ on left ventricular (LV) end-systolic pressure. Four phase-plane plots (LV dP/dt versus LV pressure [LVP] plot) of LV pressure decay obtained in a patient with aortic stenosis are shown. Curve A was recorded at rest, curve B following infusion of sodium nitroprusside, curve C following aortic valvuloplasty, and curve D following infusion of sodium nitroprusside after aortic valvuloplasty. The lower value of LV dP/dt$_{min}$ of curve B (arrow) compared with curve A results from the lower LV end-systolic pressure of curve B and is not a reflection of altered LV relaxation kinetics as evident from the perfect superimposition of curves A and B. In contrast, following the drastic alterations in LV end-systolic pressure and LV systolic loading profile after combined aortic valvuloplasty and sodium nitroprusside infusion (curve D), the low value of LV dP/dt$_{min}$ (arrow) results not only from the low LV end-systolic pressure but also from depressed LV relaxation kinetics as evident from the divergent course of curve D.

pressure decay in a patient with aortic stenosis at rest (curve A), following infusion of sodium nitroprusside (curve B), following aortic valvuloplasty (curve C), and following infusion of sodium nitroprusside after aortic valvuloplasty (curve D).[7] The lower value of LV dP/dt$_{min}$ of curve B (arrow) compared with curve A results from the lower LV end-systolic pressure of curve B and is not a reflection of altered LV relaxation kinetics as evident from the perfect superimposition of curves A and B. In contrast, following the drastic alterations in LV end-systolic pressure and LV systolic loading profile after combined aortic valvuloplasty and sodium nitroprusside infusion (curve D), the low value of LV dP/dt$_{min}$ (arrow) not only results from the low LV end-systolic pressure but also from the depressed LV relaxation kinetics as evident from the divergent course of curve D. Construction of LV relaxation pressure phase-plane plots also allows deviation of LV pressure decay from an exponential course to be appreciated. If LV relaxation pressure would decay exponentially, its course on the phase-plane plot would be linear, as the first derivative of an exponential relationship also yields an exponential relationship. As is obvious from Figure 9.1, deviations from a linear course on the phase-plane plot occur and become more evident if LV relaxation pressure decays to a low mitral valve opening pressure. Important deviations of LV relaxation pressure from an exponential decay have been described in hypertrophic cardiomyopathy, in LV hypertrophy of aortic stenosis,[7] and in LV dyssynchrony induced by coronary occlusion or intracoronary isoproterenol infusion.[8-10]

In search of an LV relaxation index that would not be afterload dependent, Weiss et al.[11] were the first to propose the time constant of LV pressure decay (tau). The time constant of LV pressure decay is derived from a high-fidelity tip-micromanometer LV pressure recording using the following formula:

$$P_t = P_0 \, e^{-t/\tau} + P_{inf}$$

where P_t equals LV pressure at a given point in time, P_0 equals LV pressure at LV dP/dt$_{min}$, and P_{inf} is the asymptote pressure to which LV pressure would decay in the absence of LV filling. Left ventricular pressure data points are obtained by digitization at 5-ms intervals. The time constant tau can be derived from an exponential fit to the LV pressure–time data points or from a linear fit to the LV pressure–LV dP/dt points (a derivative method). Three important questions should be addressed when performing these calculations: (1) Does a monoexponential curve fit adequately describe LV pressure decay? (2) Which start and end points have to be used for the curve-fitting procedure? (3) Which value has to be assigned to the asymptote pressure P_{inf}?

Does a monoexponential curve fit adequately describe LV pressure decay? Although biexponential, polynomial, and logistic models have all been proposed, a single monoexponential curve fit usually adequately describes LV pressure decay and yields a satisfactory correlation coefficient (i.e., r > 0.99). Exceptions are patients with hypertrophic cardiomyopathy, aortic stenosis, and acute myocardial ischemia. In these patients, the deviation of LV pressure decay from a monoexponential curve can easily be appreciated by the downward convexity of the dP/dt signal in the phase following peak negative dP/dt. This downward convexity is indicated in the last panel of Figure 9.2 by an arrow. In the foregoing panels, the same phase of the dP/dt signal shows a normal configuration with upward convexity.

Which start and end points have to be used for the curve-fitting procedure? The curve fit is applied to the isovolumic LV pressure data points. It starts from LV pressure at LV dP/dt$_{min}$, which coincides with aortic valve closure, and ends at an LV pressure corresponding to mitral valve opening (usually set equal to the LV end-diastolic pressure of the following beat + 5 mm Hg). Because of some deviation of LV pressure decay from an exponential decline, a higher starting point or a higher end point will erroneously prolong tau.[12] This usually has no implications except when tau values are compared under widely varying LV loading conditions. Under these conditions, the tau values are best calculated over a similar range

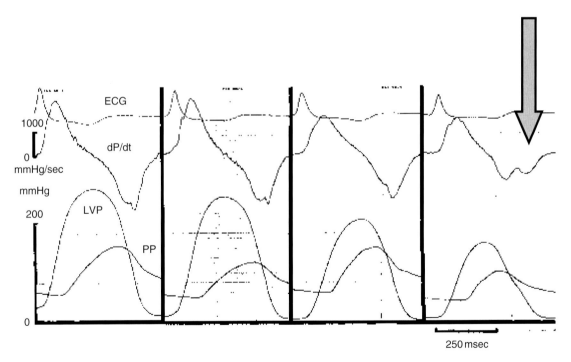

FIGURE 9.2. Deviation of left ventricular pressure (LVP) decay from an exponential course. Recordings of electrocardiogram (ECG), LV dP/dt, LVP, and peripheral artery pressure (PP) obtained in a patient with aortic stenosis at rest, during infusion of sodium nitroprusside, following aortic valvuloplasty, and during infusion of sodium nitroprusside following aortic valvuloplasty. In the first three panels there is upward convexity of the portion of the LV dP/dt signal, which follows LV minimum dP/dt, but in the last panel, as a result of the drastic LV unloading and the abbreviation of LV contraction, there is downward convexity of the same portion of the LV dP/dt signal (arrow). The latter implies a marked deviation of LV pressure decay from an exponential course.

of LV pressures by using for all curve fits a similar starting point (i.e., the lowest pressure at which LV dP/dt_{min} occurred) and end point (i.e., the highest mitral valve opening pressure).[7]

Which value has to be assigned to the asymptote pressure (P_{inf})? Asymptote pressure is the final pressure to which LV pressure would decay in the absence of LV filling. It has experimentally been determined in a nonfilling dog heart using a metal occluder implanted in the mitral position. In this experimental preparation with a rigid mitral structure, subatmospheric pressures were observed during early diastole when LV filling was impeded by closure of the metal occluder. This subatmospheric pressure amounted to — 7 mm Hg.[13] In another nonfilling dog heart preparation with preserved mitral apparatus[14] and in patients with mitral stenosis[15] during occlusion of the mitral valve with the self-positioning Inoue balloon at the time of percutaneous balloon mitral valvuloplasty, these subatmospheric pressures were not observed and P_{inf} equaled +2 mm Hg. In both experimental[13] and clinical[15] nonfilling beats, it has been demonstrated that the value of P_{inf} derived from extrapolation of a curve fit to isovolumic LV relaxation data points had no relation to the directly measured value of P_{inf}. As P_{inf} in the human heart equals +2 mm Hg, the use of a zero asymptote ($P_{inf} = 0$) seems adequate when calculating tau to assess LV relaxation kinetics in the human heart. Furthermore, in dilated and failing hearts, echocardiographic evidence of LV recoil is absent, as recently demonstrated from refined digital processing of color Doppler M-mode recordings,[16] and in these hearts the presence of subatmospheric LV asymptote pressures during early diastole in the absence of LV filling is even more unlikely. The use of a variable asymptote is therefore only recommended for a refined analysis of LV relaxation kinetics, for instance when specifically assessing pharmacologic manipulation of LV isovolumic relaxation kinetics.

Left Ventricular Diastolic Distensibility

- Left ventricular diastolic distensibility refers to the position of the LV pressure–volume (PV) relation on a PV plot.

- Increased or decreased LV diastolic distensibility implies altered position of the LV PV relation but not altered slope.
- Use of multiple LV PV loops during caval balloon occlusion improves accuracy of LV diastolic distensibility assessment.

Left ventricular diastolic distensibility refers to the position on a PV plot of the LV diastolic PV relation.[17] An increase in LV diastolic distensibility refers to a right and downward displacement of the LV diastolic PV relation, and a decrease in LV diastolic distensibility refers to a left and upward displacement of the LV PV relation (Figure 9.3, top). As such, a change in LV diastolic distensibility is less stringent than a change in diastolic LV stiffness, which implies both a change in slope of the LV diastolic PV relation and a shift in position on the PV plot. Segmental diastolic distensibility uses regional segment length or regional wall thickness instead of LV volume. Again, an increase in segmental diastolic distensibility refers to a right and downward displacement of the diastolic pressure–segment length or pressure–wall thickness relation, whereas a decrease in segmental diastolic distensibility implies a left and upward displacement of the diastolic pressure–segment length or pressure–wall thickness relation (Figure 9.3, top right and bottom). When reporting altered diastolic distensibility, changes in the slope of the diastolic PV, diastolic pressure–segment length, or diastolic pressure–wall thickness relations are not being considered.

Inference of a shift in LV diastolic distensibility after an intervention (e.g., pacing-induced angina) can be based on comparison of single diastolic LV PV, pressure–segment length, or pressure–wall thickness relations. These single relations are then considered to be representative for a given experimental or clinical condition (e.g., before and during pacing-induced angina). This use of single diastolic LV PV, pressure–segment length, or pressure–wall thickness relations is open to critique. Evaluation of displacement of single diastolic LV PV, pressure–segment length, or pressure–wall thickness relations includes both the LV rapid filling phase and the atrial contraction. During these time periods, there is no static equilibrium between instantaneous LV distend-

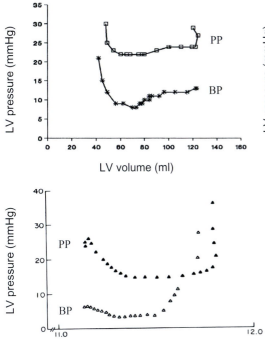
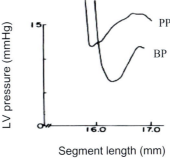

FIGURE 9.3. Left ventricular (LV) and segmental diastolic distensibility before and during pacing-induced angina. Left ventricular distensibility decreases during pacing-induced angina as evident from the upward displacement of the diastolic LV pressure–volume relation **(top left)**. Similarly, segmental distensibility also decreases during pacing-induced angina because of upward displacement of the diastolic LV pressure–segment length relation **(top right)** or diastolic LV pressure–wall thickness relation **(bottom)**. When a change in diastolic distensibility is reported, changes in the slope of the diastolic LV pressure–volume, diastolic LV pressure–segment length, or diastolic LV pressure–wall thickness relations are not being considered; BP, before pacing; PP, after pacing.

ing pressure and instantaneous LV volume. It is therefore unclear to what extent an eventual displacement of the single diastolic LV PV, pressure–segment length, or pressure–wall thickness relations results from an alteration in LV inflow or atrial kinetics or from a true change in diastolic myocardial material properties. To overcome this problem, multiple LV diastolic PV, pressure–segment length, or pressure–wall thickness relations are obtained during balloon caval occlusion (Figure 9.4).[17–20] Progressive balloon caval occlusion induces multiple LV PV loops, multiple LV pressure–segment length loops, or multiple LV pressure–wall thickness loops. The end-diastolic PV points, end-diastolic pressure–segment length points, or end-diastolic pressure–wall thickness points of these loops are situated widely apart on the respective LV diastolic PV, pressure–segment length, or pressure–wall thickness relations. Because of this wide range of the measurement points, the LV diastolic PV, pressure–segment length, or pressure–wall thickness relations are a more accurate reflection of diastolic LV distensibility than the short range evaluation derived from single LV diastolic PV, pressure–segment length, or pressure–wall thickness relations. When using multiple LV PV loops, multiple LV pressure–segment length loops, or multiple LV pressure–wall thickness loops, LV diastolic distensibility is assessed from multiple static end-diastolic LV PV, LV pressure–segment length, or LV pressure–wall thickness points and this offers the advantage of avoiding early dynamic effects of continuing LV relaxation,[21] early dynamic effects of myocardial viscous forces related to LV filling,[22] and late dynamic effects of atrial contraction.

A reduction in LV diastolic distensibility provides diagnostic evidence for diastolic LV dysfunction.[1] Left ventricular end-diastolic distensibility is reduced when LV end-diastolic pressure (>16 mm Hg)[23] or mean pulmonary venous pressure (>12 mm Hg)[24] are elevated in the presence of a normal LV end-diastolic volume index (<102 mL/m^2) or normal LV end-diastolic internal dimension index (<3.2 cm/m^2).

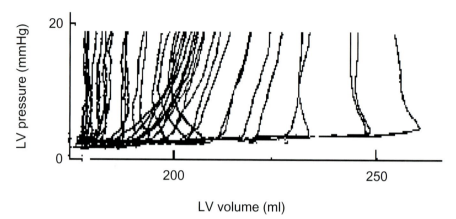

FIGURE 9.4. Left ventricular (LV) diastolic distensibility derived from multiple LV pressure–volume loops during balloon caval occlusion. When recording multiple LV pressure–volume loops during balloon caval occlusion, LV diastolic distensibility can be assessed from multiple static end-diastolic LV pressure–volume points. This offers the advantage of avoiding early dynamic effects of continuing LV relaxation, early dynamic effects of myocardial viscous forces related to LV filling, and late dynamic effects of atrial contraction.

Left Ventricular Diastolic Stiffness

- Left ventricular stiffness refers to the slope of the LV diastolic PV relation.
- Left ventricular stiffness needs to be compared at equal LV pressure levels.
- A constant of LV chamber stiffness is derived from an exponential curve fit to the diastolic LV PV points.

Left ventricular stiffness refers to a change in diastolic LV pressure relative to diastolic LV volume (dP/dV) and equals the slope of the LV diastolic PV relation. Its inverse is LV diastolic compliance (dV/dP). As the slope of the diastolic LV PV relation varies along the diastolic LV PV curve, LV stiffness values obtained under different experimental conditions can only be compared at a common level of LV filling pressures.[25] In many experimental setups (e.g., before and during pacing-induced angina), a common level of LV filling pressures cannot be defined, as the LV filling pressures diverged too far from one another as a result of the intervention. To overcome this problem, diastolic LV stiffness is no longer assessed by the slope of the diastolic LV PV relation at a common level of LV filling pressures but by the constant b of an exponential curve fit to the diastolic LV pressure (LVP)–volume (LVV) points:

$$LVP = aLVV^b + c$$

where b is the constant of chamber stiffness and a and c are the intercept and asymptote of the relation.

Such a curve fit can be applied to a single diastolic LV PV relation or to a diastolic LV PV relation constructed from multiple LV PV loops during balloon caval occlusion. The latter again offers the advantage of a more accurate curve fit, as the diastolic LV PV points are more widely apart and devoid of interference caused by early diastolic continuation of LV pressure decay, early diastolic viscous forces related to LV filling, and late diastolic atrial contraction. If a single diastolic LV PV relation is used, the diastolic LV points need to be obtained at ≤20-ms intervals from a frame-by-frame analysis of the LV angiogram and from simultaneously recorded high-fidelity tip-micromanometer LV pressure recordings.

The mathematical validity of an exponential curve fit to the diastolic LV PV relation has been challenged.[26] Nevertheless, this approach to measure LV stiffness is frequently used and can easily be achieved through logarithmic transformation of the exponential diastolic LV PV relation into a linear equation[27–29]:

$$\ln(LVP - c) = \ln a + bLVV$$

9. Invasive Evaluation Techniques

where b is the constant of chamber stiffness and a and c are the intercept and asymptote of the relation. The mean value and upper range of the constant of chamber stiffness (b) in control subjects are 0.21 and 0.27, respectively.[30] A b value >0.27 therefore provides diagnostic evidence for diastolic LV dysfunction.

Diastolic Myocardial or Muscle Stiffness

- Muscle stiffness refers to the slope of the LV diastolic stress–strain relation.
- A radial stiffness modulus overcomes geometric assumptions.
- Calculation of residual diastolic LV pressure is an elegant way to obtain similar stress levels following interventions.

Muscle stiffness (E) is the slope of the myocardial stress–strain relation and represents the resistance to stretch when the myocardium is subjected to stress. In contrast to LV stiffness, myocardial or muscle stiffness is unaffected by changes in right ventricular filling pressures or pleural pressures. Calculation of stress (σ) requires a geometric model of the left ventricle and calculation of strain (ε) an assumption of an unstressed LV dimension, which cannot be measured in vivo and is therefore usually replaced by an LV dimension at a wall stress of $1\,\mathrm{g/cm^{-2}}$. Diastolic stress within the myocardium can be split into three orthogonal components, which are usually indicated as circumferential, meridian, and radial stress. Circumferential LV diastolic wall stress is most frequently used and is usually computed with a thick wall ellipsoid model of the left ventricle to account for absence or presence of LV hypertrophy:

$$\sigma = PD/2h \times [1 - (h/D) - (D^2/2L^2)]$$

where P is LV diastolic pressure, h is echocardiographically determined diastolic LV wall thickness, and D and L are diastolic LV short axis diameter and long axis length at the midwall.[7] With this formula of diastolic wall stress and expression of the data in kN/m^2, close numerical agreement was recently observed between the value of diastolic circumferential stress calculated

for a normal human heart and the passive force observed in cardiomyocytes isolated from the same hearts when the passive force was also expressed in kN/m.[2,31] The close numerical agreement between LV diastolic wall stress and resting tension of cardiomyocytes indicates resting tension to be an important contributor to diastolic LV elastic properties in the normal human heart.

As the slope of the diastolic stress–strain relation varies, muscle stiffness under varying experimental conditions can only be compared at a common diastolic stress level. Because a common diastolic stress level is frequently absent, an exponential curve fit to the LV diastolic stress–strain data has been proposed to derive the constant of muscle stiffness (b′). After logarithmic transformation, the exponential relation between diastolic LV stress and strain is transformed into a linear equation[27–29]:

$$\ln(\sigma - c') = \ln a' + b'\varepsilon$$

where b′ is the constant of muscle stiffness and a′ and c′ are the intercept and asymptote of the relation. The mean value of the constant of muscle stiffness (b′), observed in a control group, equals 9.9 ± 3.3.[32] A b′ value >16 provides diagnostic evidence for diastolic LV dysfunction.

To overcome the geometric assumptions involved in calculating circumferential or meridian wall stress, calculation of a radial myocardial stiffness modulus (E) was introduced by Mirsky and colleagues to assess myocardial material properties.[33,34] The radial stiffness modulus was defined as follows:

$$E = \Delta\sigma_R/\Delta\varepsilon_R$$

and derived in the following way:

$$E = \Delta\sigma_R/\Delta\varepsilon_R = \Delta P/(\Delta h/h) = -\Delta P/\Delta \ln h$$

This derivation assumes the increment in radial stress ($\Delta\sigma_R$) to be equal but opposite in sign to the increment in LV diastolic pressure (ΔP) at the endocardium and the increment in radial strain ($\Delta\varepsilon_R$) to be equal to the increment in wall thickness (Δh) relative to the instantaneous wall thickness. Because $\Delta h/h = \Delta \ln h$, E equals the slope of an instantaneous P versus $\ln h$ plot.[33–36] The P versus $\ln h$ plot is obtained from the corresponding echocardiographic wall thickness and the LV

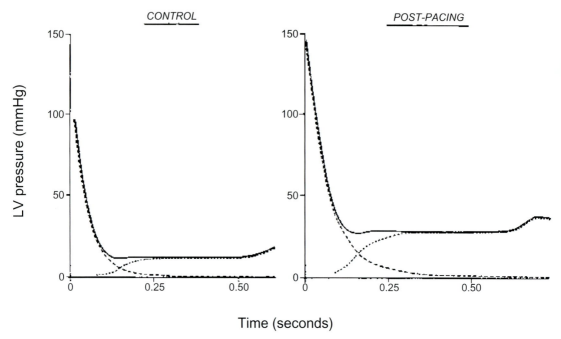

FIGURE 9.5. Diastolic left ventricular (LV) measured relaxation and residual pressures before and during pacing-induced angina. Residual diastolic LV pressure is obtained by subtracting diastolic LV relaxation pressure from measured diastolic LV pressure. Diastolic LV relaxation pressure is extrapolated from the exponential curve fit to isovolumic LV relaxation used to calculate the time constant of LV pressure decay. As residual diastolic LV pressure always equals zero at mitral valve opening, residual diastolic LV pressure shows a wide range of pressure overlap when comparing recordings obtained before and during pacing-induced angina. In contrast, because of the rise of measured LV minimum diastolic pressure during pacing-induced angina, there is little overlap of measured diastolic LV pressure before and during pacing-induced angina.

diastolic pressure recordings. Agreement between E and diastolic LV stiffness measurements derived from an exponential curve fit to multiple end-diastolic LV PV points during caval occlusion has previously been reported in patients with dilated cardiomyopathy.[37]

The slope of the myocardial stress–strain relation varies, and a myocardial stiffness modulus therefore needs to be compared at equal levels of myocardial stress. The same condition also applies to the LV stiffness modulus, which also needs to be compared at equal levels of LV pressure. Following some interventions (e.g., pacing-induced angina) this condition can no longer be satisfied because of lack of corresponding levels of myocardial stress or LV pressure. As previously explained, this obstacle can be overcome by fitting an exponential curve to the diastolic LV PV or the diastolic myocardial stress–strain relations and calculating the constant of chamber stiffness (b) or of muscle stiffness (b'). Another method proposed to overcome this problem is to define a corresponding level of LV pressure or myocardial stress in all experimental conditions by subtracting extrapolated LV relaxation pressure from measured LV pressure during the diastolic LV filling phase[38] (Figure 9.5) and by subsequently constructing diastolic LV PV or stress–strain relations using the residual diastolic LV pressure resulting from this subtraction procedure (Figure 9.6). The extrapolated LV relaxation pressure after mitral valve opening is derived from the exponential curve to isovolumic LV pressure decay used to calculate the time constant of LV pressure decay. Although residual LV relaxation pressure decay during LV filling deviates from an exponential course because of myocardial relengthening,[39,40] this approach to obtain corresponding levels of LV filling pressures or myocardial wall stresses has been applied in numerous

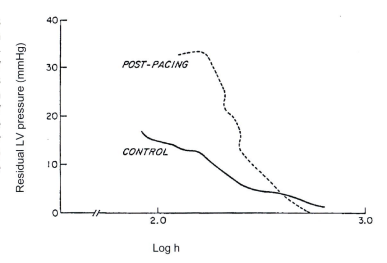

FIGURE 9.6. Radial stress–strain relations before and during pacing-induced angina derived from residual diastolic left ventricular (LV) pressure. The radial stress (LV diastolic pressure) – strain (ln$h$) relations before and during pacing-induced angina were derived from residual diastolic LV pressure and therefore share a large common range of radial stresses over which the slope (radial stiffness modulus) of the stress-strain relation can be compared.

studies ranging from experimental or clinical ischemic heart disease[33–35] to DHF.[41]

Conclusion

Diagnosis of DHF requires evidence of diastolic LV dysfunction.[1] Because of the low sensitivity of noninvasive techniques for the diagnosis of diastolic LV dysfunction, invasively obtained evidence remains the gold standard.[2] Such evidence can consist of demonstration of slow LV relaxation, reduced LV distensibility, or increased LV or myocardial stiffness. Future evaluation of noninvasive indexes of diastolic LV dysfunction[42] or of plasma markers (e.g., brain natriuretic peptide) of diastolic LV dysfunction[43] requires an obligatory comparison with an invasive assessment of LV diastolic dysfunction. Knowledge and correct application of invasively derived indices of diastolic LV function remain therefore indispensable for modern "diastology."

References

1. European Study Group on Diastolic Heart Failure. How to diagnose diastolic heart failure. Eur Heart J 1998;19:990–1003.
2. Vasan RS, Levy D. Defining diastolic heart failure: a call for standardized diagnostic criteria. Circulation 2000;101:2118–2121.
3. Mirsky I. Assessment of passive elastic stiffness of cardiac muscle: mathematical concepts, physiological and clinical considerations, direction of future research. Prog Cardiovasc Dis 1976;18:277.
4. Hirota Y. A clinical study of left ventricular relaxation. Circulation 1980;62:756–763.
5. Weisfeldt ML, Scully HE, Frederiksen J, et al. Hemodynamic determinants of maximum negative dP/dt and periods of diastole. Am J Physiol 1974; 227:613–621.
6. Gillebert TC, Lew WYW. Influence of systolic pressure profile on rate of left ventricular pressure fall. Am J Physiol 1991;261:H805–H813.
7. Paulus WJ, Heyndrickx GR, Buyl P, et al. Wide-range load shift of combined aortic valvuloplasty–arterial vasodilation slows isovolumic relaxation of the hypertrophied left ventricle. Circulation. 1990; 81:886–898.
8. Kumada T, Karliner JS, Pouleur H et al. Effects of coronary occlusion on early ventricular diastolic events in conscious dogs. Am J Physiol 1979;237:542–549.
9. Lew WYW, Rasmussen CM. Influence of nonuniformity on rate of left ventricular pressure fall in the dog. Am J Physiol 1989;256:H222–H232.
10. Skulstad H, Edvardsen T, Urheim S, et al. Post-systolic shortening in ischemic myocardium: active contraction or passive recoil? Circulation 2002;106:718–24.
11. Weiss JL, Frederiksen JW, Weisfeldt ML. Hemodynamic determinants of the time course of fall in canine left ventricular pressure. J Clin Invest 1976; 58:751–776.

12. Martin G, Gimeno JV, Cosin J et al. Time constant of isovolumic pressure fall: new numerical approaches and significance. Am J Physiol 1984;247:H283–H294.
13. Yellin EL, Hori M, Yoran C, et al. Left ventricular relaxation in the filling and nonfilling intact canine heart. Am J Physiol 1986;250:H620–H629.
14. Ohtani M, Nikolic SD, Glantz SA. A new approach to in situ left ventricular volume clamping in dogs. Am J Physiol 1991;261:H1335–H13343.
15. Paulus WJ, Vantrimpont PJ, Rousseau MF. Diastolic function of the nonfilling human left ventricle. J Am Coll Cardiol 1992;20:1524–1532.
16. Yotti R, Bermejo J, Carlos Antoranz J, et al. Noninvasive method for assessing impaired diastolic suction in patients with dilated cardiomyopathy. Circulation 2005;112:2921–2929.
17. Rankin SJ, Arentzen CE, Ring WS, et al. The diastolic mechanical properties of the intact left ventricle. Fed Proc 1980;39:141–147.
18. Kass DA, Midei M, Brinker J et al. Influence of coronary occlusion during PTCA on end-systolic and end-diastolic pressure–volume relations in humans. Circulation 1990;81:447–460.
19. Applegate RJ. Load dependence of left ventricular diastolic pressure–volume relations during short-term coronary artery occlusion. Circulation 1991;83:661–673.
20. Pak PH, Maughan WL, Baughman KL, et al. Marked discordance between dynamic and passive diastolic pressure–volume relations in idiopathic hypertrophic cardiomyopathy. Circulation 1996;94:52–60.
21. Brutsaert DL, Rademakers FE, Sys SU et al. Analysis of relaxation in the evaluation of ventricular function of the heart. Prog Cardiovasc Dis 1985;28:143–163.
22. Rankin SJ, Arentzen CE, McHale PA, et al. Viscoelastic properties of the diastolic left ventricle in the conscious dog. Circ Res 1977;41:37–45.
23. Yamakado T, Takagi E, Okubo S, et al. Effects of aging on left ventricular relaxation in humans. Circulation 1997;95:917–923.
24. Little WC, Downes TR. Clinical evaluation of left ventricular diastolic performance. Prog Cardiovasc Dis 1990;32:273–290.
25. Gaasch WH. Passive elastic properties of the left ventricle. In Gaasch WH, LeWinter M, eds. Left Ventricular Diastolic Dysfunction and Heart Failure. Malvern, PA: Lea & Febiger, 1994:143–149.
26. Yettram AL, Grewal BS, Gibson DG, et al. Relation between intraventricular pressure and volume in diastole. Br Heart J 1990;64:304–308.

27. Hess OM, Ritter M, Schneider J, et al. Diastolic function in aortic valve disease: techniques of evaluation and postoperative changes. Herz 1984;9:288–296.
28. Krayenbuehl HP, Hess OM, Monrad ES, et al. Left ventricular myocardial structure in aortic valve disease before, intermediate and late after aortic valve replacement. Circulation 1989;79:744–55.
29. Villari B, Campbell SE, Hess OM, et al. Influence of collagen network on left ventricular systolic and diastolic function in aortic valve disease. J Am Coll Cardiol 1993;22:1477–1484.
30. Krayenbuehl HP, Hess OM, Ritter M, et al. Influence of pressure and volume overload on diastolic compliance. In Grossman W, Lorell BH, eds. Diastolic Relaxation of the Heart. Boston: Martinus Nijhoff, 1987:143–150.
31. Borbély A, van der Velden J, Papp Z, et al. Cardiomyocyte stiffness in diastolic heart failure. Circulation 2005;111:774–781.
32. Krayenbuehl HP, Villari B, Campbell SE, et al. Diastolic dysfunction in chronic pressure and volume overload. In Grossman W, Lorell BH, eds. Diastolic Relaxation of the Heart. Boston: Martinus Nijhoff, 1994:283–288.
33. Bourdillon PD, Lorell BH, Mirsky I, et al. Increased regional myocardial stiffness of the left ventricle during pacing-induced angina in man. Circulation 1983;67:316–323.
34. Paulus WJ, Grossman W, Serizawa T, et al. Different effects of two types of ischemia on myocardial systolic and diastolic function. Am J Physiol 1985;248:H719–H728.
35. Bronzwaer JG, de Bruyne B, Ascoop CA, et al. Comparative effects of pacing-induced and balloon coronary occlusion ischemia on left ventricular diastolic function in man. Circulation 1991;84:211–222.
36. Bronzwaer JG, Heymes C, Visser CA, et al. Myocardial fibrosis blunts nitric oxide synthase-related preload reserve in human dilated cardiomyopathy. Am J Physiol 2003;284:H10–H16.
37. Bronzwaer JG, Zeitz C, Visser CA, et al. Endomyocardial nitric oxide synthase and the hemodynamic phenotypes of human dilated cardiomyopathy and of athlete's heart. Cardiovasc Res 2002;55:270–278.
38. Pasipoularides A, Mirsky I, Hess OM, et al. Myocardial relaxation and passive diastolic properties in man. Circulation 1986;74:991–1001.
39. Sys SU, Paulus WJ, Claes VA, et al. Post-reextension force decay of relaxing cardiac muscle. Am J Physiol 1987;253:H256–H261.

40. Kass DA, Bronzwaer JGF, Paulus WJ. What mechanisms underlie diastolic dysfunction in heart failure? Circ Res 2004;94:1533–1542.

41. Zile MR, Baicu CF, Gaasch WH. Diastolic heart failure – abnormalities in active relaxation and passive stiffness of the left ventricle. N Engl J Med 2004;350:1953–1959.

42. Smiseth OA. Assessment of ventricular diastolic function. Can J Cardiol 2001;17:1167–1176.

43. Lubien E, DeMaria A, Krishnaswamy P, et al. Utility of B-natriuretic peptide in detecting diastolic dysfunction: comparison with Doppler velocity recordings. Circulation 2002;105:595–601.

10
Echocardiographic Assessment of Diastolic Function and Diagnosis of Diastolic Heart Failure

Grace Lin and Jae K. Oh

Introduction

Asymptomatic diastolic dysfunction in the general population is common, even in patients without congestive heart failure, [1,2] and the prevalence of moderate to severe diastolic dysfunction in asymptomatic patients increases in patients >65 years old with associated hypertension and coronary artery disease.[2] The presence of diastolic dysfunction alone predicts worse outcome, with worse prognosis as the degree of diastolic dysfunction increases.[2] Thus, it is important to identify and treat underlying problems (most frequently, hypertension) in patients with diastolic dysfunction.

In population-based studies, diastolic heart failure (DHF) accounts for up to half of patients with the diagnosis of congestive heart failure [2–6]. Although DHF can be diagnosed clinically by documenting the presence of signs and symptoms of heart failure and preserved systolic function (EF ≥50%), objective evidence of diastolic dysfunction and increased filling pressure should also be demonstrated.[7–9]

Evaluation of diastolic function consists of assessing myocardial relaxation, filling pressures, and left ventricular (LV) compliance. Although diastolic dysfunction can be diagnosed invasively by cardiac catheterization,[10] this is not always feasible or practical. Both two-dimensional and Doppler echocardiography can be used to non-invasively assess diastolic function. Although systolic function and major cardiac structures are usually normal in patients with DHF, two-dimensional echocardiography is useful in identifying changes, although subtle, associated with cardiac diseases that result primarily in diastolic dysfunction. These changes include reduced motion of the mitral annulus, increased left atrial size, and frequently increased LV wall thickness. Left ventricular diastolic function is more objectively characterized by the mitral inflow pattern, pulmonary and hepatic vein Doppler velocities, tissue Doppler imaging of the mitral annulus, and color flow imaging of mitral inflow.

Two-Dimensional Echocardiography

Two-dimensional echocardiography can be used to evaluate anatomic changes of diseases that cause diastolic dysfunction, including hypertension, hypertrophic cardiomyopathy, infiltrative diseases, and restrictive cardiomyopathy. Left ventricular wall thickness is frequently increased in patients with primary diastolic dysfunction or heart failure. Myocardial relaxation is usually decreased when LV wall thickness is increased unless it is related to conditioning and exercise. However, most patients with increased wall thickness do not experience heart failure symptoms. Another important point is that increased wall thickness does not always indicate LV hypertrophy and may represent infiltrative cardiomyopathy. In cardiac amyloid, the electroencephalographic voltage is low despite increased LV wall thickness. Diastolic dysfunction results in chronically elevated LV filling pressures that lead to increased left atrial enlargement. Thickened pericardium and abnormal ventricular septal motion associated with respiratory changes in ventricular filling are features of constrictive pericarditis, another cause of DHF, which are readily identified by two-dimensional echocardiography (see Chapter 21). Right atrial pressures can be increased in diastolic dysfunction, causing inferior vena cava and hepatic vein dilatation. In addition, systolic dysfunction, valvular heart disease, LV dilatation, and other structural heart diseases can be excluded with two-dimensional echocardiography.

The atria remodel and enlarge with systolic heart failure and DHF.[11] With progressive degrees of diastolic dysfunction, left atrial size and volume increase,[12] and increased left atrial volume indexed to body surface area is predictive of future cardiovascular events, including atrial fibrillation, heart failure, myocardial infarction, stroke, and cardiovascular death, independent of other clinical and echocardiographic risk factors.[13,14]

Most commonly, left atrial volume is measured by the biplane area–length method. The left atrial area obtained by planimetry in the apical four-chamber (A1) and apical two-chamber views (A2), and the left atrial length measured from the mitral annulus to the posterior left atrial wall in either view are used in the calculation of left atrial volume[15]:

$$\text{Left atrial volume} = (0.85 \times A1 \times A2)/\text{Length}$$

The resulting left atrial volume is then indexed to body surface area. Normal left atrial volume usually excludes clinically important diastolic dysfunction, and, conversely, left atrial enlargement indicates presence of diastolic dysfunction unless it is related to increased stroke volume in individuals with trained bradycardic heart.

Doppler Echocardiography

Left Ventricular Diastolic Function

Mitral Inflow Velocities

Assessment of the transmitral velocities is usually the first Doppler evaluation of LV diastolic function and filling. At the onset of diastole, LV pressure falls below left atrial pressure during active relaxation, followed by mitral valve opening and early diastolic filling. Mitral inflow decelerates as

LV pressure rises and exceeds left atrial pressure with rapid filling and then increases again with atrial contraction. Normally, early diastolic filling accounts for 70%–80% of filling, with atrial contraction accounting for 20%–30%. Changes in the transmitral pressure gradient during diastole are demonstrated by the mitral inflow peak velocities recorded by pulsed wave Doppler and consist of early rapid filling (E wave) and late filling due to atrial contraction (A wave; Figure 10.1).[16,17] The deceleration time is the time interval from the peak E velocity until it declines to baseline, extrapolated to zero velocity. Different degrees of diastolic dysfunction correspond to specific mitral inflow patterns, which demonstrate the relationship between LV and left atrial pressures.[16,17] In normal, healthy individuals, the E/A ratio is >1.0. With delayed relaxation, the E/A ratio is reduced and deceleration time is prolonged due to slower equilibration of left atrial and LV pressures. In a noncompliant ventricle with elevated filling pressure, the E/A ratio is increased with a shorter deceleration time (see Figure 10.1).

To measure mitral inflow velocities, the ultrasound transducer is placed at the apex, and a 1–2-mm sample volume is placed at the tip of the mitral valve leaflets in the apical four-chamber view during diastole. Accurate measurement of the mitral inflow velocities is dependent on appropriate placement of the sample volume as well as the heart rate. The maximal mitral flow velocity occurs at the tips of the mitral valve; placement of the sample volume at sites other than the mitral leaflet tips may result in underestimation of the flow velocities. At higher heart rates and with first degree atrioventricular block, the mitral inflow velocities may be fused. In this situation, the deceleration time is difficult to determine, and the A velocity may be increased. If the E velocity has not declined to baseline and remains higher than 0.2 m/s, measurement of the A velocity and the E/A ratio may be inaccurate. The mitral A wave duration may also be useful in determining LV end-diastolic pressure.[18,19] In atrial fibrillation, the A wave is absent.

Pulmonary Vein Flow Velocity

Pulmonary vein flow velocity reflects left atrial filling, pressures, and compliance and can also be

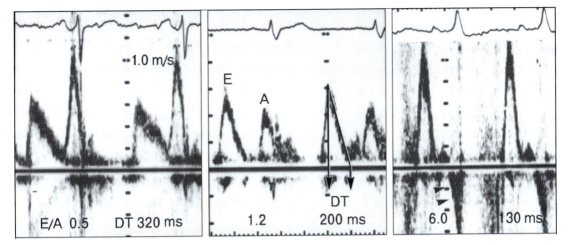

FIGURE 10.1. Pulsed wave Doppler recordings of mitral inflow velocity to determine diastolic filling pattern. These Doppler recordings represent impaired myocardial relaxation (left), normal (center), and restrictive diastolic filling pattern (right). In impaired relaxation pattern, which is an initial diastolic dysfunction, early diastolic velocity (E) is reduced and deceleration (DT) time is prolonged, usually longer than 240 ms. The late diastolic filling velocity at the time of atrial contraction (A) is augmented and higher than E. In normal mitral inflow velocity, E velocity is equal to or higher than A velocity, and deceleration time ranges from 160 to 240 ms. In the restrictive filling pattern, early diastolic velocity (E) is increased, usually higher than 1 m/s with short deceleration time of less than 160 ms, and A velocity is reduced with a resulting E/A ratio >2. Frequently, we see diastolic mitral regurgitation in the restrictive filling pattern due to increased diastolic filling pressure (arrowheads). (Reprinted with permission from Oh J, et al. Echo Manual, 2nd ed. Philadelphia: Lippincott Williams & Wilkins; 1999.)

recorded by pulsed wave Doppler. Of the four pulmonary veins, the right upper pulmonary vein is the most readily seen by transthoracic echocardiography in the apical four-chamber view (Figure 10.2A). Color flow imaging of the posterior left atrium may help visualize the color flow into the left atrium at the orifice of the right upper pulmonary vein, and a 5-mm sample volume is placed in the pulmonary vein 1 to 2 cm from the orifice, where pulmonary vein pressure begins to approximate left atrial pressures.[20] Normal pulmonary vein flow consists of biphasic systolic forward flow (PVs1, PVs2), diastolic forward flow (PVd), and atrial reversal due to atrial contraction (PVa; Figure 10.2B). The two components of systolic flow correspond to early systolic flow due to atrial relaxation (PVs1), followed by mid to late systolic flow due to increasing pulmonary venous pressure (PVs2). The two pulmonary vein systolic velocities may not be distinct even in normal patients. Diastolic forward flow occurs with the fall in left atrial pressure after mitral valve opening. Atrial reversal is a low velocity waveform that reflects flow reversal in the pulmonary vein due to atrial contraction in late diastole.[20]

Although pulmonary vein flow velocity patterns cannot be used alone to characterize diastolic function, they complement mitral inflow patterns. In normal patients, pulmonary vein systolic velocity is equal to or higher than diastolic velocity. With impaired ventricular relaxation, pulmonary vein systolic forward flow is blunted, and the majority of forward flow into the left atrium occurs during diastole, resulting in a relatively higher PVd than PVs2 (Figure 10.3). When LV filling pressures are increased, peak PVd is increased and the deceleration time of PVd is shortened.[21] Together with the mitral inflow A velocity duration, PVa reflects LV end-diastolic pressure. A PVa duration greater than the mitral A velocity predicts an LV end-diastolic pressure of 15–20 mm Hg or greater.[18,19]

Tissue Doppler Imaging of Mitral Annular Velocity

Mitral annular motion during early diastole reflects LV relaxation and is useful in the assessment and classification of diastolic dysfunction.[22–25]

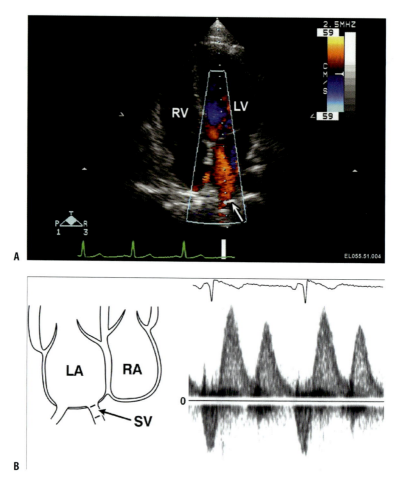

FIGURE 10.2. (A) Apical four-chamber view with color flow imaging demonstrating pulmonary venous flow from the right paraseptal vein. Sample volume (arrow) is placed in the pulmonary vein guided by the color flow imaging. RV, right ventricle; LV, left ventricle. (B) Diagram of the atria (LA, left atrium; RA, right atrium) and pulmonary vein demonstrating the optimal location of sample volume (SV) placement. See text for details. (Reprinted with permission from Oh J, et al. Echo Manual, 2nd ed. Philadelphia: Lippincott, Williams & Wilkins; 1999.)

Longitudinal mitral annular velocities can be recorded with tissue Doppler imaging from the apical four-chamber view, with a 2–5-mm sample volume placed at the medial or lateral aspect of the mitral annulus. Interrogation of the mitral annulus usually results in three waveforms, the systolic (S′) velocity of systolic annular motion, and two diastolic velocities, reflecting early (E′) and late (A′) diastolic annular motion (Figure 10.4A). Normally, the E′ velocity is equal to or higher than A′, and this ratio reverses with diastolic dysfunction as E′ decreases with impaired relaxation and in all stages of diastolic dysfunction (Figure 10.4B). E′ is less dependent on volume and loading conditions than transmitral flow velocities, although, with normal myocardial relaxation, E′ increases with higher preload. However, in patients with impaired relaxation, E′ is reduced and affected less by changes in preload.[23] Thus E′ may be combined with transmitral flow velocities to further define diastolic function. The ratio of early transmitral velocity and early diastolic mitral annular velocity, E/E′, correlates with pulmonary capillary wedge pressure measurements and is not affected by sinus tachycardia or the presence of atrial fibrillation.[25–28]

10. Echocardiographic Assessment

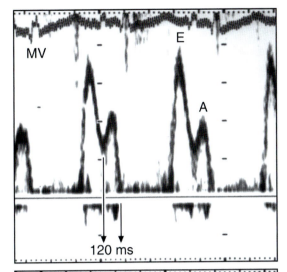

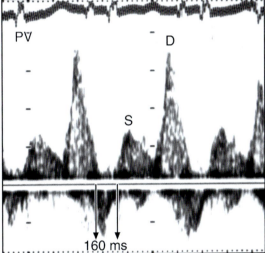

FIGURE 10.3. Pulsed wave Doppler recording of mitral inflow (MV) **(top)** and pulmonary vein (PV) **(bottom)** flow velocities. The E/A ratio is slightly less than 2 and deceleration time is 180 ms. The PV flow velocity shows predominant diastolic forward flow velocity, which indicates increased left atrial pressure. The PV atrial flow reversal is also longer (160 ms) than the duration of the A wave (120 ms), indicating that mitral flow velocity is "pseudonormalized." (Reprinted with permission from Oh J, et al. Echo Manual, 2nd ed. Philadelphia: Lippincott, Williams & Wilkins 1999.)

Propagation Velocity by Color M-Mode Echocardiography

As blood moves from the base of the left ventricle to the apex during diastole the velocity of blood flow decreases. This change in velocity of blood flow through the ventricle is called the *mitral inflow propagation velocity* and can be demonstrated by measuring the slope of the color M-mode pattern from the mitral annulus to the apex (Figure 10.5A).[29–31] With narrow sector color Doppler imaging in the apical four-chamber view, the M-mode cursor is placed in the center of the mitral inflow blood column. The color flow baseline is adjusted so that the central, highest velocity jet is blue, and color aliasing occurs at the edges of the blood column. The slope of the edge of the color M-mode, where the first aliasing velocity occurs, is measured from the mitral annulus to 4 cm from the apex. In normal hearts, early diastolic filling is rapid and the change in mitral inflow velocity from the mitral annulus to the apex is minimal, resulting in a steep slope and higher propagation velocity. In diastolic dysfunction, early diastolic filling is slower, and the slope of the color M-mode is prolonged and propagation velocity is reduced (Figure 10.5B). A propagation velocity of ≥50 cm/s is considered normal[29–30] An abnormal propagation velocity indicates impaired relaxation.[29] Propagation velocity can also be used to estimate pulmonary capillary wedge pressure when combined with isovolumic relaxation time or transmitral E velocity.[32,22] However, measurement of propagation velocity may be affected by cardiac size and preload.[34] An E to propagation velocity ratio of ≥2.5 predicts a pulmonary capillary wedge pressure of >15 mm Hg.[33]

Right Ventricular Diastolic Function

Tricuspid Inflow Velocity

Right ventricular diastolic function can be measured by recording tricuspid inflow velocities.[35] The transtricuspid gradient creates a similar inflow pattern to mitral inflow. Right ventricular diastolic filling pattern may be different from the mitral inflow pattern in the same patient. Tricuspid inflow velocities are typically lower than mitral inflow velocities, and, unlike mitral flow, tricuspid flow velocities normally vary with respiration.

Hepatic Vein Velocities

Hepatic vein velocities reflect right atrial filling, volume, and compliance. Using pulsed wave Doppler, a 2–5-mm pulsed wave sample volume

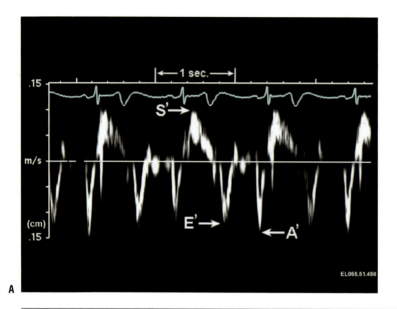

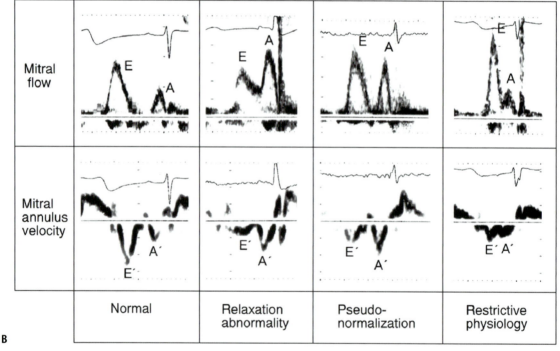

FIGURE 10.4. **(A)** Recording of pulsed tissue Doppler velocity from the septal mitral annulus. There are three major velocity components: S′, systolic velocity; E′, early diastolic velocity of the mitral annulus, which reflects myocardial relaxation; and A′, late diastolic mitral annulus velocity with atrial contraction. The peak velocity of each component is used for measurement. Each small horizontal bar indicates 200 ms, and large bar indicates 1 s. **(B)** Patterns of mitral inflow and mitral annulus velocities in various stages of diastolic dysfunction. Mitral annulus velocity was obtained from the septal side of the mitral annulus using Doppler tissue imaging. Each calibration mark in the recording of the mitral annulus velocity represents 5 cm/s. Early diastolic annulus velocity (E′) is greater than late diastolic annulus velocity (A′) in a normal pattern. In all other patterns, E′ is reduced and lower than the A′ velocity. In relaxation abnormality, E′ and A′ have a change similar to that of the E and A velocities of mitral inflow. However, when diastolic filling pressures increase (pseudonormalized and restrictive physiology), E′ remains reduced (i.e., persistent underlying relaxation abnormality) while mitral inflow E velocity increases. Hence, E/E″ is useful for estimating left ventricular filling pressures. (Reprinted with permission from Sohn et al.[22]).

10. Echocardiographic Assessment 155

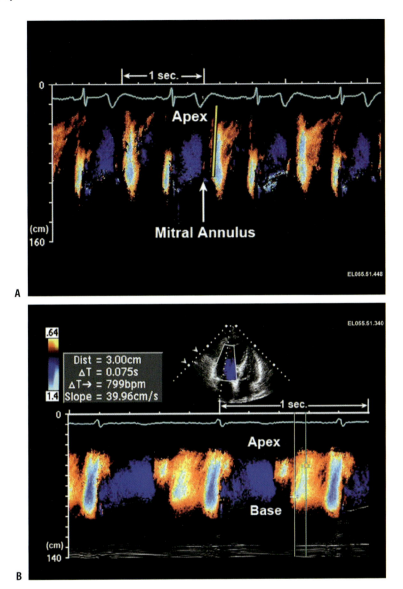

FIGURE 10.5. (A) Normal color flow propagation velocity of mitral inflow indicated by the yellow slope. (B) Color flow M-mode echocardiogram of mitral inflow velocity from a normal individual. Color flow map baseline was shifted upward to decrease the positive aliasing velocity. The manipulation of the color flow map allows demonstration of the highest velocity of the early diastolic velocity of mitral inflow. The slope of the flow propagation of mitral inflow E is measured by calculating the slope of the highest velocity. In this case, the distance the blood traveled was 3 cm, and the time it took to travel from the annulus to 3 cm apically was 75 ms. Therefore, the slope was 40 cm/s (3 cm/0.075 s), which is reduced.

is placed in the hepatic vein in the subcostal view. Combined with inferior vena cava dimension, hepatic vein velocities can be used to assess right atrial pressure.[36] Normal hepatic vein flow consists of systolic forward flow, diastolic forward flow, systolic flow reversal, and diastolic flow reversal (Figure 10.6). In normal patients, systolic forward flow velocity exceeds diastolic forward flow velocity, without significant reversal velocities.[37] The effect of elevated right ventricular filling pressure on hepatic vein flow velocities is analogous to the change in pulmonary vein flow velocity with elevated LV filling pressure. Hepatic vein systolic forward flow velocity is decreased and

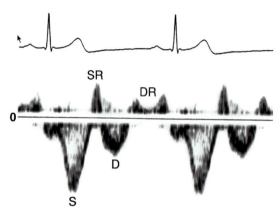

FIGURE 10.6. Pulse wave Doppler recording of hepatic vein flow velocity in a normal subject. Systolic velocity (S) is usually greater than diastolic velocity (D), with no prominent reversal flow velocity. SR, DR, systolic reversal and diastolic reversal, respectively.

diastolic forward flow velocity is increased with elevated right ventricular filling pressure. Changes in hepatic vein flow reversals and hepatic vein forward flow that occur with timing and respiration are important in the diagnosis of tricuspid regurgitation, constrictive pericarditis, tamponade, restrictive cardiomyopathy, and pulmonary hypertension.[38,39] In constrictive pericarditis, diastolic forward flow is limited, with more prominent systolic forward flow and significant diastolic flow reversal, especially during expiration. Diastolic flow reversals are also seen in pulmonary hypertension but without significant respiratory variation. Restrictive cardiomyopathy is characterized by decreased systolic forward flow and increased systolic and diastolic flow reversals with inspiration. Systolic flow reversals may occur with severe tricuspid regurgitation but is not diagnostic of severe tricuspid regurgitation.

Superior Vena Cava Velocities

Superior vena cava velocities also reflect right atrial filling and are obtained from the right supraclavicular window. A 2–5-mm pulsed wave Doppler sample volume is placed at a depth of 5–7 cm. Systolic forward flow velocity is higher than diastolic forward flow velocity in normal patients and is decreased with increasing right atrial pressure. Superior vena cava velocity is increased with inspiration, but this respiratory variation is less prominent with increased right atrial pressure.

Classification of Diastolic Function

Grading of Diastolic Dysfunction

Diastolic function is graded from 1 to 4 based on the severity of the diastolic filling pattern reflected by the mitral inflow velocities.[40] Further classification may require supplementation of the mitral inflow pattern by additional Doppler echocardiographic parameters of diastolic function, including pulmonary vein flow velocity, mitral annular velocity, and color M-mode echocardiography (Figure 10.7). Normally, diastolic filling is affected by variations in heart rate, respiration, loading conditions, and atrioventricular conduction. Impaired relaxation is usually the first manifestation of diastolic dysfunction. As diastolic function worsens, left atrial pressure rises and deceleration time shortens, giving a pseudonormalized pattern. Restrictive filling occurs as LV compliance is affected. Irreversible restrictive filling is the final stage of diastolic dysfunction. Grading of diastolic function is discussed below.

Normal

In normal patients, most of diastolic filling occurs during early diastole, with minimal contribution from atrial contraction. The E/A ratio is ≥1.5, deceleration time ranges from 160 to 230 ms, E' is ≥10 cm/s, E/E' is <8, and propagation velocity is ≥50 cm/s. Mitral annular velocities parallel the mitral inflow pattern such that E' is higher than A'. The E/A and E/E' ratios are unaffected by the Valsalva maneuver or exercise. With aging, the E velocity decreases and the A velocity increases as late diastolic filling becomes more prominent (E/A ratio <1). Similarly, changes are seen in the pulmonary vein flow velocities: diastolic forward flow decreases and more flow occurs during systolic forward flow because of atrial contraction in late diastole.[41–44]

Grade 1 Diastolic Dysfunction

With a relaxation abnormality, deceleration time and isovolumic relaxation time are prolonged. Relaxation continues into mid to late diastole and results in a lower initial transmitral gradient with subsequent relative increase in transmitral gradient at the time of atrial contraction in late diastole

10. Echocardiographic Assessment

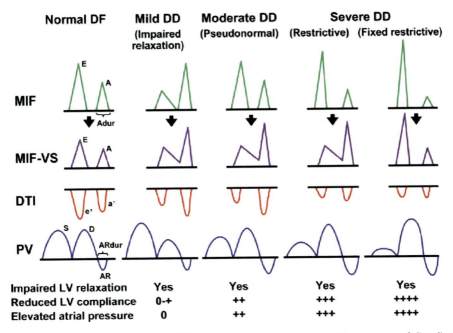

FIGURE 10.7. Schematic diagram of mitral inflow (MIF), mitral inflow with the Valsalva maneuver (MIF-VS), Doppler tissue imaging (DTI), and pulmonary vein velocities (PV) in normal diastolic function and in different stages of diastolic dysfunction. (Reprinted with permission from Redfield et al.[2])

due to higher residual left atrial pressure. Thus, E velocity is lower and the E/A ratio is <1. As with age-related changes, pulmonary diastolic forward flow decreases and pulmonary systolic forward flow increases. Mitral annular velocity (E′) decreases with a relaxation abnormality, to <7 cm/s, and propagation velocity also decreases to <50 cm/s. If LV filling pressures are normal, E/E′ is ≤8, as in normal patients.[23] As filling pressures increase, E velocity increases while E′ is not affected so that E/E′ is ≥15. If LV end-diastolic pressure is elevated in the setting of normal mean left atrial pressure, the E/A ratio is still <1, but the duration of mitral flow during atrial contraction (A wave) is shorter than the duration of the pulmonary vein atrial flow reversal.

Grade 2 (Pseudonormalized Pattern) Diastolic Dysfunction

Grade 2 diastolic dysfunction occurs when increased left atrial pressure is added to a myocardial relaxation abnormality. In this situation, E/A is >1, and deceleration time is normal, giving the appearance of normal mitral inflow. However, other features of diastolic dysfunction are present. Left atrial volume is increased, suggesting chronically elevated LV filling pressures. Markers of myocardial relaxation, E′ and propagation velocity, are abnormal, with E′ being <7 cm/s (using pulsed Doppler recording from tissue Doppler imaging) and propagation velocity being <50 cm/s. With elevated filling pressures, E/E′ is >15, and pulmonary venous A duration is longer than mitral A duration.

A pseudonormalized pattern of diastolic dysfunction can also be distinguished from a normal diastolic filling pattern by the Valsalva maneuver (see Figure 10.7). A Valsalva maneuver involves forced expiration against a closed mouth and nose that decreases LV preload. In normal patients, E and A velocity are equally diminished by decreased preload and resultant lower transmitral gradient, while deceleration time is prolonged. However, a relaxation abnormality is unmasked in patients with a pseudonormalized pattern, and the mitral inflow pattern with a Valsalva maneuver resembles grade 1 diastolic dysfunction: E/A ratio decreases by ≥0.5.[45] It should be noted, however, that an adequate Valsalva maneuver may not be possible in some patients.

Grades 3 and 4 (Restrictive Physiology) Diastolic Dysfunction

Restrictive filling occurs when there is reduced LV compliance accompanied by severely increased left atrial pressure. The changes seen in the mitral inflow pattern are due to early filling into a non-compliant left ventricle. Pressure in the stiff left ventricle rises quickly, causing a rapid deceleration of a high E velocity. There is rapid equilibration of left atrial and LV pressure, which shortens the deceleration time (<160 msec). Mitral valve opening is earlier because of high left atrial pressure, which shortens the isovolumic relaxation time (<70 msec). The contribution of atrial contraction in late diastole is limited because of the rapidly increasing LV pressure, giving a short mitral A duration and a decreased A velocity. The E/A ratio is usually >2.0, which may be even more exaggerated by low A velocity.

Pulmonary vein systolic flow is also affected. Systolic forward flow is decreased because of high left atrial pressure and diastolic forward flow is blunted by the sharp increase in LV pressure in mid to late diastole. Atrial reversal is prominent, during atrial contraction LV pressure is high, and the pulmonary venous atrial reversal duration is prolonged with a higher velocity.

Although both myocardial relaxation and compliance are abnormal, relaxation abnormalities are masked by the hemodynamic changes of the noncompliant left ventricle and elevated left atrial pressure. Again, E′ is <7 cm/s and propagation velocity is reduced, reflecting slow flow propagation, although propagation velocity may be preserved if the LV cavity size and systolic function are normal. E/E′ is generally >15, reflecting high filling pressures. A Valsalva maneuver may be attempted to lower preload and demonstrate reversibility of the restrictive filling pattern, but reversibility should not be excluded if there are no changes with this maneuver. Irreversible restrictive physiology should only be diagnosed by documentation of a persistent restrictive filling pattern.

Triphasic Mitral Inflow Pattern

Markedly prolonged myocardial relaxation can produce a triphasic mitral inflow pattern (Figure 10.8), with forward flow (L wave) during mid diastole.[46] This typically occurs in severe LV hypertrophy, such as in patients with hypertrophic cardiomyopathy and hypertension, but also in patients with ischemic heart disease. The mid diastolic relaxation abnormality is also seen by mitral annular tissue Doppler imaging (see Figure 10.8), where an L′ velocity wave occurs after E′.[46,47] It is also associated with left atrial enlargement, elevated E/E′ (>15) and increased brain natriuretic peptide, suggesting high filling pressures and significant diastolic dysfunction.[46,47]

Atrial Fibrillation

Characterization of diastolic dysfunction in atrial fibrillation is difficult, because the usual classifications based on mitral inflow pattern do not apply. The mitral E wave peak velocity and deceleration time vary with the variable cardiac cycle lengths, and the mitral A wave is absent. Pulmonary vein flow velocities are also affected; systolic forward flow is absent.

Most of the echocardiographic parameters that can be used to describe diastolic function in atrial fibrillation relate to elevated filling pressure. Peak acceleration of the mitral E velocity and shortened deceleration time are associated with increased filling pressures.[48,49] The deceleration time of the mitral E wave, E/E′, duration of the pulmonary diastolic forward flow, and deceleration time of the flow correlate with pulmonary artery wedge pressure by catheterization.[27,50] However, if the E velocity is terminated early by a shorter cardiac cycle, measurement of deceleration time may not be reliable.

Time Interval Between Onset of Mitral Inflow and Onset of Early Diastolic Mitral Annular Velocity

In normal individuals, mitral valve E velocity and mitral annular E′ velocity occur simultaneously. Normally, the mitral valve opens with rapid suction of the left ventricle so that early diastolic

10. Echocardiographic Assessment

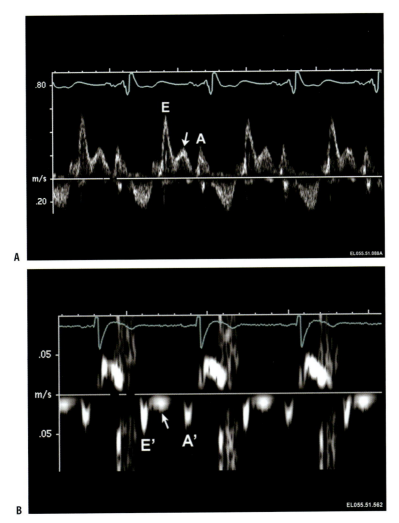

FIGURE 10.8. (A) Pulsed wave Doppler recording of mitral inflow velocity demonstrating mid diastolic flow (arrow) between E and A velocities. Mid diastolic flow velocity represents markedly delayed myocardial relaxation. This pattern usually indicates advanced diastolic dysfunction with at least moderately increased filling pressures. (B) Tissue Doppler imaging of septal mitral annulus demonstrating a mid diastolic mitral annulus velocity (arrow) that corresponds to the mid diastolic velocity shown in the mitral inflow velocity recording.

filling occurs with mitral annular motion. With impaired relaxation, mitral annular motion begins after the onset of mitral inflow, and thus E′ is delayed. Therefore, the delay between E′ and mitral E velocity can be used to characterize diastolic dysfunction, with that time delay increasing with worsening diastolic function.[51,52] The time interval between onset of mitral inflow and onset of early diastolic mitral annular velocity also correlates with pulmonary capillary wedge pressure.

Diagnosis of Diastolic Heart Failure

If a patient presents with symptoms of heart failure and systolic function is normal, DHF should be considered. It has been well demonstrated that impaired myocardial relaxation due to various causes is a major reason for DHF. This entity is distinctly different from systolic heart failure. The size of the myocytes in patients with DHF is larger than that of patients with systolic heart failure, although the fraction of collagen and fibrosis is similar in both conditions,[53] which suggests that there is concentric myocyte hypertrophy in patients with DHF. This finding is consistent with the idea that DHF is related to an abnormality of an intrinsic myocardial diastolic property.[54]

To establish the diagnosis of DHF, we need to demonstrate increased diastolic filling pressure as well as an abnormality in diastolic function. Myocardial relaxation is the initial property to become abnormal, and its impairment is usually necessary to develop increased filling pressure and DHF. Increased filling pressure and impaired myocardial relaxation can be reliably identified by comprehensive echocardiography using two-dimensional, Doppler, color flow imaging, and tissue Doppler imaging.[55] Recent advances in speckle tracking echocardiography and analysis of myocardial torsion[56,57] will undoubtedly improve our ability to evaluate diastolic as well as systolic function by echocardiography. One important clinical mimicker for myocardial DHF is constrictive pericarditis. Diastolic heart failure due to myocardial dysfunction can also be reliably differentiated from clinically similar heart failure from constrictive pericarditis by echocardiography, as discussed in Chapter 21.

Patients with diastolic dysfunction remain asymptomatic for a long period of time. Before clinically apparent heart failure, they develop symptoms only with exertion because of the increased filling pressure with exercise. Doppler echocardiographic parameters that have been shown to correlate well with pulmonary capillary wedge pressure at resting stage also estimate filling pressure with exercise. A restrictive mitral inflow filling pattern corresponds to increased filling pressures, and an E/E' of ≥15 suggests pulmonary capillary wedge pressure >20 mm Hg. In normal individuals with well-maintained diastolic function, mitral E and A velocities and mitral annular E' and A' increase proportionally with exercise with no change in the E/A or E/E' ratio, because filling pressures do not increase much with exercise.[58,59] However, patients with diastolic dysfunction usually develop a higher filling pressure with exercise and experience exertional dyspnea. The E/E' measured noninvasively during exercise has been correlated well with filling pressures measured by cardiac catheterization simultaneously with measurement of E/E' by echocardiography.[60,61] Estimation of filling pressure and evaluation of diastolic function with exercise as well as at resting stage will help identify patients with diastolic dysfunction earlier to prevent or at least slow down its progression to symptomatic DHF.

References

1. Fischer M, et al. Prevalence of left ventricular diastolic dysfunction in the community: results from a Doppler echocardiographic-based survey of a population sample. Eur Heart J 2003;24(4):320–328.
2. Redfield MM, et al. Burden of systolic and diastolic ventricular dysfunction in the community: appreciating the scope of the heart failure epidemic. JAMA 2003;289(2):194–202.
3. Hogg K, Swedberg K, McMurray J. Heart failure with preserved left ventricular systolic function: epidemiology, clinical characteristics, and prognosis. J Am Coll Cardiol 2004;43(3):317–327.
4. Vasan RS, et al. Congestive heart failure in subjects with normal versus reduced left ventricular ejection fraction: prevalence and mortality in a population-based cohort. J Am Coll Cardiol 1999;33(7):1948–1955.
5. Senni M, et al. Congestive heart failure in the community: a study of all incident cases in Olmsted County, Minnesota, in 1991. Circulation 1998;98(21):2282–2289.
6. Dauterman K, Massie B, Gheorghiade M. Managing the patient with advanced heart failure. Am H J 1998;135:S310–S319.
7. Hunt SA. ACC/AHA 2005 Guideline Update for the Diagnosis and Management of Chronic Heart Failure in the Adult: A Report of the American College of Cardiology/American Heart Association Task Force on Practice Guidelines (Writing Committee to Update the 2001 Guidelines for the Evaluation and Management of Heart Failure). J Am Coll Cardiol 2005;46(6):e1–82.
8. European Study Group on Diastolic Heart Failure. How to diagnose diastolic heart failure. Eur Heart J 1998;19(7):990–1003.
9. Vasan RS, Levy D. Defining diastolic heart failure: a call for standardized diagnostic criteria. Circulation 2000;101(17):2118–2121.
10. Zile MR, et al. Heart failure with a normal ejection fraction: is measurement of diastolic function necessary to make the diagnosis of diastolic heart failure? Circulation 2001;104(7):779–782.

11. Khan A, et al. The cardiac atria are chambers of active remodeling and dynamic collagen turnover during evolving heart failure. J Am Coll Cardiol 2004;43(1):68–76.

12. Tsang TSM, et al. Left atrial volume as a morphophysiologic expression of left ventricular diastolic dysfunction and relation to cardiovascular risk burden. Am J Cardiol 2002;90(12):1284–1289.

13. Liang H, et al. Comparison of usefulness of echocardiographic Doppler variables to left ventricular end-diastolic pressure in predicting future heart failure events. Am J Cardiol 2006;97(6):866–871.

14. Tsang TSM, et al. Prediction of risk for first age-related cardiovascular events in an elderly population: the incremental value of echocardiography. J Am Coll Cardiol 2003;42(7):1199–1205.

15. Ren J, et al. Two-dimensional echocardiographic determination of left atrial emptying volume: a noninvasive index in quantifying the degree of nonrheumatic mitral regurgitation. J Am Coll Cardiol 1983;729–736.

16. Appleton C, Hatle L, Popp R. Relation of transmitral flow velocity patterns to left ventricular diastolic function: new insights from a combined hemodynamic and Doppler echocardiographic study. J Am Coll Cardiol 1988;12:426–440.

17. Oh JK, et al. The noninvasive assessment of left ventricular diastolic function with two-dimensional and Doppler echocardiography. J Am Soc Echocardiogr 1997;10:246–270.

18. Yamamoto K, et al. Assessment of left ventricular end-diastolic pressure by Doppler echocardiography: contribution of duration of pulmonary venous versus mitral flow velocity curves at atrial contraction. J Am Soc Echocardiogr 1997; 10(1):52–59.

19. Rossvoll O, Hatle L. Pulmonary venous flow velocities recorded by transthoracic Doppler ultrasound: relation to left ventricular diastolic pressures. J Am Coll Cardiol 1993;21(7):1697–1700.

20. Appleton C. Hemodynamic determinants of Doppler pulmonary venous flow velocity components: new insights from studies in lightly sedated dogs. J Am Coll Cardiol 1997;30:1562–1574.

21. Kinnaird T, Thompson C, Munt B. The deceleration time of pulmonary venous diastolic flow is more accurate than the pulmonary artery occlusion pressure in predicting left atrial pressure. J Am Coll Cardiol 2001;37:2025–2030.

22. Sohn D, et al. Assessment of mitral annular velocities by Doppler tissue imaging in the evaluation of left ventricular diastolic function. J Am Coll Cardiol 1997;30:474–480.

23. Nagueh S, et al. Hemodynamic determinants of the mitral annulus diastolic velocities by tissue Doppler. J Am Coll Cardiol 2001;37:278–285.

24. Nagueh S, et al. Doppler tissue imaging: a noninvasive technique for evaluation of left ventricular relaxation and estimation of filling pressures. J Am Coll Cardiol 1997;30:1527–1533.

25. Ommen S, et al. Clinical utility of Doppler echocardiography and tissue Doppler imaging in the estimation of left ventricular filling pressures. Circulation 2000;102:1788–1794.

26. Sohn D, et al. Evaluation of left ventricular diastolic function when mitral E and A waves are completely fused: role of assessing mitral annulus velocity. J Am Soc Echocardiogr 1999;12(3):203–208.

27. Sohn D, et al. Mitral annulus velocity in the evaluation of left ventricular diastolic function in atrial fibrillation. J Am Soc Echocardiogr 1999;12(11): 927–931.

28. Nagueh SF, et al. Doppler estimation of left ventricular filling pressure in sinus tachycardia: a new application of tissue Doppler imaging. Circulation 1998;98(16):1644–1650.

29. Brun P, et al. Left ventricular flow propagation during early filling is related to wall relaxation: a color M-mode Doppler analysis. J Am Coll Cardiol 1992;20:420–432.

30. Takatsuji H, et al. A new approach for evaluation of left ventricular diastolic function: Spatial and temporal analysis of left ventricular filling flow propagation by color M-mode Doppler echocardiography. J Am Coll Cardiol 1996;27(2):365–371.

31. de Boeck B, et al. Colour M-mode velocity propagation: a glance at intra-ventricular pressure gradients and early diastolic ventricular performance. Eur J Heart Fail 2005;7(1):19–28.

32. Gonzales-Vilchez F, et al. Comparison of Doppler echocardiography, color M-mode Doppler, and Doppler tissue imaging for the estimation of pulmonary capillary wedge pressure. J Am Soc Echocardiogr 2002;15:1245–1250.

33. Gonzales-Vilchez F, et al. Combined use of pulsed and color M-mode Doppler echocardiography for the estimation of pulmonary capillary wedge pressure: an empirical approach based on an analytical relation. J Am Coll Cardiol 1999;34:515–523.

34. Takeda K, et al. Dependence of flow propagation velocity on cardiac size: observations from patients with dilated cardiomyopathy and hypertrophic cardiomyopathy [abstr]. J Am Coll Cardiol 2002;39:383A–384A.

35. Spencer K, Weinert L, Lang R. Effect of age, heart rate, and tricuspid regurgitation on the Doppler echocardiographic evaluation of right ventricular diastolic function. Cardiology 1999;92(1):59–64.

36. Ommen S, et al. Assessment of right atrial pressure with 2-dimensional and Doppler echocardiography: a simultaneous catheterization and

echocardiographic study. Mayo Clin Proc 2000; 75(1):24–9.

37. Appleton C, Hatle L, Popp R. Superior vena cava and hepatic vein Doppler echocardiography in healthy adults. J Am Coll Cardiol 1987;10(5):1032–1039.

38. Burstow D, et al. Cardiac tamponade: characteristic Doppler observation. Mayo Clin Proc 1989;64(3):312–324.

39. Mancuso L, et al. Constrictive pericarditis versus restrictive cardiomyopathy: the role of Doppler echocardiography in differential diagnosis. Int J Cardiol 1991;31(3):319–327.

40. Nishimura R, Tajik AJ. Evaluation of diastolic filling of the left ventricle in health and disease: Doppler echocardiography is the clinician's Rosetta stone. J Am Coll Cardiol 1997;30(1):8–18.

41. Kitzman DW, et al. Age-related alterations of Doppler left ventricular filling indexes in normal subjects are independent of left ventricular mass, heart rate, contractility and loading conditions. J Am Coll Cardiol 1991;18(5):1243–1250.

42. Spirito P, Maron BJ. Influence of aging on Doppler echocardiographic indices of left ventricular diastolic function. Br Heart J 1988;59(6):672–679.

43. Klein AL, et al. Effects of age on left ventricular dimensions and filling dynamics in 117 normal persons. Mayo Clinic Proc 1994;69(3):212–224.

44. Oh J, et. al. Diastolic heart failure can be diagnosed by comprehensive two-dimensional and Doppler echocardiography. J Am Coll Cardiol 2006;47(3):500–506.

45. Hurrell D, et al. Utility of preload alteration in assessment of left ventricular filling pressure by Doppler echocardiography: a simultaneous catheterization and Doppler echocardiographic study. J Am Coll Cardiol 1997;30(2):459–467.

46. Ha J-W, et al. Triphasic mitral inflow velocity with mid diastolic filling: clinical implications and associated echocardiographic findings. J Am Soc Echocardiogr 2004;17(5):428–431.

47. Ha J-W, et al. Triphasic mitral inflow velocity with mid-diastolic flow: the presence of mid-diastolic mitral annular velocity indicates advanced diastolic dysfunction. Eur J Echocardiogr 2006;7(1):16–21.

48. Nagueh SF, Kopelen HA, Quinones MA. Assessment of left ventricular filling pressures by Doppler in the presence of atrial fibrillation. Circulation 1996;94(9):2138–2145.

49. Hurrell D, et al., Short deceleration time of mitral inflow E velocity: prognostic implication with atrial

fibrillation from transthoracic Doppler indexes of mitral and pulmonary venous flow velocity. J Am Coll Cardiol 1998;30:19–26.

50. Chirillo M, et al. Estimating mean pulmonary wedge pressure in patients with chronic atrial fibrillation from transthoracic Doppler indexes of mitral and pulmonary venous flow velocity. J Am Coll Cardiol 1997;30(1):19–26.

51. Rivas-Gotz C, et al. Time interval between onset of mitral inflow and onset of early diastolic velocity by tissue Doppler: a novel index of left ventricular relaxation: experimental studies and clinical application. J Am Coll Cardiol 2003;42(8):1463–1470.

52. Hasegawa H, et al. Diastolic mitral annular velocity during the development of heart failure. J Am Coll Cardiol 2003;41(9):1590–1597.

53. van Heerebeek L, et al. Myocardial structure and function differ in systolic and diastolic heart failure. Circulation 2006;113:1966–1973.

54. Zile M, et al. Diastolic heart failure—abnormalities in active relaxation and passive stiffness of the left ventricle. N Engl J Med 2004;350(19):1953–1959.

55. Oh J, Hatle L, et al. Diastolic heart failure can be diagnosed by comprehensive two-dimensional and Doppler echocardiography. J Am Coll Cardiol 2006;47(3):500–506.

56. Helle-Valle T, et al. New noninvasive method for assessment of left ventricular rotation: speckle tracking echocardiography. Circulation 2005;112:3149–3156.

57. Notomi Y, et al. Assessment of left ventricular torsional deformation by Doppler tissue imaging: validation study with tagged magnetic resonance imaging. Circulation 2005;111:1141–1147.

58. Ha J-W, et al. Effects of treadmill exercise on mitral inflow and annular velocities in healthy adults. Am J Cardiol 2003;91(1):114–115.

59. Ha J-W, et al. Diastolic stress echocardiography: a novel noninvasive diagnostic test for diastolic dysfunction using supine bicycle exercise Doppler echocardiography. J Am Soc Echocardiogr 2005;18(1):63–68.

60. Talreja D, Nishimura R, Oh J. Noninvasive parameters of diastolic function reflect invasively measured filling pressures during exercise [abstr 2235]. Circulation 2004;110(17):III-474.

61. Burgess MI, Jenkins C, Sharman JE, Marwick TH. Diastolic stress echocardiography: hemodynamic validation and clinical significance of estimation of ventricular filling pressure with exercise. J Am Coll Cardiol 2006;47(9):1891–1900.

11
Magnetic Resonance Imaging

Frank E. Rademakers and Jan Bogaert

Introduction

The diagnosis of diastolic heart failure requires a combination of clinical, laboratory, and technical findings, providing evidence of the existence of heart failure, the absence of (significant) systolic abnormalities, and the presence of diastolic dysfunction. As the latter cannot be "captured" with a single physiologic parameter, a combination of parameters and findings is used. Although invasive techniques can be employed to establish the primary diagnosis, a noninvasive method is preferred for follow-up of patients and evaluation of treatment. Echocardiography, because of its wide availability, low cost, and ease of access is the preferred noninvasive method. Cardiovascular magnetic resonance (CMR) is an alternative noninvasive modality that can provide similar parameters as echocardiography but that is also capable of adding some unique information.[1] Moreover, CMR is very accurate and reproducible and uniquely suited for the follow-up of individual patients. The following topics are discussed in this chapter:

- Technique
- Information also available from echocardiography
- Unique CMR parameters
- Future contributions

Technique

Cardiovascular magnetic resonance provides morphologic, functional, and flow information as well as tissue characterization by utilization of a series of dedicated acquisition schemes or sequences (several recent textbooks provide further details on these aspects, which are beyond the scope of this chapter). Since the development of steady-state free-precession sequences, the distinction between morphologic and functional acquisitions has slightly faded, as this technique provides a bright blood image of the moving heart with a very high spatial (1.3 × 1.3–mm in-plane and 5-mm slice thickness) and a reasonable temporal resolution (20 ms; Figure 11.1). If needed, additional T1- and T2-weighted images can be acquired for morphology and tissue characterization (Figure 11.2); images can also be acquired after administration of a contrast agent (gadolinium diethylenetriaminepentaacetate) either in three dimensions to look for general cardiac and vascular features or for perfusion (first pass), late enhancement (Figure 11.3), and distinctive tissue features.

The specific advantage of CMR over echocardiography is the ability of acquiring images in any selected plane or along the specific cardiac axes, which makes it possible to thoroughly study cardiac morphology and function, irrespective patient build or habitus. A routine CMR examination in the setting of heart failure will acquire the following images: cine (same slice over the cardiac cycle) with a set of contiguous short axis slices, covering the entire heart from base to apex, and a set of long axis slices (two, three, and four chamber).

By contouring the epi- and endocardial borders of the different cavities, these provide left and right heart volumes (end-diastolic volume, end-systolic volume, stroke volume, ejection fraction) and left ventricular mass. Because images from the entire cardiac cycle are available, emptying and filling rates can be calculated as well.[2-4]

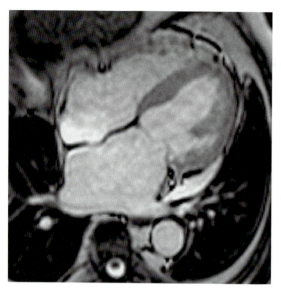

FIGURE 11.1. A 66-year old man with renal transplant and diastolic heart failure. SSFP cine MRI in the horizontal long-axis, at end diastole (**left**) and end systole (**right**). Note a moderately severe biatrial enlargement, and a small pericardial effusion laterally of the left ventricle. The systolic function was only slightly diminished (LV ejection fraction 54%).

Qualitative (visual) assessment of regional function (wall displacement and thickening) is possible, but also quantitative wall thickening (from the contours using the chord technique) is easily available with the existing software tools. Atrial volume and global function can similarly be assessed. Such functional imaging can be repeated during dobutamine administration to look for viability (response to low dose dobutamine) or ischemia (decrease in deformation of the wall at high dose). The three-dimensional nature of the data permits reconstruction of the heart and quantification of the global and regional shape of the cavities (sphericity, radii of curvature).[5]

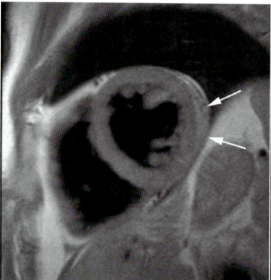 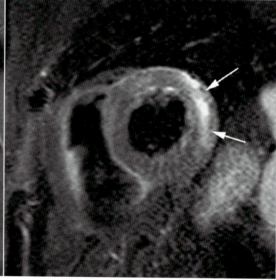

FIGURE 11.2. Acute (peri)myocarditis in a 39-year old man with retrosternal chest pain, increased cardiac enzymes (troponins) and normal coronary arteries. (**Left**) T1-weighted FSE in mid-ventricular cardiac short-axis. (**Right**) T2-weigthed STIR FSE in the same position. Especially the T2-weighted STIR-FSE image shows a curvilinear hyper-intense rim in the lateral LV wall, located in the epicardial layers (arrows).

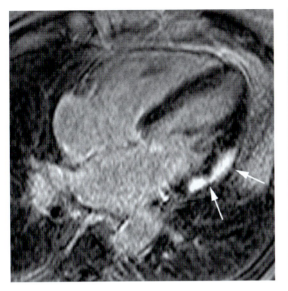
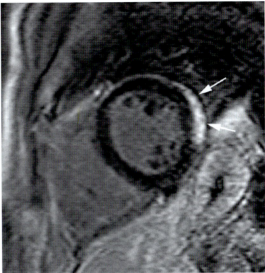

FIGURE 11.3. Acute (peri)myocarditis in a 39-year old man with retrostenal chest pain, increased cardiac enzymes (troponins) and normal coronary arteries. Cardiac horizontal long-axis (**left**), and short-axis (**right**) contrast-enhanced T1-weighted 3D fast field- echo image obtained 16 and 18 min after injection of 0.2 mmol/kg of Gd-DPTA shows strong enhancement in the outer myocardial layers of the laterobasal LV wall (arrows).

By placing the interrogating plane at the level of the atrioventricular valves, the outlet valves, or the venous connections (caval veins,[6] subhepatic veins, pulmonary veins) and using a specific flow sensitive sequence, flow at these sites during the cardiac cycle is studied much as with pulsed wave Doppler in echocardiography.[7] A difference is that CMR provides velocities (meters per second) as well as volume flow (milliliters per second)[8,9] and is less angle dependent.[10] Flow in the cavities can be quantified as well,[11] giving insight into the presence and distribution of flow divergence and vortices. Adjusting the maximal velocity encoding, the low velocities in the myocardial wall can be obtained as with myocardial velocity imaging.[12] Although mostly velocities through the image plane are interrogated, CMR intrinsically can obtain all three components of the true velocity vector,[13] but this requires several subsequent acquisitions and a significant amount of postprocessing.

After administration of gadolinium-chelated contrast media in a peripheral vein, the passage of the contrast through the right heart, the left heart, and the myocardium can be followed and semiquantitated, providing information about regional myocardial perfusion and, if repeated during administration of adenosine, perfusion reserve. Specific imaging with nulling of the signal of the normal myocardium some 10–20 min after gadolinium administration allows visualization of areas of late contrast captation or late enhancement, which corresponds to either infarcted tissue or zones of inflammation/fibrosis (Figure 11.4).

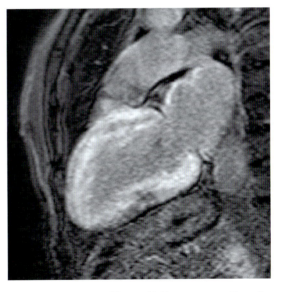

FIGURE 11.4. A 75-year-old man with biopsy proven senile cardiac amyloidosis. Cardiac horizontal long-axis contrast-enhanced T1-weighted 3D fast field-echo image obtained 18 min after injection of 0.2 mmol/kg of Gd-DTPA shows strong myocardial enhancement which is most pronounced in subendo- and subepicardium. (Courtesy, Dr. I. Crevits, Roeselare, Belgium.)

Using a specific prepulse, the myocardium can be marked with a line or grid pattern at end diastole that deforms with the myocardium on which it is inscribed[14,15]; this myocardial tagging can be applied to any image plane, and, when performed on a series of short and long axis images, the full spectrum of myocardial deformation can be quantified as myocardial strains. Using a local myocardial coordinate system, the normal strains (thickening, circumferential, and longitudinal shortening) as well as the shear strains (circumferential-radial, radial-longitudinal, and circumferential-longitudinal, i.e., torsion) can be obtained throughout the entire ventricle.[16]

Finally, using diffusion tensor imaging, fiber orientations within the myocardial mass can be visualized and quantified. Although obtaining this diffusion tensor is much easier in the ex vivo[17] than in the moving in vivo situation,[18,19] such information about regional fiber orientation can be combined with tagging to calculate fiber mechanics.

Magnetic resonance is contraindicated when vascular clips are present in the brain or when metal fragments have entered the eye. Implanted pacemakers, implantable cardioverter defibrillators, and neurostimulators are also contraindications, although more recent models are far less influenced by the magnetic field and radiofrequency energy; several patients with such devices have been examined with magnetic resonance without any negative consequences, but the formal advice remains very strict; beside interference with the device itself, a magnetic resonance examination can induce electrical currents in the connecting pacemaker and implantable cardioverter defibrillator leads, causing heating of the tip (with possible tissue damage and increased resistance) as well as severe arrhythmias. Vascular clips outside the brain (coronary artery bypass graft), valve prostheses, coronary stents, and orthopedic implants are not contraindications. When in doubt, consult the existing device lists.

Complementary to Echocardiography

As indicated in the previous section, CMR can provide a whole range of parameters that are identical or nearly identical to those obtained with echocardiography (interpretation of these parameters is covered in Chapter 10 and therefore is not expanded on in this section). As such, CMR is a valid alternative for those patients who do not have adequate image quality to reliably obtain these parameters. Moreover, the three-dimensional nature of CMR, its excellent contrast between cavity (blood) and myocardium, and its high spatial and adequate temporal resolutions have made this technique the gold standard for assessing volumes and mass.[20] Because several of the systolic and diastolic function parameters are volume derived, it is clear that CMR constitutes not only a valid alternative to echocardiography but could be the first choice technique if small changes in volume, mass, or any derived parameter are expected and are needed to evaluate progression of disease or reaction to therapy or could indicate another step in the treatment algorithm. These parameters can be grouped as indices of systolic and of diastolic performance; the former are needed to illustrate the absence of systolic dysfunction and the latter to quantify the presence and origin of filling abnormalities.

Systolic Performance

The classic parameters of end-diastolic and end-systolic volumes, stroke volume and ejection fraction, have been mentioned. Global and regional wall thickening can contribute to exclude underlying ischemic heart disease, although other conditions, such as myocarditis and idiopathic dilated cardiomyopathy, can show a significant heterogeneous behavior.

Diastolic Performance

Flow patterns across the mitral[21] and tricuspid[22] valves can be obtained and interpreted with respect to relative volume flow during early versus late atrial filling[8]; the absolute values have been less well validated, however, and cannot be just extrapolated from the echo values because they constitute volume flow in milliliters per second rather than velocities in centimeters per second. Similarly, derived parameters such as acceleration and deceleration of the E wave have to be used cautiously because of lack of validation. Duration of flow, on the contrary, for example of atrial

11. Magnetic Resonance Imaging

versus pulmonary vein retrograde flow, can be interpreted as for the corresponding Doppler parameters.

Left atrial volume has been suggested as a long-term parameter for atrial filling pressures,[23] much as hemoglobin A1 for blood glucose levels. Because CMR can accurately quantify atrial volumes, follow-up of patients using this volumetric factor could be an interesting use of the technique.[24]

Pulmonary vein flow can be easily measured at any of the four pulmonary vein orifices in cardiac transplant patients.[25] In patients with overall limited echo quality, pulmonary vein flow is often difficult to evaluate, and the correct interpretation of the mitral inflow signal often requires a good quality pulmonary vein trace.

Differentiation between restrictive and constrictive pathology requires obtaining inflow signals during the respiratory cycle, but also for patients with pulmonary disease it is often interesting to observe such respiratory variation. With the advent of real-time flow measurements, CMR is now capable of obtaining such traces[26] and facilitating the interpretation of the left- and right-sided inflow and venous patterns.

Using the peak velocities across any valve or orifice, CMR can provide estimates of gradients and the derived values (right ventricular systolic pressures, valve gradients, and calculated areas) using the same Bernoulli and continuity equations as in echocardiography. Because volume flows across valves (both antegrade and retrograde) can be obtained with high accuracy, valvular insufficiencies and shunts between the left and right heart can be quantitated. Such abnormalities can be quite important in the differential diagnosis of diastolic dysfunction and can constitute a specific target for treatment of symptoms of dyspnea and fatigue, which are also typical for diastolic heart failure.

Specific to Cardiovascular Magnetic Resonance

Several morphologic and functional parameters can be obtained uniquely with CMR and can contribute to the differential diagnosis of diastolic heart failure.

Morphology

Atrial volume has been mentioned, as echocardiography can also measure it, but CMR is much better suited to do so reliably and with high study reproducibility.[27] The use of near-real-time three-dimensional echo techniques constitutes a significant improvement in this respect to echocardiography, but the technique is not yet widely available and is subject to good image quality. Left ventricular myocardial mass is a similar parameter of long-term importance for compliance and diastolic function that can be more reliably quantified with CMR and that provides, together with the functional parameters, a powerful tool for evaluation of treatment effects.[28]

The pericardium can be well visualized on CMR, and its thickness can be evaluated on a regional basis. Although calcifications are much better seen with computed tomography, the visualization of the pericardial structure itself (Figure 11.5) combined with the motion pattern of the underlying myocardium or cavity is a powerful tool. If needed, tagging can be applied to further illustrate the fusion of the pericardial layers and the restriction of cardiac motion, which is the cause of the filling abnormalities.

Flow Patterns

When constriction is suspected, the venous left- and right-sided flow patterns can be easily measured (Figure 11.6). They can also be measured during respiratory variation and after a fluid challenge, if required. As the mitral and tricuspid valves lie in nearly the same plane, flows across these valves can be measured simultaneously,[29] allowing better comparison of changing left- and right-sided flows during respiration or other interventions.

Function

Of particular interest in this pathology is the motion pattern of the interventricular septum,[30] which shows an inspiratory early diastolic flattening and even shape reversal toward the left caused by the sudden alterations in transseptal pressure gradients due to exaggerated right-sided filling on

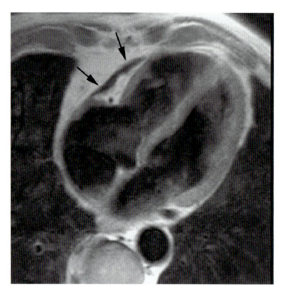

FIGURE 11.5. Constrictive pericarditis in a 68-year old man presenting with right heart failure and pericardial calcifications on his chest-x-ray and computed tomography (not shown). Axial **(left)** and short-axis **(right)** T1-weighted FSE (FastSpinEcho) MR images show low-signal irregular thickening of the pericardium along the basal part of the RV free wall and right atrioventricular groove.

inspiration in constriction.[31] This septal motion can be quantified (Figures 11.7 to 11.9) and represents an easily obtained and powerful tool in the differential diagnosis of hemodynamically important pericardial disease.[32]

With tagging, myocardial strains can be measured throughout the cardiac cycle.[16] Besides systolic strains, diastolic strains can also be calculated[33] Wall thinning and circumferential and longitudinal lengthening can be used both as global but more importantly as regional parameters of diastolic mechanics.[34] Shear strains, including torsion, can be measured in this way. Torsion is an important mechanical feature of the thick-walled oval-shaped left ventricle[35,36] and permits a high ejection fraction (70%) for a more limited fiber shortening (15%) as well as near-equalization of fiber strains throughout the wall. Disappearance of torsion or untwisting is a key feature of diastolic performance[37,38] and occurs to a large extent before filling and during or even before isovolumic relaxation.[39] As such it provides a functional, mechanical basis for the presence of restoring or suction forces and can be used as a

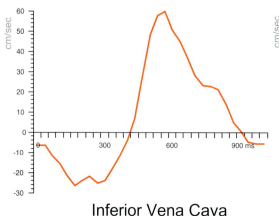

Inferior Vena Cava

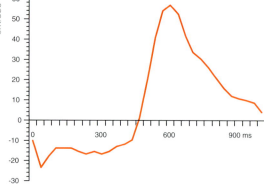

Tricuspid Valve

FIGURE 11.6. Example of restrictive inflow pattern: the negative flow corresponds to systolic reversal flow (small insufficiency); the positive flow is the fusion between a larger early diastolic and a smaller atrial antegrade flow in the caval vein and across the tricuspid valve.

11. Magnetic Resonance Imaging

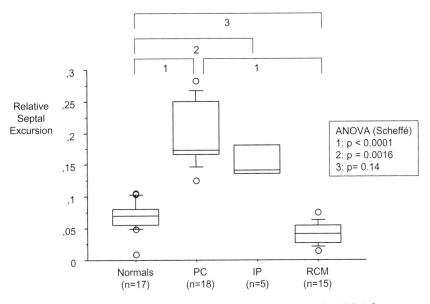

FIGURE 11.7. Relative septal excursion in normals and patients with constrictive pericarditis (PC), inflammatory pericarditis (IP) and restrictive cardiomyopathy RCM). (Adapted from Francone et al.[32] Eur Radiol 2005.)

Constrictive Pericarditis

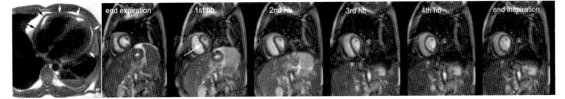

FIGURE 11.8. Influence of respiration on septal shape: constrictive pericarditis. **Far Left** horizontal long axis image showing pericardial thickening. **Breathing Series**: influence of respiration on septal shape going from end-expiration to end-inspiration, showing images from the heart beats inbetween (hb: heart beat).

RCM (Cardiac Amyloidosis)

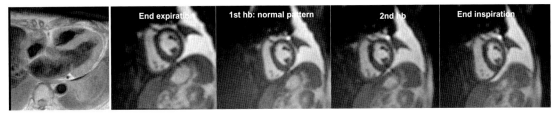

FIGURE 11.9. Influence of respiration on septal shape: restrictive cardiomyopathy. **Far Left**: horizontal long axis image showing myocardial hypertrophy. **Breathing Series**: influence of respiration on septal shape going from end-expiration to end-inspiration, showing images from the heart beats inbetween (hb: heart beat).

and quantification of cardiac laminar structure. Magn Reson Med 2005;54:850–859.

18. Reese TG, Wedeen VJ, Weisskoff RM. Measuring diffusion in the presence of material strain. J Magn Reson B 1996;112:253–258.

19. Tseng WY, Reese TG, Weisskoff RM, Wedeen VJ. Cardiac diffusion tensor MRI in vivo without strain correction. Magn Reson Med 1999;42:393–403.

20. Hauser TH, McClennen S, Katsimaglis G, Josephson ME, Manning WJ, Yeon SB. Assessment of left atrial volume by contrast enhanced magnetic resonance angiography. J Cardiovasc Magn Reson 2004;6:491–497.

21. Dendale PA, Franken PR, Waldman GJ, Baur LH, Vandamme S, van der Geest RJ, et al. Regional diastolic wall motion dynamics in anterior myocardial infarction: analysis and quantification with magnetic resonance imaging. Coron Artery Dis 1995;6: 723–729.

22. Helbing WA, Niezen RA, Le Cessie S, van der Geest RJ, Ottenkamp J, de Roos A. Right ventricular diastolic function in children with pulmonary regurgitation after repair of tetralogy of Fallot: volumetric evaluation by magnetic resonance velocity mapping. J Am Coll Cardiol 1996;28:1827–1835.

23. Sachdev V, Shizukuda Y, Brenneman CL, Birdsall CW, Waclawiw MA, Arai AE, et al. Left atrial volumetric remodeling is predictive of functional capacity in nonobstructive hypertrophic cardiomyopathy. Am Heart J 2005;149:730–736.

24. Therkelsen SK, Groenning BA, Svendsen JH, Jensen GB. Atrial and ventricular volume and function in persistent and permanent atrial fibrillation, a magnetic resonance imaging study. J Cardiovasc Magn Reson 2005;7:465–473.

25. Freimark D, Silverman JM, Aleksic I, Crues JV, Blanche C, Trento A, et al. Atrial emptying with orthotopic heart transplantation using bicaval and pulmonary venous anastomoses: a magnetic resonance imaging study. J Am Coll Cardiol 1995;25: 932–936.

26. Paelinck BP, Lamb HJ, Bax JJ, Van der Wall EE, de Roos A. MR flow mapping of dobutamine-induced changes in diastolic heart function. J Magn Reson Imaging 2004;19:176–181.

27. Sievers B, Kirchberg S, Franken U, Bakan A, Addo M, John-Puthenveettil B, et al. Determination of normal gender-specific left atrial dimensions by cardiovascular magnetic resonance imaging. J Cardiovasc Magn Reson 2005;7:677–683.

28. Hoffmann U, Globits S, Stefenelli T, Loewe C, Kostner K, Frank H. The effects of ACE inhibitor therapy on left ventricular myocardial mass and diastolic filling in previously untreated hyperten-

sive patients: a cine MRI study. J Magn Reson Imaging 2001;14:16–22.

29. Kroft LJ, de Roos A. Biventricular diastolic cardiac function assessed by MR flow imaging using a single angulation. Acta Radiol 1999;40:563–568.

30. Harasawa H, Li KS, Nakamoto T, Coghlan L, Singleton HR, Dell'Italia LJ, et al. Ventricular coupling via the pericardium: normal versus tamponade. Cardiovasc Res 1993;27:1470–1476.

31. Giorgi B, Mollet NR, Dymarkowski S, Rademakers FE, Bogaert J. Clinically suspected constrictive pericarditis: MR imaging assessment of ventricular septal motion and configuration in patients and healthy subjects. Radiology 2003;228:417–424.

32. Francone M, Dymarkowski S, Kalantzi M, Rademakers FE, Bogaert J. Assessment of ventricular coupling with real-time cine MRI and its value to differentiate constrictive pericarditis from restrictive cardiomyopathy. Eur Radiol 2005;1–8.

33. Fonseca CG, Dissanayake AM, Doughty RN, Whalley GA, Gamble GD, Cowan BR, et al. Three-dimensional assessment of left ventricular systolic strain in patients with type 2 diabetes mellitus, diastolic dysfunction, and normal ejection fraction. Am J Cardiol 2004;94:1391–1395.

34. Azevedo CF, Amado LC, Kraitchman DL, Gerber BL, Osman NF, Rochitte CE, et al. Persistent diastolic dysfunction despite complete systolic functional recovery after reperfused acute myocardial infarction demonstrated by tagged magnetic resonance imaging. Eur Heart J 2004;25:1419–1427.

35. Sorger JM, Wyman BT, Faris OP, Hunter WC, McVeigh ER. Torsion of the left ventricle during pacing with MRI tagging. J Cardiovasc Magn Reson 2003;5:521–530.

36. Lorenz CH, Pastorek JS, Bundy JM. Delineation of normal human left ventricular twist throughout systole by tagged cine magnetic resonance imaging. J Cardiovasc Magn Reson 2000;2:97–108.

37. Buchalter MB, Rademakers FE, Weiss JL, Rogers WJ, Weisfeldt ML, Shapiro EP. Rotational deformation of the canine left ventricle measured by magnetic resonance tagging: effects of catecholamines, ischaemia, and pacing. Cardiovasc Res 1994;28: 629–635.

38. Rademakers FE, Buchalter MB, Rogers WJ, Zerhouni EA, Weisfeldt ML, Weiss JL, et al. Dissociation between left ventricular untwisting and filling. Accentuation by catecholamines. Circulation 1992;85:1572–1581.

39. Rosen BD, Gerber BL, Edvardsen T, Castillo E, Amado LC, Nasir K, et al. Late systolic onset of regional LV relaxation demonstrated in three-dimensional space by MRI tissue tagging. Am J

11. Magnetic Resonance Imaging

Physiol Heart Circ Physiol 2004;287:H1740–H1746.

40. Fuchs E, Muller MF, Oswald H, Thony H, Mohacsi P, Hess OM. Cardiac rotation and relaxation in patients with chronic heart failure. Eur J Heart Fail 2004;6:715–722.

41. Nagel E, Stuber M, Burkhard B, Fischer SE, Scheidegger MB, Boesiger P, et al. Cardiac rotation and relaxation in patients with aortic valve stenosis. Eur Heart J 2000;21:582–589.

42. Nagel E, Stuber M, Lakatos M, Scheidegger MB, Boesiger P, Hess OM. Cardiac rotation and relaxation after anterolateral myocardial infarction. Coron Artery Dis 2000;11:261–267.

43. Oxenham HC, Young AA, Cowan BR, Gentles TL, Occleshaw CJ, Fonseca CG, et al. Age-related changes in myocardial relaxation using three-dimensional tagged magnetic resonance imaging. J Cardiovasc Magn Reson 2003;5:421–430.

44. Chen J, Liu W, Zhang H, Lacy L, Yang X, Song SK, et al. Regional ventricular wall thickening reflects changes in cardiac fiber and sheet structure during contraction: quantification with diffusion tensor MRI. Am J Physiol Heart Circ Physiol 2005;289:H1898–H1907.

45. Helm PA, Younes L, Beg MF, Ennis DB, Leclercq C, Faris OP, et al. Evidence of structural remodeling in the dyssynchronous failing heart. Circ Res 2006;98:125–132.

46. Lamb HJ, Beyerbacht HP, van Der LA, Stoel BC, Doornbos J, Van der Wall EE, et al. Diastolic dysfunction in hypertensive heart disease is associated with altered myocardial metabolism. Circulation 1999;99:2261–2267.

47. Beyerbacht HP, Lamb HJ, van Der LA, Vliegen HW, Leujes F, Hazekamp MG, et al. Aortic valve replacement in patients with aortic valve stenosis improves myocardial metabolism and diastolic function. Radiology 2001;219:637–643.

48. Spindler M, Saupe KW, Christe ME, Sweeney HL, Seidman CE, Seidman JG, et al. Diastolic dysfunction and altered energetics in the alphaMHC403/+ mouse model of familial hypertrophic cardiomyopathy. J Clin Invest 1998;101:1775–1783.

12
Natriuretic Peptides in the Diagnosis of Diastolic Heart Failure

Michał Tendera and Wojciech Wojakowski

Introduction

Heart failure can occur in the presence of both normal and compromised left ventricular (LV) systolic function. In the presence of compromised systolic function, appropriate signs and symptoms make it relatively easy to make the diagnosis of heart failure. However, because of the nonspecific nature of clinical findings, especially the symptoms of heart failure, when LV systolic function is normal, the diagnosis becomes more difficult. Although most of the time the presence of diastolic heart failure (DHF) can be confirmed by echocardiographic demonstration of impaired ventricular function in diastole, in clinical practice DHF often remains the diagnosis of exclusion.[1,2] This is true because the echocardiographic criteria for the diagnosis of diastolic dysfunction are still being developed and validated. Assessment of LV diastolic function is complex, involving measurement of heart rate and load-dependent variables, so an additional simple, inexpensive test that helps to diagnose LV diastolic dysfunction is needed. Given the robust and compelling evidence that measurement of plasma levels of cardiac natriuretic peptides provides useful diagnostic information in patients with heart failure with decreased LV ejection fraction (LVEF), the approach seems valid also for patients with suspected diastolic LV dysfunction.[2]

The widespread use of measuring natriuretic peptides (brain natriuretic peptide [BNP] or N-terminal prohormone BNP [NT-pro-BNP]) in the evaluation of a patient with acute dyspnea and their high negative predictive value, allowing the exclusion of cardiac causes of dyspnea, stimulated the attempts to use BNP measurements when heart failure with normal systolic function (DHF) is suspected. The rationale for this approach is to simplify the process of decision making, especially in the emergency department (Figure 12.1).[3] The Breathing Not Properly Multinational Study investigated 1,586 patients presenting with acute dyspnea to the emergency department. It showed that measurement of BNP with the cut-off value of 100 pg/mL improved diagnostic accuracy when combined with clinical judgment (diagnostic accuracy 74% for clinical judgment alone; 81.2% in patients with BNP >100 pg/mL; 81.5% when the two were combined — area under the curve [AUC], 0.93; 95% CI, 0.92–0.94).[2,4,5]

Structure and Mechanisms of Natriuretic Peptides

Increased synthesis and release of cardiac natriuretic peptides is one of the pivotal biochemical markers of neurohormonal activation in response to volume overload. Secretion of natriuretic peptides reflects the function of the heart as the endocrine organ. The primary stimulus for the release of atrial natriuretic peptide (ANP) and BNP is the stretch of cardiomyocytes. Brain natriuretic peptide is a neurohormone synthesized and released from the myocardium as a response to pressure overload, volume expansion, and increased filling pressure of the LV. Direct upregulation of expression of the BNP gene directly by angiotensin II is another mechanism involved in its increased synthesis.[3,6] The secretion of BNP is an independent predictor of increased LV end-diastolic pressure and increased pulmonary capillary wedge pressure.[7] An increase in BNP can be also induced by right ventricular overload secondary to pulmonary embolism[8] and left atrium overload in chronic mitral regurgitation.[9] Atrial cardiomyocytes are the primary source of circulating ANP (biologically active c-ANP and inactive NT-pro-ANP) whose levels increase acutely within minutes after a rise in atrial pressure. In the setting of LV systolic dysfunction and hypertrophy, ANP can be synthesized in both atria and ventricles. The activation of natriuretic peptide secretion is a regulatory mechanism counteracting the activation of the renin-angiotensin-aldosterone and sympathetic nervous systems. The receptors for BNP coupled with guanylate cyclase were identified on cardiomyocytes, endothelial cells, smooth muscle cells, and adipocytes

and also in the kidneys and lungs. The binding of BNP leads to increase of intracellular cyclic guanosine monophosphate levels.[10,11]

Circulating inactive 108–amino acid peptide pro-BNP undergoes proteolytic cleavage by the enzyme corin into active peptide (amino acids 77–108) and inactive NT-pro-BNP (amino acids 1–76) in equimolar amounts.[12] Both peptides can be reliably measured using high-sensitivity assays and an automated platform in the hospital laboratories for NT-pro-BNP and BNP and point-of-care immunofluorometric assay for BNP. Amino-terminal pro-BNP has a sixfold longer plasma half-life than BNP (120 vs. 20 min), and plasma levels of this inactive peptide are higher than those of BNP. Amino-terminal pro-BNP also displays lower intraindividual variability; however, both peptides have high biologic variability, which may influence the diagnostic value, especially in asymptomatic patients.[10] Both BNP and

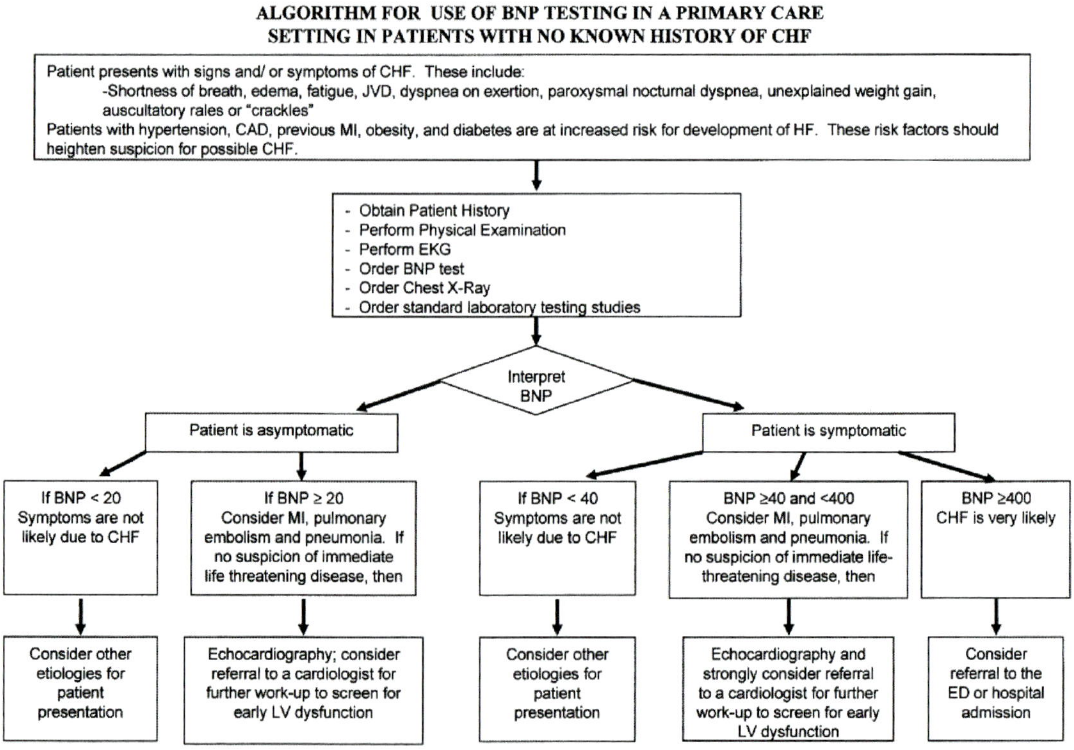

ALGORITHM FOR USE OF BNP TESTING IN A PRIMARY CARE SETTING IN PATIENTS WITH NO KNOWN HISTORY OF CHF

Patient presents with signs and/ or symptoms of CHF. These include:
-Shortness of breath, edema, fatigue, JVD, dyspnea on exertion, paroxysmal nocturnal dyspnea, unexplained weight gain, auscultatory rales or "crackles"
Patients with hypertension, CAD, previous MI, obesity, and diabetes are at increased risk for development of HF. These risk factors should heighten suspicion for possible CHF.

- Obtain Patient History
- Perform Physical Examination
- Perform EKG
- Order BNP test
- Order Chest X-Ray
- Order standard laboratory testing studies

Interpret BNP

Patient is asymptomatic

Patient is symptomatic

If BNP < 20 Symptoms are not likely due to CHF

If BNP ≥ 20 Consider MI, pulmonary embolism and pneumonia. If no suspicion of immediate life threatening disease, then

If BNP < 40 Symptoms are not likely due to CHF

BNP ≥40 and <400 Consider MI, pulmonary embolism and pneumonia. If no suspicion of immediate life-threatening disease, then

BNP ≥400 CHF is very likely

Consider other etiologies for patient presentation

Echocardiography; consider referral to a cardiologist for further work-up to screen for early LV dysfunction

Consider other etiologies for patient presentation

Echocardiography and strongly consider referral to a cardiologist for further work-up to screen for early LV dysfunction

Consider referral to the ED or hospital admission

FIGURE 12.1. Algorithm for using brain natriuretic peptide (BNP) testing in the primary care setting. CAD, coronary artery disease; CHF, congestive heart failure; ED, emergency department; EKG, electrocardiogram; HF, heart failure; JVD, jugular venous disten-sion; LV, left ventricular; MI, myocardial infarction. (Reprinted from Maisel A. The coming of age of natriuretic peptides: the emperor does have clothes! J Am Coll Cardiol 2006;47:61–64, with permission of the American College of Cardiology Foundation.)

12. Natriuretic Peptides

TABLE 12.1. Mechanisms of natriuretic peptide actions.

Increased urine output[10]
Increased urinary sodium excretion[14]
Relaxation of the vascular smooth muscle cells[10]
Antagonism of the renin-angiotensin-aldosterone system (decreased plasma renin activity, inhibition of aldosterone release)[14]
Antagonism of the sympathetic nervous system[10]
Antimitotic activity[10]
Lipolysis[15]

NT-pro-BNP were more sensitive than ANP in detecting LV systolic and diastolic dysfunctions and are presently used in the clinical setting. Significantly fewer data pertain to the role of C-type natriuretic peptide (CNP), which in contrast to ANP and BNP is produced primarily in vascular endothelium and less abundantly expressed in brain and kidney. C-type natriuretic peptide is vasoactive and involved in vascular remodeling. The levels of CNP are increased in heart failure but have no significant association with LV systolic function.[13] Table 12.1 summarizes the effects of upregulation of the natriuretic peptide system.

When measuring the levels of natriuretic peptides for diagnostic purposes, one should also bear in mind the mechanisms of their release other than heart failure. Table 12.2 summarizes the factors influencing the release of BNP and NT-pro-BNP.

Renal dysfunction can significantly alter the optimum cut-off level of BNP and NT-pro-BNP for diagnosis of heart failure, especially in the emergency setting. Data from the Augsburg MONICA register suggest that, in 469 randomly selected patients with a history of acute myocardial infarction, renal dysfunction was associated with more significant increases in the BNP and NT-pro-BNP levels, and the peptides levels were negatively correlated with glomerular filtration rate. Importantly, the adjustment of the BNP and NT-pro-BNP cut-off values used for detection of LV systolic dysfunction according to the presence of renal dysfunction increased the predictive power and specificity of both markers. Furthermore, in patients with renal impairment and no LV dysfunction, plasma levels of BNP and NT-pro-BNP may be elevated up to twofold the normal limit. Mild to moderate renal dysfunction seems to affect the levels of both markers to a comparable degree, whereas end-stage renal failure seems to be associated with a significant elevation of NT-pro-BNP.[32,33]

Another factor that influences the levels of BNP is obesity, probably by increased receptor-mediated uptake in the adipose tissue. In patients with heart failure the body mass index was independently negatively correlated with BNP levels. Obese patients with systolic LV dysfunction had 28%–40% lower levels of BNP than lean subjects with the same severity of heart failure, and 40% of obese patients had BNP levels below the cut-off value for diagnosis of heart failure.[15] This observation was also true for the general population of subjects without heart failure. As confirmed in a large population (n = 3,389) of participants in the Framingham Study, obese subjects had lower plasma levels of BNP and NT-pro-ANP than lean controls.[28]

TABLE 12.2. Factors that influence brain natriuretic peptide and N-terminal prohormone brain natriuretic peptide levels.

Cardiac factors
Acute coronary syndromes (increase/increased risk)[16]
Stable coronary artery disease with exercise-inducible ischemia (increase)[17]
Chronic mitral regurgitation (increase)[9]
Atrial fibrillation and ventricular arrhythmias (increase)[10,18]
Right ventricular overload (increase)[19]
Heart rate[10]
Aortic stenosis (increase)[20]
Amyloidosis with cardiac involvement (increase)[21]
Hypertrophic cardiomyopathy (increase)[22]
Factors affecting cardiac filing pressure (medications, sodium and water intake, posture)[10]
Treatment with anthracyclines (increase)[23]
Anemia in patients with diastolic heart failure (inverse correlation in males)[24]
Noncardiac factors
Age (positive correlation)[10,25–27]
Sex[25,26]
Obesity (inverse correlation)[15,28,29]
Chronic obstructive pulmonary disease (increase)[8]
Pulmonary embolism (increase)[8,30]
Acute respiratory distress syndrome (increase)[31]
Renal dysfunction (increase)[32,33]
Hypertension with left ventricular hypertrophy (increase)[34]
Metabolic syndrome (hyperinsulinemia, dyslipidemia, obesity) (inverse correlation)[34]
Genetic determinants[35]

A similar relationship between body mass index and NT-pro-BNP was found in the Dallas Heart Study.[29] Amino-terminal pro-BNP levels are also inversely correlated with obesity coexisting with dyslipidemia and hyperinsulinemia, so the definition of cut-off values, at least for diagnosis of asymptomatic LV dysfunction, may be problematic because of the high prevalence and various components of metabolic syndrome in the general population.[34] Definitions of normal values should be based on sex, age, and coexisting metabolic and clinical conditions rather than on uniform normal limits.[10] The presence of stable coronary artery disease with exercise-inducible ischemia, especially in patients with a history of myocardial infarction, may be associated with higher levels of BNP independent of LV dysfunction.[17] Therefore, caution is recommended when using BNP levels to diagnose asymptomatic diastolic dysfunction based on moderately increased BNP levels in patients with known coronary artery disease.

Choice of Natriuretic Peptide in the Clinical Setting

There is agreement that BNP and NT-pro-BNP have comparably high diagnostic accuracies and negative prognostic values in decompensated heart failure and asymptomatic LV systolic dysfunction and are superior to measurements of other natriuretic peptides. It seems true also for diastolic dysfunction based on a prospective comparison of c-ANP, N-ANP, and BNP, which showed that BNP is superior to ANP in the detection of diastolic dysfunction and was validated by echocardiography and cardiac catheterization, at least in a population with a high prevalence of LV dysfunction.[11] The clinical utility of BNP measurement is more evident in the setting of symptomatic diastolic dysfunction, because the symptoms of heart failure are associated with increased LV filling pressure, which is a pivotal stimulus for BNP release. Diastolic dysfunction associated with dyspnea on exertion is in most cases due to impaired relaxation that may not lead to a significant increase in LV filling pressure at rest, and therefore the BNP may be a suboptimal diagnostic tool in this setting.[2]

Diastolic Dysfunction in the General Population

Lubien et al.[36] studied BNP levels in 294 patients referred for echocardiographic evaluation of LV function and focused on 119 cases of diastolic dysfunction and three altered filling patterns: impaired relaxation, pseudonormalization, and restrictive-like filling. The BNP levels were significantly higher in patients with diastolic dysfunction than in controls (286 vs. 33 pg/mL). There was an incremental rise in BNP levels with increasing severity of diastolic dysfunction. Patients with impaired relaxation had the smallest, those with the restrictive-like filling pattern had the greatest, and those with pseudonormalization had intermediate relative increases in BNP. Moreover, symptomatic patients had higher BNP levels than asymptomatic patients in all three subgroups. The BNP levels were significantly higher in patients with diastolic dysfunction and no history of heart failure than in asymptomatic patients with normal diastolic function (263 vs. 33 pg/mL). The BNP levels increased most significantly in patients with an E/A ratio >1.5 and deceleration time less than 160 s. Receiver operating characteristic (ROC) analysis revealed that an AUC of 0.91 characterized the ability of BNP measurement to detect diastolic dysfunction in patients with normal LVEF (>50%) and absence of any segmental wall motion abnormalities. The test's accuracy was highest when used to diagnose restrictive filling pattern (AUC 0.98), but was insufficient for differentiation between the three forms of diastolic dysfunction. In the logistic regression model, BNP at a relatively low cut-off level of 62 pg/mL was an independent predictor of diastolic dysfunction (OR 26.8 [95% CI] 12.5–57.4).[36]

A community-based study carried out in Olmsted County, Minnesota, with 2,042 randomly selected residents evaluated the incidence of asymptomatic systolic and diastolic dysfunction and revealed that 24.6% of the screened population had various degrees of diastolic dysfunction. When the high-risk subgroup was identified by the presence of cardiovascular disease and age ≥65 years, the incidence of diastolic dysfunction was substantially higher, reaching 52% (36% had mild and 16% moderate to severe diastolic dysfunction). The study confirmed in a large population the previously published observations that plasma BNP levels increase in subjects with any form of diastolic dysfunction and correlate with its severity (r = 0.38) in a whole population with normal systolic function as well as in subgroups (males [r = 0.35], females [r = 0.29], aged <65 years [r = 0.098] and ≥65 years [r = 0.28]; all respective *p* values significant). The ROC AUC for detection of any preclinical LV dysfunction (systolic and moderate to severe diastolic) in the whole screened cohort was 0.79 and 0.73–0.74 for females and males, respectively, with a BNP cut-off level o 25.9 pg/mL for the detection of moderate to severe LV diastolic dysfunction. This study, carried out in a relatively large general population, sheds some light on the performance of BNP testing as a screening tool for detection of asymptomatic diastolic dysfunction. It proved to be suboptimal in diagnosing moderate diastolic dysfunction (AUC <0.70). The highest discriminatory efficiency of BNP testing to diagnose moderate or severe diastolic dysfunction was confined to the group of subjects aged ≥65 years in the general population and to high-risk populations. Given the results of the ROC analysis, the use of BNP cut-off values based on a ROC curve as a screening test would be associated with 29%–38.8% of screened patients requiring echocardiography for definite diagnosis. When the age- and sex-adjusted upper normal levels are employed, fewer screened patients would be referred for echocardiography (10%–34%), but, on the other hand, 41%–61% of patients with moderate to severe diastolic function would be missed. Therefore, BNP measurement is not particularly useful for screening asymptomatic patients to detect preclinical diastolic dysfunction. This study also shows that for asymptomatic subjects with a lesser degree of diastolic impairment, which is associated with substantially increased mortality and morbidity, BNP testing has very low accuracy to detect the dysfunction, questioning the usefulness of this approach. On the other hand, for patients with exertional dyspnea, assessment of BNP following an exercise test that can induce an increase in LV filling pressure seems reasonable given the strong correlation between these parameters.[1,2,37]

A subgroup of participants in the international WHO MONICA epidemiologic program recruited in the MONICA Augsburg study was screened for associations between asymptomatic diastolic dysfunction and plasma BNP levels.[38] The echocardiography carried out in 1,678 subjects (827 males and 851 females) aged 27–75 years revealed abnormalities in LV diastolic function; however, neither clinical signs nor symptoms of heart failure were present in this randomly selected age-stratified cohort. In this population free from symptoms of heart failure, the prevalence of diastolic dysfunction was 3.3%. The mean plasma levels of BNP were significantly higher in subjects with diastolic dysfunction (median 12 pg/mL) than in the control population (median 6.2 pg/mL) but lower than in subjects with systolic dysfunction defined as LVEF <45% (median 19.9 pg/mL). Importantly, the BNP levels were higher in subjects with diastolic dysfunction coexisting with LV hypertrophy than in both controls and patients with diastolic dysfunction without hypertrophy, who had BNP levels comparable with controls. The following parameters showed significant correlations with BNP levels: age, body mass index, systolic blood pressure, LV mass index, LVEF, left atrial size, and diastolic dysfunction. However, only age, body mass index, LV mass index, and LVEF were independent predictors of plasma BNP levels.

The ROC analysis revealed that random BNP sampling had acceptable specificity and sensitivity only in subjects with diastolic dysfunction and LV hypertrophy (AUC with 95% CI 0.82 [0.71–0.93]; specificity, 85.7%, sensitivity, 73.3%; and a cut-off value of 12.8 pg/mL) but was suboptimal in subjects without LV hypertrophy (0.63 [0.55–0.72]; specificity, 60.5%; sensitivity, 54.5%). Interestingly, because of the high negative predictive value (97.6% for diastolic dysfunction and 99.9% for diastolic dysfunction coexisting with LV hypertrophy), the BNP levels below the cut-off value can be used to rule out both conditions with a high level of probability. The BNP cut-off value for diastolic dysfunction with LV hypertrophy was very close to the value for LV hypertrophy without diastolic dysfunction, again suggesting that random BNP sampling in the asymptomatic general population is not an optimal screening diagnostic tool for identification of subjects with isolated diastolic dysfunction.[38]

Performance of BNP testing as a part of community screening to detect diastolic dysfunction is largely dependent on the prevalence of this condition in a given population. The patients referred for screening are preselected based on the assessment of clinical risk factors and other factors that can influence the BNP results (e.g., obesity).[3,10]

Diastolic Heart Failure

The study of Tschope et al.,[39] which compared 68 subjects with diastolic dysfunction and symptoms of heart failure (New York Heart Association [NYHA] classes I to III) to 50 controls, included a comprehensive search for diastolic dysfunction, including left and right cardiac catheterization, echocardiography and bicycle ergometry. Subjects with diastolic dysfunction and normal LVEF ($\geq$50%) had significantly higher levels of plasma NT-pro-BNP levels (mean 189.5 pg/mL) than controls without diastolic abnormalities (51.8 pg/mL). Amino terminal pro-BNP concentration correlated with the severity of diastolic abnormalities (Spearman's r = 0.67), being lowest in subjects with impaired relaxation, increased in pseudonormal filling, and highest in subjects with a restrictive filling pattern. Levels of NT-pro-BNP were positively correlated with NYHA class (Spearman's r = 0.48). The ROC analyses of the accuracy of NT-pro-BNP to diagnose isolated diastolic dysfunction revealed that this parameter was more reliable than E/A ratio and tissue Doppler imaging and only marginally less accurate than LV end-diastolic pressure measured during cardiac catheterization (AUC for NT-pro-BNP, 0.83; for LV end-diastolic pressure, 0.84; and for tissue Doppler imaging and E/A ratio, 0.81). The diagnostic utility of NT-pro-BNP to diagnose isolated diastolic dysfunction in this population is further confirmed by its high negative predictive value of 93%–94% for the cut-off level of 110–120 pg/mL, which is close to the values of the invasive measurements (LV end-diastolic pressure, pulmonary capillary wedge pressure at rest and after exercise, time constant of LV pressure decay [tau], and dP/dt$_{min}$) and echocardiographic parameters (E/A ratio, E′/A′ ratio, and isovolumetric relaxation time). For this cut-off value, the specificity and sensitivity of NT-pro-BNP levels were 72% and 90%, respectively. There were significant although at best moderate correlations between NT-pro-BNP levels determined with invasive measurements (LV end-diastolic pressure, dP/dt$_{min}$, pulmonary capillary wedge pressure at rest and after exercise) and those determined with echocardiography (E′/A′). In a multivariable regression analysis including such variables as sex, age, dyspnea, diabetes, hypertension, LV mass index, coronary artery disease, and body mass index, NT-pro-BNP level was the only independent predictor of diastolic dysfunction (OR 1.2 [1.1–1.4]). In contrast to asymptomatic subjects in the general population, the utility of NT-pro-BNP levels to detect diastolic dysfunction was independent of LV mass index.[38,39]

Some data pertaining to the role of natriuretic peptides were derived from a population of subjects with newly diagnosed heart failure and normal LVEF assessed in rapid access heart failure clinics in London. The diagnosis of diastolic dysfunction was based on the presence of symptoms suggestive of heart failure according to European Society of Cardiology (ESC) Guidelines, an LVEF $\geq$45%, and the results of an echocardiographic examination that included assessment of the E/A ratio (<1.0 in subjects <50 years and <0.5 in subjects >50 years), E wave deceleration time (Ed) (>220 ms in subjects <50 years and >280 ms in subjects >50 years), and isovolumic relaxation time (>100 ms in subjects <50 years and >105 ms in subjects >50 years). The BNP levels measured using point-of-care assay revealed significantly higher plasma levels in patients with heart failure and diastolic abnormalities than in subjects without heart failure (101 vs. 54 pg/mL) but markedly lower than in patients with systolic LV dysfunction (539 pg/mL).[40]

Diastolic Heart Failure and Hypertension

Hypertension is associated with an increased risk of DHF, which may be associated with frequent occurrence of LV hypertrophy in hypertensive subjects. On the other hand, cardiomyocyte hypertrophy is an established stimulus for the release of natriuretic peptides. Therefore, it would be reasonable to expect elevated levels of natriuretic peptides in patients with DHF coexisting with hypertension and LV hypertrophy.[10]

Yamaguchi et al.[41] investigated the changes in the plasma ANP and BNP levels in a population of patients with a history of acute decompensa-

12. Natriuretic Peptides

tion of heart failure due to LV diastolic dysfunction at least 1 year prior to enrollment. The study included only stable patients in NYHA classes I to III and no acute coronary syndromes at the time of blood sampling. In patients with DHF the plasma levels of ANP and BNP were significantly elevated, but in subjects in NYHA class I only BNP levels were significantly higher than in the control group consisting of patients with hypertension and no symptoms of heart failure (96 vs. 31 pg/mL). Comparison of patients with hypertension and LV hypertrophy with and without DHF yielded interesting results. The indices of LV remodeling and hypertrophy (end-systolic dimension, end-diastolic dimension, thickness of interventricular septum and LV posterior wall, LV mass index) were comparable in both groups; therefore, variations in BNP levels could not be attributed to LV hypertrophy alone.[41] The plasma ANP levels were elevated in the DHF group. Left atrial enlargement was also more frequent in these patients, which can explain the increase, because atria are the main source of circulating ANP. The principal finding from this study is that the BNP levels are elevated in patients with a history of pulmonary edema regardless of LV hypertrophy, even in subjects in NYHA class I.[41]

Decompensated Diastolic Heart Failure

A large cohort of 1,586 patients with shortness of breath was enrolled into a multinational Breathing Not Properly study that analyzed the presence of DHF. Diastolic dysfunction was diagnosed in 165 patients (36.5% of patients with established diagnosis of heart failure) using echocardiography performed 30 days after initial presentation. The median BNP levels at the time of emergency admission were significantly elevated in patients with heart failure and normal systolic function compared with patients whose dyspnea was due to causes other than heart failure (413 vs. 34 pg/mL) but lower than in patients with heart failure associated with LV systolic dysfunction (821 pg/mL).[5]

In this large cohort of patients presenting to an emergency department with shortness of breath, the measurement of BNP levels in the acute setting had excellent accuracy in differentiating between non–heart failure patients and patients with both systolic and diastolic heart failure (ROC analysis; AUC = 0.90 with 90% sensitivity for the cut-off value of 100 pg/mL, accuracy 81%). The BNP measurements were unable to differentiate between systolic heart failure (SHF) and heart failure with normal systolic function (AUC = 0.66). A significant overlap was noted for the given cut-off level with a vast majority of patients with normal systolic function having BNP levels above 100 pg/mL. In this study, the sensitivity for detecting SHF was 95%, but the specificity for DHF was only 14%. Even for incremental cut-off values of 200, 300, and 400 pg/mL, the accuracy of differentiation between SHF and DHF was low (65%–67%), and the specificity for detecting DHF did not exceed 50% (27%–50%).

On the other hand, BNP measurement combined with echocardiography is a much more attractive tool in the emergency setting, especially to rule out the DHF as a reason for dyspnea. The negative predictive value in patients with normal LVEF was 96% for BNP levels <100 pg/mL.[5]

In acutely decompensated heart failure, the principal mechanism responsible for symptoms is elevation of LV filling pressure, regardless of the type of heart failure, so a considerable overlap between the levels of BNP in both DHF and SHF is easy to explain.[42] Available evidence shows that BNP/NT-pro-BNP testing is a useful and cost-effective diagnostic tool to assess patients with acute dyspnea. Both BNP and NT-pro-BNP tests have high negative predictive values and acceptable sensitivities and can improve the patients' triage, speed up the initiation of appropriate treatment, and perhaps save costs by preventing unnecessary hospitalizations.[10]

Combined Diastolic and Systolic Heart Failure

There is significant variability among plasma BNP and NT-pro-BNP levels in patients with SHF. One of the reasons may be DHF coexisting with systolic dysfunction. As observed in isolated diastolic dysfunction, the BNP levels increase significantly in patients with compensated (NYHA classes I

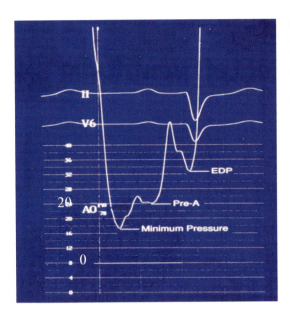

FIGURE 13.1. Left ventricular pressure recording from a patient with hypertrophic cardiomyopathy. Notice the increased left ventricular diastolic pressures and the steep rise in left ventricular pressure with left atrial contraction. EDP, end-diastolic pressure. (Reprinted from Nagueh et al.,[48] with permission of the American Heart Association.)

pressure. The diastolic LV pressure prior to left atrial contraction is referred to as "pre-A" LV pressure and can be used as a surrogate of mean left atrial pressure. Late diastolic LV pressures include the "A wave rise" that occurs after left atrial contraction and the most frequently reported end-diastolic pressure. In addition to the above LV diastolic pressures, it is possible to measure "mean LV diastolic pressure" with high fidelity pressure catheters. If available, mean LV diastolic pressure can also be used as a surrogate of mean left atrial pressure.[5]

When LV diastolic function is reduced, LV late diastolic pressures are frequently the earliest pressure recordings to become abnormally elevated. Later, mean left atrial pressure and its surrogates become elevated. It is therefore important to identify the echo-Doppler correlates of each subset of pressures. Furthermore, the presence of a normal left atrial pressure, whether by direct invasive measurement or noninvasive prediction, should not be used to infer normal diastolic function. In fact, the presence and severity of diastolic dysfunction can be reliably identified through exercise measurements of pressures, whether by invasive or noninvasive methods.[6]

Mitral Inflow

Flow across the mitral valve is primarily influenced by the transmitral pressure gradient.[7] The higher the gradient, the higher the flow rate and Doppler velocities. In the presence of normal LV relaxation, an early diastolic positive left atrial to LV pressure gradient exists because of low LV minimal pressure (for a Doppler recording of mitral inflow, see Figure 13.2). However, with reduced LV relaxation rate, flow can be maintained only with increased left atrial pressure. Therefore, an increased transmitral early diastolic or E velocity is indicative of increased left atrial pressure in the presence of myocardial disease.

In late diastole, another positive left atrial–LV pressure gradient develops because of left atrial contraction resulting in late diastolic or A velocity. The latter velocity is dependent on left atrial systolic function and left atrial preload and afterload. A higher preload results in an increased A velocity, as in patients with impaired LV relaxation and normal left atrial pressure, where the reduced early diastolic flow leads to reduced left atrial emptying in early diastole and an increase in left atrial volume prior to its contraction. On

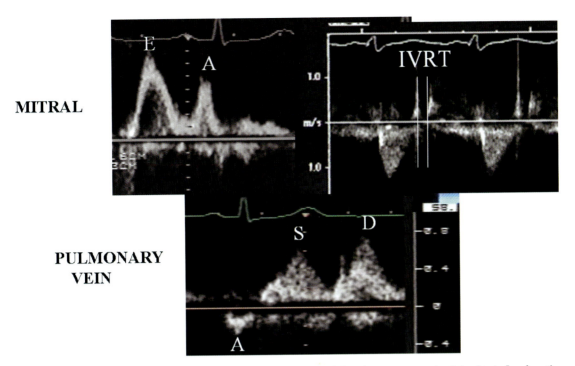

FIGURE 13.2. Doppler recording of mitral inflow (top), isovolumic relaxation time (recorded with continuous wave Doppler by placing the sample volume midway between the left ventricular outflow tract and the mitral valve tips) and pulmonary venous flow (bottom). In pulmonary venous signal, A refers to flow from the left atrium to the pulmonary veins due to left atrial contraction. A, mitral late diastolic velocity; D, diastolic velocity; E, mitral peak early diastolic velocity; S systolic velocity.

the other hand, an increase in late diastolic LV pressure, which determines left atrial afterload, results in a reduced peak A velocity as well as shorter duration and shorter deceleration time.[8]

In summary, with impaired LV relaxation, the E/A ratio is reduced and the rate of rise of the E velocity is reduced, which can be measured as a prolonged acceleration time and a reduced acceleration rate. Likewise, with impaired LV relaxation and normal left atrial pressure, the decay of the E velocity is prolonged and can be measured as a prolonged deceleration time and a decreased deceleration rate. As left atrial pressure increases, the E/A ratio approaches 1 along with shorter acceleration time and deceleration time intervals. A further increase in left atrial pressure results in an even higher E/A ratio, which can exceed 2 with steep acceleration and deceleration rates and very short deceleration times (≤160 ms). This is the "restrictive LV filling pattern" and is predictive of highly increased left atrial pressure, often >25 mm Hg. Several studies have now confirmed the reduced survival of patients with congestive heart failure and depressed EF who continue to have restrictive LV filling despite adequate medical therapy or manipulations to decrease LV preload.[9,10]

The application of mitral E and A velocities for the estimation of LV filling pressures is most reliable in the presence of LV systolic dysfunction and depressed EF.[11,12] In the presence of normal EF, additional Doppler data are needed, as discussed later. Furthermore, there are diagnostic and therapeutic implications to the preload-dependent nature of transmitral velocities. From a diagnostic perspective, a pseudonormal mitral inflow pattern can be uncovered during the strain phase of the Valsalva maneuver as the rise in intrathoracic pressure leads to decreased venous return and a decline in left atrial pressure and therefore an impaired relaxation pattern.[11] From a therapeutic perspective, changes in mitral inflow velocities can be used to track changes in LV filling in response to therapy for congestive heart failure (Figure 13.3).

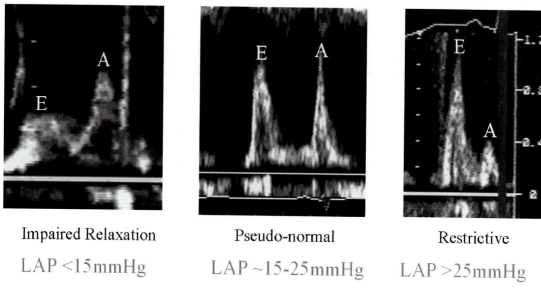

FIGURE 13.3. Effect of changes in left atrial pressure on mitral inflow velocities. (**Left**) Impaired relaxation. (**Right**) Pseudonormal.

Pulmonary Venous Flow

Flow from the pulmonary veins into the left atrium follows the pressure gradient between the two. In early systole, a lower left atrial pressure is present due to left atrial relaxation, which results in an S1 wave. This signal is most reliably recorded by transesophageal echocardiography. Later, another systolic wave is recorded, S2, which appears related to right ventricular contraction leading to a rise in pulmonary vein pressure[13] and mitral annular descent leading to a lower left atrial pressure. Antegrade flow into the left atrium occurs also in diastole because of a decrease in left atrial pressure with left atrial emptying (see Figure 13.2). Therefore, in the presence of impaired LV relaxation, the reduced diastolic emptying of the left atrium leads to predominant left atrial filling in systole. It is possible to express the relation between systolic and diastolic pulmonary venous flow in several ways, namely, the ratio of peak systolic velocity to peak diastolic velocity, the ratio of systolic time velocity integral (TVI) to diastolic TVI, and systolic filling fraction where systolic TVI is divided by total antegrade flow TVI (the sum of systolic and diastolic TVI). An increase in left atrial pressure leads to predominant diastolic left atrial filling or reduced systolic filling fraction.[14]

Another measurement obtained from pulmonary venous diastolic flow is the deceleration time of the diastolic velocity. This time interval is related to left atrial compliance and left atrial pressure, such that an increase in left atrial pressure is associated with a short deceleration time. Some studies have shown the utility of this approach for patients undergoing cardiac surgery[15] and in the setting of myocardial infarction.[16] In other studies, deceleration time of pulmonary venous diastolic velocity was of value only in patients with depressed EF[12] and no significant mitral valve pathology.

An atrial reversal or Ar signal is frequently recorded from the pulmonary veins (>70% in the outpatient setting) that can provide important insights into left atrial systolic function and LV late diastolic pressures. The Ar flow is caused by a higher left atrial pressure in comparison with pulmonary venous pressure. In the presence of normal left atrial contractility and increased LV end-diastolic pressure, atrial contraction leads to an increased velocity (>30 cm/s) with a prolonged duration. The Ar prolonged duration is readily apparent when compared with the transmitral A duration and a difference of >35 ms is a reliable indicator of increased LV end-diastolic pressure (Figure 13.4) irrespective of LVEF.[12,17–19]

13. Left Ventricular Filling Pressures

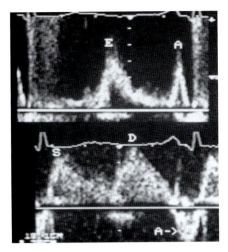

PV-Ad = 170ms
MV-Ad = 120ms

FIGURE 13.4. Mitral inflow (**top**) and pulmonary venous flow (**bottom**) from a patient with increased left ventricular end-diastolic pressure. Note the prolonged duration of pulmonary venous A compared with the mitral A duration.

Isovolumic Relaxation Time

Isovolumic relaxation time (IVRT) refers to the time interval between aortic valve closure and mitral valve opening. It was recorded by a combination of phonocardiography and M-mode echocardiography[20,21] prior to the introduction of Doppler technology. Currently, IVRT is usually recorded by pulse wave or continuous wave Doppler by placing a sample volume between the mitral valve leaflets and the LV outflow tract in an apical long or apical five-chamber view. In our experience, IVRT by continuous wave Doppler is the more reliable and reproducible signal (see Figure 13.2). Isovolumic relaxation time is dependent on left atrial pressure, LV end-systolic pressure, and rate of LV relaxation. An increase in LV systolic pressure and/or a slowed rate of LV relaxation results in a prolonged IVRT, whereas an increase in left atrial pressure has the opposite effect. The complete relation can be expressed as: LA pressure = LV end-systolic pressure $\times$ $e^{-IVRT/\tau}$, where τ is the time constant of LV relaxation.[22] Although IVRT has been used to predict filling pressures in multiple regression models, particularly in patients with depressed EF,[23,24] it is possible to combine IVRT with preload-independent Doppler indices of LV relaxation to predict LV filling pressures (see later). Therefore, it is advantageous to routinely acquire IVRT as part of the comprehensive Doppler examination of patients referred for echocardiographic evaluation of LV diastolic function.

New Indices of Left Ventricular Relaxation for Prediction of Left Ventricular Filling Pressures

Early Diastolic Flow Propagation Velocity by Color M-Mode Echocardiography

Because of its high temporal and spatial resolution, color M-mode echocardiography is used to record early diastolic flow propagation velocity (Vp). Studies in animals and patients[25] have suggested that Vp is preload independent and as such can be primarily used as a measurement of LV relaxation.[25-28] Furthermore, combining it with transmitral E velocity to correct for the influence of LV relaxation on mitral E can be used to predict LV filling pressures such that E/Vp is directly proportional to left atrial pressure.[29] Later studies revealed that Vp is load dependent in patients with both normal[30] and depressed[31] EF. Furthermore, Vp appears to have a stronger relation with LV end-systolic volume than with LV relaxation,[32] and a number of patients with normal EF and LV volumes but with impaired LV relaxation can have a normal Vp. Therefore, caution should be exercised when using the ratio of E to Vp for the prediction of LV filling pressures in patients with normal EF. On the other hand, this ratio can be helpful for patients with depressed EF.[12]

Early Diastolic Mitral Annulus Velocity by Tissue Doppler Echocardiography

Early diastolic mitral annulus velocity (Ea) can be recorded as peak (by pulse Doppler echocardiography) or mean (by two-dimensional color Doppler echocardiography) velocity using tissue Doppler imaging of the mitral annulus. Early diastolic mitral annulus velocity has been shown in a number of studies to behave as an index of LV relaxation. It decreases with age,[33,34] has a significant relation with LV relaxation in animal[35,36] and

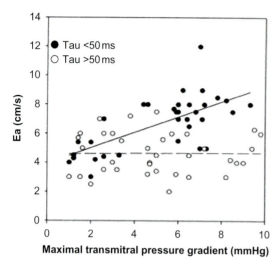

FIGURE 13.5. Relation between transmitral pressure gradient and mitral annulus Ea velocity with data divided according to tau. Note the direct relation with normal or enhanced left ventricular relaxation and the lack of a significant relation with prolonged tau. (Reprinted from Nagueh et al.,[35] with permission of the American College of Cardiology Foundation.)

related to LV filling pressure and the transmitral pressure gradient (Figure 13.5) as shown in animal[35,36,42] and human[43] studies. However, in the presence of impaired LV relaxation, filling pressures have a minimal effect on Ea.[35,36,42] Accordingly, the E/Ea ratio (Figures 13.6 and 13.7) has been successfully used for the estimation of LV filling pressures[34,39,44] in the presence of cardiac disease whether EF was normal or depressed, in the presence of sinus tachycardia[45] or atrial fibrillation,[46] in cardiac transplant patients,[47] and in patients with hypertrophic cardiomyopathy.[48] Figures 13.8 and 13.9 show examples of the E/Ea ratio being used for the estimation of LV filling pressures. Some researchers used septal Ea,[37,39] whereas we and others have used lateral Ea or an average of Ea recorded at septal, lateral, anterior, and inferior mitral annular areas. In our experience, an average of septal and lateral Ea is superior to either alone in the presence of regional dysfunction,[12,49] whereas either septal or lateral Ea may be used in idiopathic dilated cardiomyopathy.[12]

human[37–39] studies and is related to β-adrenergic receptor density,[40] extent of interstitial fibrosis,[40] and local myocardial cytokine levels.[41] Its relation with LV filling pressures is more complicated. In the presence of normal LV relaxation, Ea is directly

From a practical point, when Ea velocities are measured, one should utilize pulsed wave Doppler, because this was the modality applied in the validation studies. Also, different cut-off values of E/Ea should be applied based on LVEF and

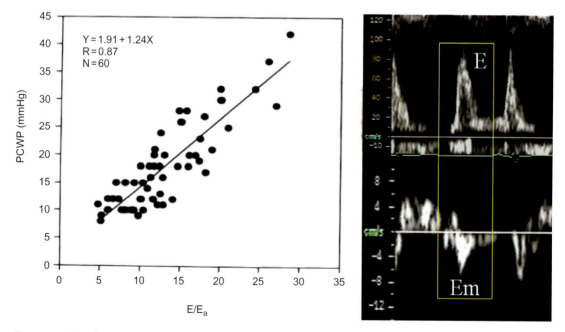

FIGURE 13.6. Plot of correlation between mean wedge pressure and E/Ea (or Em) ratio. (Reprinted from Nagueh et al.,[34] with permission of the American College of Cardiology Foundation.)

13. Left Ventricular Filling Pressures

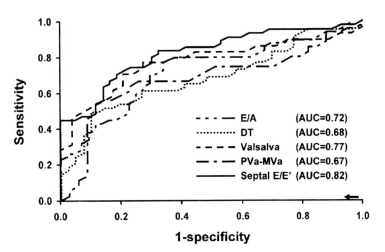

FIGURE 13.7. Receiver operating characteristic curve showing the accuracy of the E/Ea ratio in identifying elevated left ventricular mean diastolic pressure. Note that the septal E/Ea ratio has the largest area. DT, deceleration time. PVa-MVa refers to the difference in the duration between pulmonary venous A velocity and mitral A velocity. (From Ommen et al.[39])

whether one is using septal, lateral, or average Ea.[12] In general, a ratio of >15 is reliably associated with a left atrial pressure of >15 mm Hg, whereas a ratio of <8 is associated with a normal left atrial pressure.[39] In the range between 8 and 15, other parameters are needed to verify the status of left atrial pressure. Limitations of the E/Ea ratio include mitral valve diseases such as moderate to severe mitral annular calcification and constrictive pericarditis.[50]

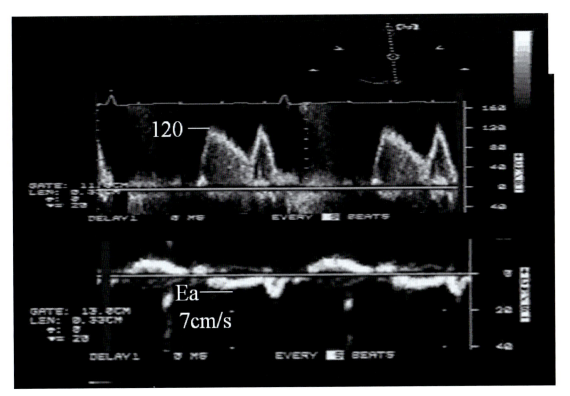

FIGURE 13.8. An example of the cardiac etiology of dyspnea. Mitral inflow and Tissue Doppler (TD) velocities from a 53-year-old patient with hypertension and shortness of breath. Note the reduced Ea velocity and the increased E/Ea ratio of 17.

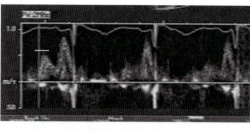

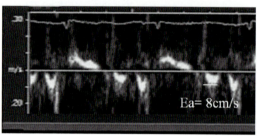

$E/Ea = 55/8$
$= 6.9$

$Ea = 8 cm/s$

FIGURE 13.9. An example of a noncardiac etiology of dyspnea. Mitral inflow and TD velocities from a 70-year-old patient with obstructive airway disease. Note that the Ea velocity is reduced appropriately for age and the E/Ea ratio is 6.9, which is indicative of normal/reduced filling pressures.

Timing the onset of Ea can provide yet another Doppler measurement of LV relaxation. With impaired LV relaxation, Ea velocity is not only reduced but also delayed. This becomes particularly apparent when compared with the onset of mitral E velocity. In normal hearts, E and Ea can occur simultaneously, and Ea can even precede mitral E velocity. As LV relaxation is impaired, Ea is delayed in comparison with mitral E and the time interval E–Ea has been shown in animal[42,51] and human[51] studies to have a strong relation with LV relaxation (Figure 13.10). Furthermore, when combined with IVRT and LV end-systolic pressure (derived noninvasively as $0.9 \times$ systolic blood pressure by sphygmomanometer cuff), it can be used to estimate mean left atrial pressure[51] with the equation: left atrial pressure = $LV_{\text{end-systolic pressure}} \times e^{-IVRT/(T_{E-Ea})}$, where T_{E-Ea} is used as a surrogate of the time constant of LV relaxation. Alternatively, tau can be derived using the regression equation[51] tau = $32 + 0.7$ (T_{E-Ea}).

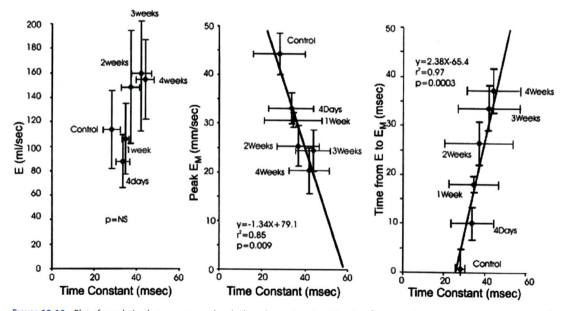

FIGURE 13.10. Plot of correlation between tau and early diastolic transmitral flow rate **(left)**, peak E_M velocity **(middle)**, and time from E to E_M **(right)**. The highest correlation was between tau and time from E to E_M ($r^2 = 0.97$). (Reprinted from Hasegawa et al.,[42] with permission of the American College of Cardiology Foundation.)

Other Echocardiographic Correlates of Left Ventricular Filling Pressures

Useful clues about LV filling pressures can be gleaned from two-dimensional echocardiography. For example, in the presence of pathologic LV hypertrophy, the expected mitral inflow pattern in the presence of a normal left atrial pressure is one of impaired relaxation. Therefore, a pseudonormal or restrictive filling pattern is indicative in and of itself of increased left atrial pressure.

Left atrial volume is another important two-dimensional measurement. In the absence of atrial dysrhythmia and mitral valve disease, LV diastolic dysfunction via increased left atrial pressure leads to left atrial dilatation.[52] A number of left atrial volumes can be measured, including maximal volume (at end systole), minimal volume (at end diastole), and emptying volume (the difference between maximal and minimal volumes). Because there is minimal incremental information in left atrial minimal volume and left atrial emptying volume over left atrial maximal volume for the purpose of predicting LV filling pressures, only left atrial maximal volume measurement is usually needed. In that regard, left atrial anteroposterior diameter measurement is inadequate, because an increased left atrial volume can be associated with only a minimal change in left atrial anteroposterior dimension.

Patients with LV diastolic dysfunction and pulmonary congestion symptoms usually have increased pulmonary arterial pressures. Therefore, the presence of increased pulmonary arterial systolic and/or diastolic pressure in the absence of pulmonary parenchymal and vascular disease can be used to infer that LV filling pressures are increased. Pulmonary arterial systolic pressure can be derived using the tricuspid regurgitation jet, and pulmonary arterial diastolic pressure can be derived using the pulmonary regurgitation jet.[53] Pulmonary arterial systolic pressure is estimated as 4 (peak tricuspid regurgitation jet velocity by continuous wave in m/s)^2 + right atrial pressure. Pulmonary arterial diastolic pressure is estimated as 4 (end-diastolic pulmonary regurgitation jet velocity by continuous wave in m/s)^2 + right atrial pressure (Figure 13.11). Right atrial pressure can in turn be estimated using inferior

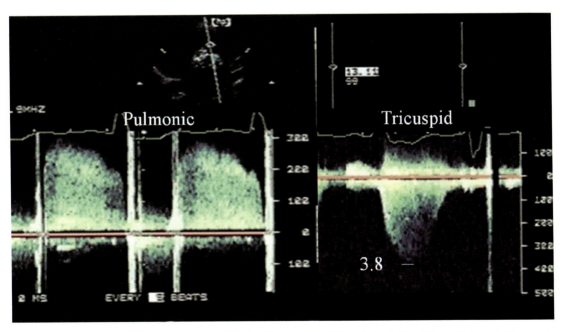

FIGURE 13.11. Example of pulmonary regurgitation and tricuspid regurgitation jets for the estimation of pulmonary arterial diastolic pressure (end-diastolic velocity approximately 2 m/s) and pulmonary arterial systolic (peak tricuspid regurgitation velocity approximately 3.8 m/s) pressure, respectively.

vena caval diameter and its change with respiration as well as hepatic venous flow.

Mitral and aortic regurgitation signals by continuous wave Doppler can be used for the estimation of left atrial pressure and LV end-diastolic pressure, respectively, provided proper alignment is feasible and no or minimal angulation (<20°) is present.[54] Left atrial pressure can be estimated as left atrial pressure = systolic blood pressure — 4 (peak velocity of mitral regurgitation jet by continuous wave Doppler in m/s)^2. Left ventricular end-diastolic pressure is estimated as aortic diastolic pressure — 4 (end-diastolic velocity of aortic regurgitation jet by continuous wave Doppler in m/s)^2.

Problems with the latter approach include angulation between Doppler beam and regurgitant jets, leading to an underestimation of velocity and an overestimation of filling pressures. In addition, peripheral blood pressure recordings may not be an accurate reflection of central aortic and LV systolic pressures. Therefore, mitral and aortic regurgitation jets should be used in conjunction with other Doppler measurements as discussed earlier.

Estimation of Left Ventricular Filling Pressures According to Left Ventricular Ejection Fraction

As outlined earlier, in patients with depressed EF, mitral and pulmonary venous flow Doppler signals are reasonably accurate without the need for additional flow velocity measurements. However, when EF is normal in the presence of cardiac disease, only the Ar–A duration remains clinically useful. In this subgroup, the E/Ea ratio remains somewhat helpful but with lower cut-off values than for patients with depressed EF.[12] In our experience, E/Vp is not useful in this population; however, inferences drawn from left atrial volume and pulmonary arterial pressures remain valid.

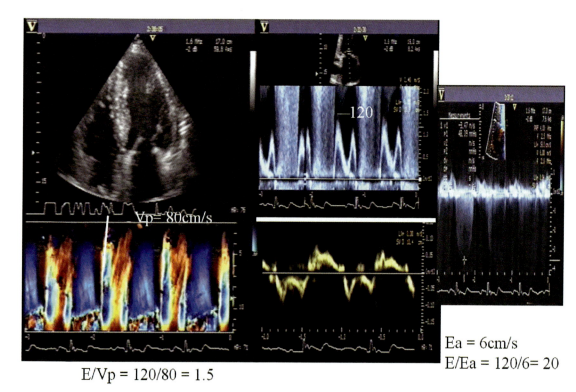

FIGURE 13.12. Mitral inflow, propagation velocity (Vp), and tricuspid regurgitation jet from a patient with exertional dyspnea and normal ejection fraction. Note the normal Vp velocity and the borderline ratio of E/Vp. However, the enlarged left atrium, the increased E/Ea ratio, and the increased peak velocity of the tricuspid regurgitation jet (3.5 m/s) are all indicative of increased filling pressures.

Figure 13.12 illustrates a case with normal EF and increased filling pressures in which the E/Vp ratio was of borderline value, whereas the E/Ea ratio and the peak velocity of the tricuspid regurgitation jet were both indicative of increased filling pressures.

Doppler Estimation of Filling Pressures in Sinus Tachycardia

In sinus tachycardia, many of the principles discussed earlier still hold. However, the merging of mitral E and A velocities represents a challenge. We have identified three patterns of mitral inflow (Figure 13.13) that can serve as a useful starting point in the exercise of predicting LV filling pressures, taking into account LVEF. In particular, pattern C is usually associated with increased filling pressures, whereas pattern B can be associated with normal filling pressures. However, the most accurate prediction is reached when annular Ea velocity is measured (see Figure 13.13) and the E/Ea ratio is used.[45] Worth noting is that in situations in which there is complete merging of mitral E and A velocities, it is still possible to detect a distinct annular Ea and to use the E/Ea ratio.[45,55]

Doppler Estimation of Filling Pressures in Atrial Fibrillation

Atrial fibrillation poses a frequent and important challenge to the Doppler methodology. Because of atrial fibrillation, mitral A and pulmonary venous Ar velocities are not present. Likewise, left atrial volumes and pulmonary venous systolic filling fraction have limited roles. In addition, one has to deal with the effect of varying cycle lengths on the Doppler measurements. Despite these limitations, it is still possible to apply some of the principles discussed. With depressed EF, the deceleration time of the mitral diastolic velocity can provide accurate information quite similar to that obtained in patients in sinus rhythm,[56,57] where a shorter deceleration time is associated with increased

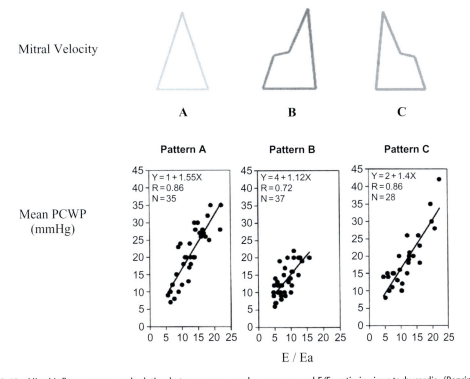

FIGURE 13.13. Mitral inflow patterns and relation between mean wedge pressure and E/Ea ratio in sinus tachycardia. (Reprinted from Nagueh et al.,[45] with permission of the American Heart Association.)

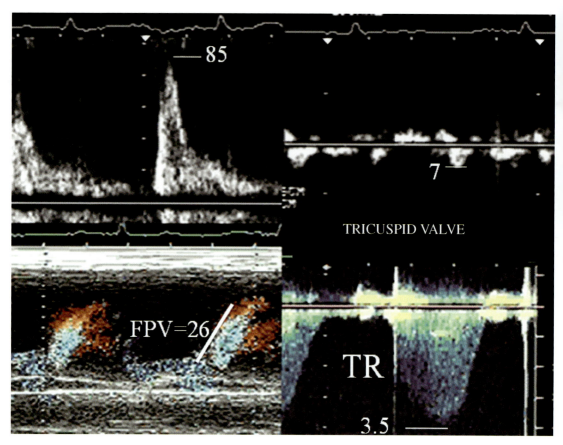

FIGURE 13.14. Mitral inflow, color M-mode early diastolic flow propagation velocity, TD of mitral annulus, and tricuspid regurgitation (TR) jet by continuous wave Doppler echocardiography from a patient with atrial fibrillation and increased filling pressures. Note the increased ratios of E to Vp and E to Ea. The pulmonary arterial systolic pressure is at least 49 mm Hg.

filling pressures. In addition, measurement of the peak acceleration rate of the mitral diastolic velocity in conjunction with IVRT is very useful.[56] Although the data gathered from 10 consecutive cycles is the most accurate, it is possible to use data from only 5 cycles or a single cycle with an RR cycle length that corresponds to the average heart rate.[56] It is also of value to examine the variability of Doppler measurements in mitral inflow (velocity and acceleration rate) with RR cycle length. Patients with increased filling pressures usually have less variation in mitral velocities for a given change in RR cycle length[56]

Additional methods of potential utility include the deceleration time of pulmonary venous diastolic velocity, which was shown in one study to have an inverse strong relation with filling pressures,[58] the E/Vp ratio,[56] and the E/Ea ratio,[46] albeit with modest correlations between the ratios and filling pressures. Figure 13.14 shows Doppler recordings filling a patient with atrial fibrillation and increased filling pressures.

Doppler Estimation of Left Ventricular Filling Pressures in Patients with Mitral Valve Disease

In patients with depressed EF and significant mitral regurgitation, mitral inflow and the E/Ea ratio can still be used. However, with normal EF, mitral inflow velocities, left atrial volumes, pulmonary venous systolic filling fraction, and E/Ea ratio are not accurate.[59,60] However, in the latter

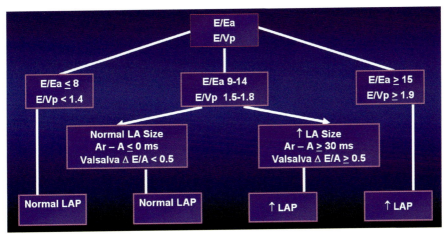

FIGURE 13.15. Diagnostic algorithm for the estimation of left ventricular filling pressures in patients with normal EF. (Reprinted from Nagueh and Zoghbi,[62] with permission of the American College of Cardiology Foundation.)

group of patients, the Ar–A duration remains helpful in predicting LV end-diastolic pressure.[61]

For patients with mitral regurgitation and mitral stenosis, irrespective of EF and cardiac rhythm (sinus or atrial fibrillation), the combination of IVRT and T_{E-Ea} time interval as described earlier appears promising not only for the prediction of mean wedge pressure but also for tracking changes after valve repair or replacement.[60]

Conclusion

The existing body of literature supports the valuable role of Doppler echocardiography in the estimation of LV filling pressures,[62] including in patients with normal EF (Figure 13.15). In fact, echocardiography can be viewed as a noninvasive pulmonary arterial catheter[63–65] when one considers the broad spectrum of hemodynamic data it can provide, including LV stroke volume, cardiac output, and right atrial and pulmonary arterial pressures.

References

1. Hillis GS, Moller JE, Pellikka PA, et al. Noninvasive estimation of left ventricular filling pressure by E/E' is a powerful predictor of survival after acute myocardial infarction. J Am Coll Cardiol 2004;43:360–367.
2. Dokainish H, Zoghbi WA, Lakkis NM, et al. Incremental predictive power of B-type natriuretic peptide and tissue Doppler echocardiography in the prognosis of patients with congestive heart failure. J Am Coll Cardiol 2005;45:1223–1226.
3. Redfield MM, Jacobsen SJ, Burnett JC Jr, et al. Burden of systolic and diastolic ventricular dysfunction in the community: appreciating the scope of the heart failure epidemic. JAMA 2003;289:194–202.
4. Udelson JE, Cannon RO 3rd, Bacharach SL, et al. Beta-adrenergic stimulation with isoproterenol enhances left ventricular diastolic performance in hypertrophic cardiomyopathy despite potentiation of myocardial ischemia. Comparison to rapid atrial pacing. Circulation 1989;79:371–382.
5. Yamamoto K, Nishimura RA, Redfield MM. Assessment of mean left atrial pressure from the left ventricular pressure tracing in patients with cardiomyopathies. Am J Cardiol 1996;78:107–110.
6. Ha JW, Oh JK, Pellikka PA, et al. Diastolic stress echocardiography: a novel noninvasive diagnostic test for diastolic dysfunction using supine bicycle exercise Doppler echocardiography. J Am Soc Echocardiogr 2005;18:63–68.
7. Ishida Y, Meisner JS, Tsujioka K, et al. Left ventricular filling dynamics: influence of left ventricular relaxation and left atrial pressure. Circulation 1986;74:187–196.
8. Tenenbaum A, Motro M, Hod H, et al. Shortened Doppler-derived mitral A wave deceleration time: an important predictor of elevated left ventricular filling pressure. J Am Coll Cardiol 1996;27:700–705.

9. Pozzoli M, Traversi E, Cioffi G, et al. Loading manipulations improve the prognostic value of Doppler evaluation of mitral flow in patients with chronic heart failure. Circulation 1997;95:1222–1230.

10. Temporelli PL, Corra U, Imparato A, et al. Reversible restrictive left ventricular diastolic filling with optimized oral therapy predicts a more favorable prognosis in patients with chronic heart failure. J Am Coll Cardiol 1998;31:1591–1597.

11. Nishimura RA, Tajik AJ. Evaluation of diastolic filling of left ventricle in health and disease: Doppler echocardiography is the clinician's Rosetta stone. J Am Coll Cardiol 1997;30:8–18.

12. Rivas-Gotz C, Manolios M, Thohan V, et al. Impact of left ventricular ejection fraction on estimation of left ventricular filling pressures using tissue Doppler and flow propagation velocity. Am J Cardiol 2003; 91:780–784.

13. Smiseth OA, Thompson CR, Lohavanichbutr K, et al. The pulmonary venous systolic flow pulse—its origin and relationship to left atrial pressure. J Am Coll Cardiol 1999;34:802–809.

14. Kuecherer HF, Muhiudeen IA, Kusumoto FM, et al. Estimation of mean left atrial pressure from transesophageal pulsed Doppler echocardiography of pulmonary venous flow. Circulation 1990;82:1127–1139.

15. Kinnaird TD, Thompson CR, Munt BI. The deceleration time of pulmonary venous diastolic flow is more accurate than the pulmonary artery occlusion pressure in predicting left atrial pressure. J Am Coll Cardiol 2001;37:2025–2030.

16. Yamamuro A, Yoshida K, Hozumi T, et al. Noninvasive evaluation of pulmonary capillary wedge pressure in patients with acute myocardial infarction by deceleration time of pulmonary venous flow velocity in diastole. J Am Coll Cardiol 1999;34:90–94.

17. Rossvoll O, Hatle LK. Pulmonary venous flow velocities recorded by transthoracic Doppler ultrasound: relation to left ventricular diastolic pressures. J Am Coll Cardiol 1993;21:1687–1696.

18. Appleton CP, Galloway JM, Gonzalez MS, et al. Estimation of left ventricular filling pressures using two-dimensional and Doppler echocardiography in adult patients with cardiac disease. J Am Coll Cardiol 1993;22:1972–1982.

19. Yamamoto K, Nishimura RA, Chaliki HP, et al. Determination of left ventricular filling pressure by Doppler echocardiography in patients with coronary artery disease: critical role of left ventricular systolic function. J Am Coll Cardiol 1997;30:1527–1533.

20. Kalmanson D, Veyrat C, Bernier A, et al. Opening snap and isovolumic relaxation period in relation to mitral valve flow in patients with mitral stenosis. Significance of A2–OS interval. Br Heart J 1976;38:135–146.

21. Palomo AR, Quinones MA, Waggoner AD, et al. Echo-phonocardiographic determination of left atrial and left ventricular filling pressures with and without mitral stenosis. Circulation 1980;61:1043–1047.

22. Thomas JD, Flachskampf FA, Chen C, et al. Isovolumic relaxation time varies predictably with its time constant and aortic and left atrial pressure: implications for the noninvasive evaluation of ventricular relaxation. Am Heart 1992;124:1305–1313.

23. Pozzoli M, Capomolla S, Pinna G, et al. Doppler echocardiography reliably predicts pulmonary artery wedge pressure in patients with chronic heart failure with and without mitral regurgitation. J Am Coll Cardiol 1996;27:883–893.

24. Nagueh SF, Kopelen HA, Zoghbi WA. Feasibility and accuracy of Doppler echocardiographic estimation of pulmonary artery occlusive pressure in the intensive care unit. Am J Cardiol 1995;75:1256–1262.

25. Garcia MJ, Smedira NG, Greenberg NL, et al. Color M-mode Doppler flow propagation velocity is a preload insensitive index of left ventricular relaxation: animal and human validation. J Am Coll Cardiol 2000;35:201–208.

26. Brun P, Tribouilloy C, Duval AM, et al. Left ventricular flow propagation during early filling is related to wall relaxation: a color M-mode Doppler analysis. J Am Coll Cardiol 1992;20:420–432.

27. Stugaard M, Smiseth OA, Risoe C, et al. Intraventricular early diastolic filling during acute myocardial ischemia, assessment by multigated color M-mode Doppler echocardiography. Circulation 1993;88:2705–2713.

28. Takatsuji H, Mikami T, Urasawa K, et al. A new approach for evaluation of left ventricular diastolic function: spatial and temporal analysis of left ventricular filling flow propagation by color M-mode Doppler echocardiography. J Am Coll Cardiol 1996; 27:365–371.

29. Garcia MJ, Ares MA, Asher C, et al. An index of early left ventricular filling that combined with pulsed Doppler peak E velocity may estimate capillary wedge pressure. J Am Coll Cardiol 1997;29:448–454.

30. Graham RJ, Gelman JS, Donelan L, et al. Effect of preload reduction by haemodialysis on new indices of diastolic function. Clin Sci (Lond) 2003;105:499–506.

31. Troughton RW, Prior DL, Frampton CM, et al. Usefulness of tissue Doppler and color M-mode indexes of left ventricular diastolic function in predicting outcomes in systolic left ventricular heart failure (from the ADEPT Study). Am J Cardiol 2005;96:257–262.

32. Ohte N, Narita H, Akita S, et al. Striking effect of left ventricular systolic performance on propagation velocity of left ventricular early diastolic filling flow. J Am Soc Echocardiogr 2001;14:1070–1074.

33. Rodriguez L, Garcia M, Ares M, et al. Assessment of mitral annular dynamics during diastole by Doppler tissue imaging: comparison with mitral Doppler inflow in subjects without heart disease and in patients with left ventricular hypertrophy. Am Heart J 1996;131:982–987.

34. Nagueh SF, Middleton KJ, Kopelen HA, et al. Doppler tissue imaging: a noninvasive technique for evaluation of left ventricular relaxation and estimation of filling pressures. J Am Coll Cardiol 1997;30:1527–1533.

35. Nagueh SF, Sun H, Kopelen HA, et al. Hemodynamic determinants of the mitral annulus diastolic velocities by tissue Doppler. J Am Coll Cardiol 2001;37:278–285.

36. Firstenberg MS, Greenberg NL, Main ML, et al. Determinants of diastolic myocardial tissue Doppler velocities: influences of relaxation and preload. J Appl Physiol 2001;90:299–307.

37. Sohn D-W, Chai I-H, Lee D-J, et al. Assessment of mitral annulus velocity by Doppler tissue imaging in the evaluation of left ventricular diastolic function. J Am Coll Cardiol 1997;30:474–480.

38. Oki T, Tabata T, Yamada H, et al. Clinical application of pulsed Doppler tissue imaging for assessing abnormal left ventricular relaxation. Am J Cardiol 1997;79:921–928.

39. Ommen SR, Nishimura RA, Appleton CP, et al. Clinical utility of Doppler echocardiography and tissue Doppler imaging in the estimation of left ventricular filling pressures: a comparative simultaneous Doppler-catheterization study. Circulation 2000;102:1788–1794.

40. Shan K, Bick RJ, Poindexter BJ, et al. Relation of tissue Doppler–derived myocardial velocities to myocardial structure and beta-adrenergic receptor density in humans. J Am Coll Cardiol 2000;36:891–896.

41. Kalra DK, Ramchandani M, Zhu X, et al. Relation of tissue Doppler–derived myocardial velocities to serum levels and myocardial gene expression of tumor necrosis factor-alpha and inducible nitric oxide synthase in patients with ischemic cardiomyopathy having coronary artery bypass grafting. Am J Cardiol 2002;90:708–712.

42. Hasegawa H, Little WC, Ohno M, et al. Diastolic mitral annular velocity during the development of heart failure. J Am Coll Cardiol 2003;41:1590–1597.

43. Firstenberg MS, Levine BD, Garcia MJ, et al. Relationship of echocardiographic indices to pulmonary capillary wedge pressures in healthy volunteers. J Am Coll Cardiol 2000;36:1664–1669.

44. Kim YJ, Sohn DW. Mitral annulus velocity in the estimation of left ventricular filling pressure: prospective study in 200 patients. J Am Soc Echocardiogr 2000;13:980–985.

45. Nagueh SF, Mikati I, Kopelen HA, et al. Doppler estimation of left ventricular filling pressure in sinus tachycardia. Circulation 1998;98:1644–1650.

46. Sohn DW, Song JM, Zo JH, et al. Mitral annulus velocity in the evaluation of left ventricular diastolic function in atrial fibrillation. J Am Soc Echocardiogr 1999;12:927–931.

47. Sundereswaran L, Nagueh SF, Vardan S, et al. Estimation of left and right ventricular filling pressures after heart transplantation by tissue Doppler imaging. Am J Cardiol 1998;82:352–357.

48. Nagueh SF, Lakkis NM, Middleton KJ, et al. Doppler estimation of left ventricular filling pressures in patients with hypertrophic cardiomyopathy. Circulation 1999;99:254–261.

49. Nagueh SF, Rao L, Soto J, et al. Haemodynamic insights into the effects of ischaemia and cycle length on tissue Doppler–derived mitral annulus diastolic velocities. Clin Sci (Lond) 2004;106:147–154.

50. Ha JW, Oh JK, Ling LH, et al. Annulus paradoxus: transmitral flow velocity to mitral annular velocity ratio is inversely proportional to pulmonary capillary wedge pressure in patients with constrictive pericarditis. Circulation 2001;104:976–978.

51. Rivas-Gotz C, Khoury DS, Manolios M, et al. Time interval between onset of mitral inflow and onset of early diastolic velocity by tissue Doppler: a novel index of left ventricular relaxation: experimental studies and clinical application. J Am Coll Cardiol 2003;42:1463–1470.

52. Tsang TS, Barnes ME, Gersh BJ, et al. Left atrial volume as a morphophysiologic expression of left ventricular diastolic dysfunction and relation to cardiovascular risk burden. Am J Cardiol 2002;90:1284–1289.

53. Quinones MA, Otto CM, Stoddard M, et al. Recommendations for quantification of Doppler echocardiography: a report from the Doppler Quantification Task Force of the Nomenclature and Standards

Committee of the American Society of Echocardiography. J Am Soc Echocardiogr 2002;15:167–184.

54. Nishimura RA, Tajik AJ. Determination of left-sided pressure gradients by utilizing Doppler aortic and mitral regurgitant signals: validation by simultaneous dual catheter and Doppler studies. J Am Coll Cardiol 1988;11:317–321.

55. Sohn DW, Kim YJ, Kim HC, et al. Evaluation of left ventricular diastolic function when mitral E and A waves are completely fused: role of assessing mitral annulus velocity. J Am Soc Echocardiogr 1999;12:203–208.

56. Nagueh SF, Kopelen HA, Quinones MA. Doppler estimation of left ventricular filling pressure in patients with atrial fibrillation. Circulation 1996;94:2138–2145.

57. Temporelli PL, Scapellato F, Corra U, et al. Estimation of pulmonary wedge pressure by transmitral Doppler in patients with chronic heart failure and atrial fibrillation. Am J Cardiol 1999;83:724–727.

58. Chirillo F, Brunazzi MC, Barbiero M, et al. Estimating mean pulmonary wedge pressure in patients with chronic atrial fibrillation from transthoracic Doppler indexes of mitral and pulmonary venous flow velocity. J Am Coll Cardiol 1997;30:19–26.

59. Bruch C, Stypmann J, Gradaus R, et al. Usefulness of tissue Doppler imaging for estimation of filling pressures in patients with primary or secondary pure mitral regurgitation. Am J Cardiol 2004;93:324–328.

60. Diwan A, McCulloch M, Lawrie G, et al. Doppler estimation of left ventricular filling pressures in patients with mitral valve disease. Circulation 2005;111:3281–3289.

61. Rossi A, Cicoira M, Golia G, et al. Mitral regurgitation and left ventricular diastolic dysfunction similarly affect mitral and pulmonary vein flow Doppler parameters: the advantage of end-diastolic markers. J Am Soc Echocardiogr 2001;14:562–568.

62. Nagueh SF, Zoghbi WA. Clinical assessment of LV diastolic filling by Doppler echocardiography. ACC Curr J Rev 2001;10:45–49.

63. Nagueh SF. Noninvasive evaluation of hemodynamics by Doppler echocardiography. Curr Opin Cardiol 1999;14:217–224.

64. Oh JK. Echocardiography as a noninvasive Swan-Ganz catheter. Circulation 2005;111:3192–3194.

65. Stein JH, Neumann A, Preston LM, et al. Echocardiography for hemodynamic assessment of patients with advanced heart failure and potential heart transplant recipients. J Am Coll Cardiol 1997;30:1765–1772.

Section 3
Epidemiology, Prognosis, and Treatment

14
Epidemiology of Diastolic Heart Failure

Michał Tendera and Wojciech Wojakowski

Introduction

Heart failure is a major public health problem, and, given the data showing a significant increase in the number of heart failure–related hospitalizations, it can be regarded as an emerging epidemic. Heart failure is the most frequent cause of hospitalization in patients aged 65 years and older. It accounts for more than 1 million hospitalizations per year in the United States.[1–3]

The epidemiology of heart failure with reduced left ventricular ejection fraction (LVEF) is relatively well known, at least in European and North American populations.[2,4,5] Recently, consistent epidemiologic data regarding the incidence and prevalence of heart failure with normal LVEF became available, despite different definitions, diagnostic modalities, and populations included in the studies. Much more is also known with regard to diastolic heart failure (DHF) as well as prevalence of asymptomatic diastolic dysfunction. The next problem encountered when gathering epidemiologic data on DHF from large population studies is the use of simple screening criteria. Some of the numerous causes of heart failure with normal LVEF other than primary diastolic dysfunction, for example, infiltrative and restrictive cardiomyopathies, pulmonary hypertension, atrial septal defect, pericardial disease, and arrhythmogenic right ventricular cardiomyopathy, may be missed because they require more thorough diagnostic processes.[6]

Epidemiologic data obtained within the past 20 years, since the concept of heart failure with normal LVEF was introduced, show that its prevalence is 30%–74% (median 45%) (Figure 14.1).[5,7,8] It should be noted, however, that the diagnostic criteria for DHF varied substantially among those studies, and some of them used only echocardiography to measure the LVEF whereas others have used current Doppler echocardiographic criteria to assess the diastolic function. Population-based studies showed that at least 40%–50% of all patients with heart failure have a normal or near-normal LVEF and that DHF is most common among patients older than 75 years.[5,9]

Incidence

Because the majority of epidemiologic data are derived from hospital discharge records, they might not accurately describe the incidence of heart failure with normal LVEF.[10] Data from the Olmsted County, Minnesota, cohort-based study, which used a uniform medical data reporting system (the Rochester Epidemiology Project), showed no significant reduction in the incidence of heart failure (without differentiating according to LVEF) during the period of 1979–2000. In addition, the age-adjusted incidence of heart failure was higher in males (378/100,000 persons) than in females (289/100,000 persons).[10]

In 216 patients from the Olmsted County area with newly diagnosed heart failure, 43% had normal LVEF. Exclusion of patients with significant valvular disease reduced the number slightly to 41%. After stratification according to age, the highest incidence of both heart failure with normal LVEF and heart failure with reduced LVEF was

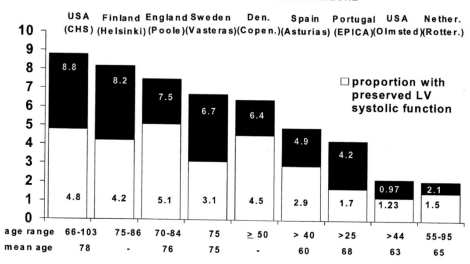

FIGURE 14.1. Prevalence of heart failure in cross-sectional, population-based, echocardiographic studies. (Reprinted from Hogg K, et al. Heart failure with preserved left ventricular systolic function: epidemiology, clinical characteristics, and prognosis. J Am Coll Cardiol 2004;43:317–327, with permission of the American College of Cardiology Foundation.)

found in patients aged 70–89 years compared with younger subjects. Furthermore, the higher incidence of heart failure with normal LVEF than heart failure with reduced LVEF was noted in very elderly patients (age >90 years). The group of patients with heart failure with normal LVEF was characterized by a higher proportion of women (69%), more advanced age (mean age 77 years), higher prevalence of atrial fibrillation (29%), lower prevalence of coronary heart disease (31%), previous myocardial infarction (15%), and less left bundle branch block (0%) compared with patients with heart failure and an LVEF <50% (women, 41%; mean age, 74 years; atrial fibrillation, 24%; coronary artery disease, 53%, previous myocardial infarction, 42%; and left bundle branch block, 12%). Interestingly, there was no difference between the two populations in the prevalence of hypertension and chronic obstructive pulmonary disease. In logistic regression analysis two factors were independently associated with normal LVEF in patients with newly diagnosed heart failure: female sex and age >90 years. Limitations of this study include low number of patients and the fact that 39% had no echocardiographic evaluation of LVEF.[11] The higher incidence of heart failure with normal LVEF in elderly patients may be associated with the age-related loss of LV compliance and long-standing effect of arterial hypertension.

Prevalence

Recently published data derived from 6,076 consecutive patients hospitalized with decompensated heart failure in Olmsted County, Minnesota, showed that prevalence of heart failure with normal LVEF significantly increased over the 15-year observation period (1987–2001). The definition of heart failure with normal LVEF used in this study included the symptoms of heart failure and LVEF ≥50%. The results of echocardiographic examinations were available for 76% of patients enrolled in this study. The demographic characteristics of the study population were diversified. There were more women and obese subjects in the group with normal LVEF. In addition, patients with normal LVEF were older and had higher body mass indexes and lower hemoglobin levels than those with reduced LVEF.

Prevalence of heart failure with normal LVEF was 40% in patients <50 years and significantly higher (49%) in patients ≥65 years. After adjustment for age difference the prevalence rates of obesity, hypertension, and atrial fibrillation were significantly higher in subjects with heart failure with normal LVEF than in those with reduced LVEF. On the other hand, coronary heart disease and valvular heart disease were more prevalent in patients with reduced LVEF, showing that different etiologies may be responsible for the two forms of heart failure. Secular trends in the prevalence rate of heart failure with normal LVEF and heart failure with reduced LVEF are different. There was an increase from 38% to 54% in the prevalence rate of heart failure with normal LVEF over a 15-year period in contrast to no change of the prevalence rate of heart failure with reduced LVEF (Figure 14.2). Similar findings come from a comparison of studies carried out earlier (1970–1995) and more recent data (1998–2003), which shows an increase from median incidence rate of 40% to 54%. A study carried out in a Spanish tertiary hospital showed a consistent increase in the prevalence of normal LVEF in 1,482 patients hospitalized with heart failure. In comparison to 1991–1996, when the prevalence of heart failure with normal LVEF was 37%, it increased to 47% in the period 2000–2001 [12]. The findings are also consistent with an increasing prevalence of all heart failure cases, especially in older subjects (1%–2% in the general population vs, 10% in elderly patients).[5,8,13,14]

There are several potential reasons for the increased prevalence of heart failure with normal LVEF in population- and referral-based studies:

- Increased prevalence of comorbidities.[13,15]
  ○ Hypertension
  ○ Diabetes
  ○ Atrial fibrillation
- Higher proportion of elderly patients included in hospital-based studies[16]
- Differences between referral-based and community-based studies (more thorough diagnostic process and more data available in referral-based studies)
- Growing awareness of heart failure with normal LVEF among physicians and other health care workers[17]
- New diagnostic methods and more frequent use of echocardiography, cardiac catheterization, and natriuretic peptides
- Diagnostic criteria (some studies used a threshold of LVEF ≥40%–50% to define normal/preserved LVEF)

A recently published prospective study involving the population of Olmsted County, Minnesota, further extends the knowledge about the epidemiology of heart failure with normal LVEF. The study enrolled 556 consecutive patients admitted with heart failure in the hospital and outpatient clinics of the Mayo Clinic, and the patients were followed up prospectively. Echocardiography was performed, including assessment of LVEF, Doppler measurement of the mitral inflow, and the velocity of the mitral annulus. In

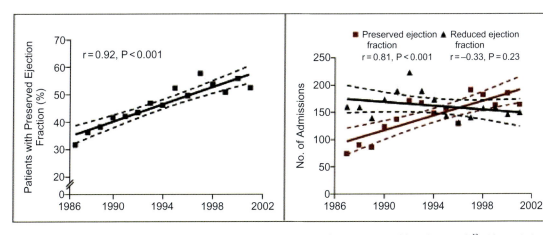

FIGURE 14.2. Trends in the prevalence of heart failure with preserved ejection fraction. Reprinted from Owan et al.,[13] with permission of the Massachusetts Medical Society.)

addition, plasma brain natriuretic peptide levels were measured. Of the screened heart failure patients, 55% had a normal LVEF and 44% had isolated diastolic dysfunction. This population of heart failure patients with normal LVEF was older (mean age, 77 years) and included more women (57%) than those with heart failure and a reduced LVEF (mean age, 73 years; 42% women). In patients with heart failure and normal LVEF, there was mild diastolic dysfunction in 7%, moderate in 63%, severe in 8%, and normal in 10% of cases. Interestingly, in patients with heart failure and reduced LVEF, mild diastolic dysfunction was present in 4%, moderate in 56%, and severe in 23%, and a relatively low number of patients had normal diastolic function (5%). This group of patients was more likely to develop moderate and severe diastolic dysfunction than patients with heart failure and normal LVEF (OR, 1.67; 95% CI, 1.11–2.51).[18]

In the MONICA Augsburg study, which assessed the cardiovascular risk factors in a randomly selected sample of the Augsburg population, the prevalence of diastolic abnormalities documented by echocardiography was approximately 11%. It was highest among older subjects and in those with LV hypertrophy, prior myocardial infarction, hypertension, diabetes, and obesity. In addition, the prevalence further increased if additional risk factors were present. Furthermore, diastolic dysfunction was more frequent in males than in females.

The Multicenter EFECT (Enhanced Feedback for Effective Cardiac Treatment) study, carried out in Ontario, Canada, assessed 2,802 patients hospitalized between 1999 and 2001 with a primary diagnosis of heart failure and analyzed the prevalence of normal LVEF. All patients presented with newly diagnosed heart failure according to the Framingham diagnostic criteria. The prevalence of heart failure with normal LVEF was 31%. The patients with a normal LVEF were more likely to be female and were older than those with decreased LVEF. There was also a higher incidence of hypertension, atrial fibrillation, and chronic obstructive pulmonary disease and lower rates of ischemic heart disease and peripheral arterial disease in the normal LVEF group.[19] Both the Olmsted County and the EFECT studies refer to patients with decompensated heart failure severe enough to warrant hospitalization, so one has to be cautious when extrapolating the data to other populations.[13]

Data from the Euro Heart Failure Survey shed some light on the prevalence of heart failure with normal LVEF in Europe. Of 6,806 patients hospitalized with signs or symptoms of heart failure, 46% had normal or mildly depressed LVEF. In this study, however, the term preserved left ventricular function (PLVF) was used, and this population included patients with an LVEF ≥40% as well as those with normal LVEF. Therefore, its population was heterogeneous. Consistent with previously discussed studies, patients with PLVF were older than those with decreased LVEF. The prevalences of hypertension and atrial fibrillation were also higher in the PLVF group in contrast to the lower prevalence of coronary artery disease. In addition, as in other studies, there were more women in the PLVF group than in the population with reduced LVEF.[20]

Most other available study results agree with those discussed above with regard to prevalence of normal LVEF in patients with heart failure. Comparable findings were reported by Smith et al.,[21] who found a 48% prevalence of normal LVEF (LVEF ≥40%) in 413 patients with heart failure. Furthermore, of the 4,549 participants in the National Heart, Lung, and Blood Institute Cardiovascular Health Study, 52% of patients with prevalent heart failure had a normal LVEF.[22]

Besides hospital and outpatient clinic-based studies, there are reports on the prevalence of heart failure with normal LVEF among randomly selected subjects from the general population without established diagnosis of heart failure. Redfield et al.[23] reported that in a cross-sectional study of 2,042 residents of Olmsted County, Minnesota, the prevalence of heart failure was 2.2%, and among heart failure patients 44% had a normal LVEF. Importantly, in subjects without a previous diagnosis of heart failure, there was a significant increase in all-cause mortality. Moreover, in the general population, 5.6% of subjects with normal LVEF also had either moderate or severe diastolic dysfunction. The prevalence of diastolic dysfunction increased with age, history of coronary artery disease, diabetes, and obesity but was not different between sexes. This was the first study to document the prevalence of various

14. Epidemiology of Diastolic Heart Failure

degrees of diastolic dysfunction validated by Doppler echocardiography in a general population without an established diagnosis of heart failure.[23]

Subpopulations

Women

Most epidemiologic studies assessing the prevalence and incidence of heart failure with normal LVEF are consistently showing that this condition is more frequent in women presenting with heart failure.[5] Nevertheless, only a few studies were designed to assess the prevalence in the sexes separately. The retrospective cohort study including the patients from the National Heart Failure (NHF) Project showed that of 19,710 patients discharged with the primary diagnosis of heart failure 35% had a normal LVEF. In this population of 6,700 patients with normal LVEF, 79% were women. In comparison, of patients with heart failure and reduced LVEF, only 49% were women. This study included only patients aged ≥65 years and those with documented LVEF. The population with heart failure with normal LVEF was significantly older by 1.5 years than those with reduced LVEF. After adjustment for age, comorbidities, and medical history, female sex was an independent predictor of normal LVEF in heart failure patients (RR, 1.71; 95% CI, 1.63–1.78).[24]

Similar data came from the Framingham study, which showed that 73% of women with a new diagnosis of heart failure had a normal LVEF compared with 33% of males, and the Olmsted County study reported that 57%–70% of patients with heart failure with normal LVEF were women.[11,18,25] Additionally, data from the New York Heart Failure Registry show that of 619 patients hospitalized in 24 medical centers in New York City because of heart failure with normal LVEF, 73% were women.[26] Importantly, the association between female sex and normal LVEF was also found in patients without arrhythmia and hypertension, so the sex-related differences in LV adaptation to hypertension and atrial fibrillation may at best explain only part of this strong predominance of women in the population of patients with heart failure and normal LVEF.[24]

Comorbidities

Analyses of comorbidities in patients admitted with heart failure reveal significantly higher prevalences of hypertension and atrial fibrillation[5,13] and lower incidences of coronary heart disease and myocardial infarction.[5,13,19,20]

Hypertension

The cohort study of 19,710 patients in the NHF Project showed in a multivariate analysis that hypertension was significantly associated with the presence of normal LVEF in heart failure patients (OR, 1.31 [1.23–1.41]; RR, 1.20 [1.15–1.26]).[24] This is consistent with and confirms the observations of other studies showing a higher prevalence of hypertension in patients with heart failure with normal LVEF, such as the Olmsted County, Minnesota, and the EFECT studies.[5,13,19,27] However, recently published data on the heart failure patients in the Olmsted County and the Cardiovascular Health Study showed no differences in the prevalences of hypertension between heart failure with normal LVEF and heart failure with reduced LVEF patients.[18,22] The association between hypertension and heart failure with normal LVEF seems to be partially dependent on ethnicity, so it needs to be validated in different populations.[5]

Atrial Fibrillation

Similar to hypertension, atrial fibrillation is in the majority of studies more frequent in patients with heart failure with normal LVEF than in those with reduced LVEF. The NHF Project investigators found that a history of atrial fibrillation is significantly correlated with the presence of normal LVEF in heart failure patients when entered into a multivariate analysis (OR, 1.39 [1.29–1.49]; RR, 1.23 [1.18–1.29]).[24] This observation was consistently confirmed in numerous studies investigating the prevalence of heart failure with normal LVEF.[13,19,20, 27] The causal link between atrial fibrillation and heart failure with normal LVEF may be bidirectional. Atrial fibrillation can precipitate symptoms of heart failure leading to hospital admission. On the other hand, patients with heart failure are more likely to have this condition. Atrial fibrillation is present in approximately 16%

of heart failure patients with reduced and 25% with normal LVEF as shown in the IN-CHF Registry.[28] Data from the CHARM study, which involved 7,599 patients randomized to treatment with candesartan or placebo, showed that atrial fibrillation was present in 17% of patients with reduced LVEF (≤40%) and in 19% of patients with preserved LVEF (>40%). The presence of atrial fibrillation was associated with an increased risk of cardiovascular morbidity and mortality in both groups, and the relative increase in risk was significantly higher in patients with preserved LVEF.[29]

Coronary Artery Disease

In contrast to hypertension and atrial fibrillation, coronary artery disease and history of acute myocardial infarction are less frequent in patients with heart failure with normal LVEF compared with patients with heart failure and reduced LVEF. This probably reflects the different pathogenesis and etiology of the two forms of heart failure. Multivariate analysis in a large population of heart failure patients showed that the presence of CAD is associated with a reduced LVEF in heart failure patients compared with those with normal LVEF (OR, 0.69 [0.63–0.77]; RR, 0.80 [0.76–0.86]. The same seems true for the history of myocardial infarction (OR, 0.42 [0.40–0.46]; RR, 0.57 [0.55–0.60] as a correlate of normal LVEF in a multivariate model).[24] Both coronary artery disease and history of myocardial infarction are less frequently found in heart failure with normal LVEF patients than in heart failure patients with reduced LVEF in virtually all of the epidemiologic studies. It seems that peripheral artery disease, smoking, and stroke are also less frequent in patients with heart failure with normal LVEF.[5,13,18–20,22]

Diabetes

Data regarding the prevalence of diabetes in heart failure with normal LVEF patients is somewhat less consistent across the studies, showing either no difference or a lower frequency of diabetes in this population of heart failure patients.[18] Recently published data on more than 6,000 patients showed no differences in the prevalence of diabetes in heart failure with normal LVEF patients compared with those with reduced LVEF (33% vs.

34%). The Cardiovascular Health Study also found no difference in the prevalences of diabetes in groups with reduced and normal LVEF and heart failure.[22] Conversely, the Ontario study of 2,802 patients showed a lower prevalence of diabetes in heart failure with normal LVEF patients than in those with reduced LVEF (31% vs. 38%).[13] Comparable results were published by the NHF investigators, showing that diabetes was present in 37% of heart failure with normal LVEF and in 40% with reduced LVEF.[24] These findings may be consistent with the high prevalence of diabetes in the general population of heart failure patients. Moreover, diabetes can be involved in both the progression of coronary artery disease and the increased risk of myocardial infarction, thus increasing the risk of heart failure with reduced LVEF, as well as in compromised LV compliance leading to diastolic failure and heart failure with normal LVEF.

Diseases of the Respiratory System

Most patients seeking medical advice for either de novo heart failure symptoms or exacerbation of chronic heart failure frequently have coexisting pulmonary and upper respiratory tract conditions such as chronic obstructive pulmonary disease (COPD) and respiratory tract infections. Epidemiologic studies showed a higher prevalence of COPD in patients with heart failure with normal LVEF than in those with reduced LVEF, although in both groups the condition was relatively frequent (34% vs. 31%).[24,30] The more recent Olmsted County, Minnesota, study showed no differences in the prevalence of COPD between these groups).[18] Importantly, patients with an established diagnosis of COPD may have unrecognized heart failure. A study by Rutten et al.[31] showed that among 405 patients with COPD at least 20% have had heart failure, which in half of them was heart failure with normal LVEF.

Other Coexisting Diseases

Data regarding the prevalence of other diseases in patients with heart failure with normal LVEF compared with heart failure with reduced LVEF is far less convincing than in the case of hypertension and atrial fibrillation. Further studies should assess the frequencies of renal impairment, anemia, smoking, hyperlipidemia, and dementia.[5]

Limitations of the Epidemiological Studies Investigating the Prevalence of Heart Failure with Normal Ejection Fraction

Available data on the incidence of heart failure with normal LVEF must be interpreted in the perspective of potential bias and inaccuracy associated with imperfect diagnostic criteria and lack of exclusion of other causes of symptoms that may be misdiagnosed as heart failure, especially in older studies. Newer diagnostic methods, such as measuring natriuretic peptides (brain natriuretic peptide and N-terminal prohormone brain natriuretic peptide) may be helpful for exclusion of the cardiac causes of dyspnea. Importantly, the data from a national survey of the prevalence, incidence, primary care burden, and treatment of heart failure in Scotland show that the most frequent non–heart failure symptoms that were the reasons of seeking medical advice (lower respiratory tract infection, breathlessness, COPD, atrial fibrillation) might have exacerbated the coexisting heart failure or resembled the heart failure symptoms, leading to selection bias in studies investigating the incidence and prevalence of heart failure with normal LVEF.[30] To diagnose DHF, three criteria must be met: (1) presence of signs or symptoms of heart failure, (2) presence of a normal LVEF, and (3) evidence of LV diastolic dysfunction. In most studies the first two criteria are met but lack direct evidence of diastolic dysfunction or LV concentric remodeling. The Euro Heart Failure Survey showed that only 64% of heart failure patients underwent LVEF evaluation. Implementation of the ESC Guidelines for the Diagnosis and Treatment of Chronic Heat Failure and the wider use of echocardiography to assess the LVEF may further increase the reported prevalence of heart failure with normal LVEF.[2,20]

Conclusion

Approximately half of the patients diagnosed with heart failure have a normal LVEF. Most of these patients have mild or moderate diastolic dysfunction. The prevalence of heart failure with normal LVEF is increasing by 1% per year, and the associated mortality remains high and unchanged over time. The survival of heart failure patients with normal LVEF is similar or only slightly better than for those with heart failure and decreased LVEF. The population of patients with heart failure with normal LVEF is characterized by a higher proportion of women and a more advanced age. In contrast to patients with heart failure with reduced LVEF, who are more likely to have coronary artery disease, prior myocardial infarction, and peripheral artery disease, patients with heart failure with normal LVEF are more frequently hypertensive and have atrial fibrillation and COPD. The high incidence of heart failure with normal LVEF in both community-based and referral-based patient populations suggest that it may become a predominant form of heart failure especially in the elderly.

References

1. Hunt SA, et al. ACC/AHA 2005 Guideline Update for the Diagnosis and Management of Chronic Heart Failure in the Adult: a report of the American College of Cardiology/American Heart Association Task Force on Practice Guidelines (Writing Committee to update the 2001 guidelines for the evaluation and management of heart failure). J Am Coll Cardiol 2005;46:1–82.
2. Swedberg K, for the Writing Committee of the Task Force for the Diagnosis and Treatment of CHF of the European Society of Cardiology Guidelines for the Diagnosis and Treatment of Chronic Heart Failure: full text (update 2005). Eur Heart J 2005;26:1115–1140.
3. de Frances CJ, Podgornik MN. 2004 National Hospital Discharge Survey. Adv Data 2006;371:1–19.
4. McMurray JJ, Pfeffer MA. Heart failure. Lancet 2005;365(9474):1877–1889.
5. Hogg K, Swedberg K, McMurray J. Heart failure with preserved left ventricular systolic function. Epidemiology, clinical characteristics and prognosis. J Am Coll Cardiol 2004;43(3):317–327.
6. Oh JK, et al. Diastolic heart failure can be diagnosed by comprehensive two-dimensional and Doppler echocardiography. J Am Coll Cardiol 2006;47(3):500–506.
7. Thomas MD, et al. The epidemiological enigma of heart failure with preserved systolic function. Eur J Heart Fail 2004;6(2):125–136.
8. Vasan RS, Benjamin EJ, Levy D. Prevalence, clinical features and prognosis of diastolic heart failure: an epidemiologic perspective. J Am Coll Cardiol 1995; 26(7):1565–1574.

9. Aurigemma GP, Gaasch WH. Clinical practice. Diastolic heart failure. N Engl J Med 2004;351(11): 1097–1105.
10. Roger VL, et al. Trends in heart failure incidence and survival in a community-based population. JAMA 2004;292:344–350.
11. Senni M, et al. Congestive heart failure in the community. a study of all incident cases in Olmsted County, Minnesota, in 1991. Circulation 1998;98:2282–2289.
12. Shamagian LG, et al. The death rate among hospitalized heart failure patients with normal and depressed left ventricular ejection fraction in the year following discharge: evolution over a 10-year period. Eur Heart J 2005;26:2251–2258.
13. Owan TE, et al. Trends in prevalence and outcome of heart failure with preserved ejection fraction. N Engl J Med 2006;355:251–259.
14. Tendera M. Epidemiology, treatment, and guidelines for the treatment of heart failure in Europe. Eur Heart J Suppl 2005;7(Suppl J):J5–J9.
15. Owan TE, Redfield MM. Epidemiology of diastolic heart failure. Prog Cardiovasc Dis 2005;47(5):320–332.
16. Aurigemma GP. Diastolic heart failure—a common and lethal condition by any name. N Engl J Med 2006;355(3):308–310.
17. Banerjee P, Clark AL, Cleland JG. Diastolic heart failure: a difficult problem in the elderly. Am J Geriatr Cardiol 2004;13(1):16–21.
18. Bursi F, et al. Systolic and diastolic heart failure in the community. JAMA 2006;296(18): 2209–2216.
19. Bhatia RS, et al. Outcome of heart failure with preserved ejection fraction in a population-based study. N Engl J Med 2006;355:260–269.
20. Lenzen MJ, et al. Differences between patients with a preserved and a depressed left ventricular function: a report from the EuroHeart Failure Survey. Eur Heart J 2004;25:1214–1220.
21. Smith GL, et al. Outcomes in heart failure patients with preserved ejection fraction mortality, readmission, and functional decline. J Am Coll Cardiol 2003;41:1510–1518.
22. Liao L, et al. Costs for heart failure with normal vs reduced ejection fraction. Arch Intern Med 2006; 166:112–118.
23. Redfield MM, et al. Burden of systolic and diastolic ventricular dysfunction in the community: appreciating the scope of the heart failure epidemic. JAMA 2003;289(2):194–202.
24. Masoudi FA, et al. Gender, age, and heart failure with preserved left ventricular systolic function. J Am Coll Cardiol 2003;41:217–223.
25. Vasan RS, et al. Congestive heart failure in subjects with normal versus reduced left ventricular ejection fraction: prevalence and mortality in a population-based cohort. J Am Coll Cardiol 1999;33:1948–1955.
26. Klapholz M, et al. Hospitalization for heart failure in the presence of a normal left ventricular ejection fraction: results of the New York Heart Failure Registry 2004;43:1432–1438.
27. Varela Roman A, et al. Heart failure in patients with preserved and deteriorated left ventricular ejection fraction. Heart 2005;91:489–494.
28. Tarantini L, Faggiano P, Senni M. Clinical features and prognosis associated with a preserved left ventricular systolic function in a large cohort of congestive heart failure outpatients managed by cardiologists. Data from the Italian Network on Congestive Heart Failure. Ital Heart J 2002;3:656–664.
29. Olsson LG, et al. Atrial fibrillation and risk of clinical events in chronic heart failure with and without left ventricular systolic dysfunction: results from the Candesartan in Heart Failure—Assessment of Reduction in Mortality and Morbidity (CHARM) Program. J Am Coll Cardiol 2006;47:1997–2004.
30. Murphy NF, et al. National survey of the prevalence, incidence, primary care burden, and treatment of heart failure in Scotland. Heart 2004;90: 1129–1136.
31. Rutten FH, et al. Unrecognized heart failure in elderly patients with stable chronic obstructive pulmonary disease. Eur Heart J 2005;26(18):1887–1894.

15
Prognosis in Diastolic Heart Failure

Piotr Ponikowski, Ewa A. Jankowska, and Waldemar Banasiak

Introduction

The clinical syndrome of heart failure can arise over a wide spectrum of left ventricular (LV) ejection fractions (LVEFs). Despite this, studies have typically focused on heart failure with reduced LVEF, and only recently has heart failure in the settings of normal and preserved LVEF (HFPEF) attained a wider interest. It has become evident that this pathology is becoming more prevalent in the modern aging communities and soon may be responsible for the majority of heart failure burden.[1–5] The natural history of HFPEF is still not well-characterized, but it seems that once this diagnosis is confirmed it is associated with high morbidity and mortality.[4–7]

The purpose of this chapter is to summarize the available evidence on the prognosis of patients with HFPEF. Different terms are used in the studies characterizing patients with heart failure signs and symptoms who do not have evidence of reduced/impaired LVEF (diastolic heart failure, heart failure with preserved systolic function, HFPEF, etc.). We have decided to use the broad term HFPEF, which also appears to be preferred by the current guidelines of the European Society of Cardiology[8] and the American College of Cardiology/American Heart Association.[9] For patients with heart failure and reduced LVEF, we use the traditional term systolic heart failure (SHF).

Mortality

Evidence emerging from the most recent epidemiologic studies confirms that HFPEF is associated with a high risk of mortality. The great diversity in the criteria used to establish a diagnosis of HFPEF, the populations, and the settings of the studies explains the wide variation in reported mortality rates (1-year mortality rates range from 1.3% to 28%).[4,5] The prognosis for patients with HFPEF is much worse than for age-matched controls, but whether it is less grim than for those with SHF remains a matter of debate.[10–21]

There has been a commonly held belief that mortality is inversely related to systolic LV function in a broad spectrum of patients with heart failure, and LVEF has been traditionally considered as one of the strongest prognosticators of poor outcome in the heart failure syndrome. Already in 1990, Cohn et al.[20] demonstrated than in heart failure patients who entered into the Veterans Administration Cooperative Study trial, those with a normal LVEF (≥45%) tended to have a significantly better prognosis than patients with SHF (annual mortality rate, 8% vs. 19%; $p = 0.0001$). In the same year, Aronow et al. performed a prospective study with elderly patients (mean age, 82 years) with heart failure associated with coronary artery disease. Survival rates significantly differed among those with preserved and impaired LVEF (1-year and 3-year mortality rates, 22% vs. 47% and 46% vs. 78%, respectively). Interestingly, 10 years later, on the basis of another prospective study of older subjects with heart failure associated with prior myocardial infarction, these authors reported very similar data: elderly patients with SHF (LVEF <50%) had more than two times higher mortality rates than those with HFPEF. Of note is the very poor outcome in both groups of elderly subjects.

Curtis et al. analyzed 7,788 outpatients with stable heart failure enrolled in the Digitalis

Investigation Group (DIG) trial and demonstrated that the association of LVEF and mortality changes substantially across the full spectrum of LVEF. Mortality decreased in a nearly linear fashion across successively higher LVEF groups until LVEF reached 45% (for a mean follow-up of 37 months, all-cause mortality rates were 51.7% for an LVEF of ≤15%; 41.7% for an LVEF of 16%–25%; 31.4% for an LVEF of 26%–35%; and 25.6% for an LVEF of 36%–45%). Interestingly, among subjects with an LVEF >45%, mortality rates were comparable and lower (although still very high) than for patients with SHF (23.3% for an LVEF of 46%–55% and 23.5% for an LVEF of >55%, respectively). Patients with a reduced LVEF were at an increased absolute risk of death due to arrhythmia and worsening of heart failure compared with patients with HFPEF, but these were the leading causes of death in all LVEF groups.

The CHARM (Candesartan in Heart Failure — Assessment of Reduction in Mortality and Morbidity) Program was designed to assess the effects of the angiotensin receptor blocker candesartan on cardiovascular mortality and morbidity in a broad spectrum of congestive heart failure patients irrespectively of the LVEF. In this trial, the risk of all-cause death declined gradually with an increasing LVEF up to 45%. This was primarily due to a close relationship between LVEF and cardiovascular death and its individual components: sudden death, death due to heart failure progression, and fatal myocardial infarction. The hazard ratio for all-cause mortality increased by 39% for every 10% reduction in EF below 45% even when adjusted for covariates. The absolute change in rate per 100 patient-years for each 10% reduction in LVEF was greatest for sudden death and heart failure–related death. The LVEF was a poor predictor of cardiovascular death in patients with an LVEF of >45%. In contrast, the rate of noncardiovascular death did not vary by LVEF.

The results of these two analyses, derived from highly selected trial-like heart failure populations, may not be simply representative of broader heart failure populations. However, another interesting study should be mentioned. In a cross-sectional survey of 2,042 randomly selected residents of Olmsted County, Minnesota, aged 45 years and older, Redfield et al. reported a prevalence of validated heart failure of 2.2%. Nearly half of the heart failure subjects had an LVEF of >50%. In a multivariate analysis, preserved LVEF was an independent predictor of better outcome, with a 19% lower risk of all-cause mortality per each 5% increase in LVEF. Applying rigorous echocardiographic criteria, the authors demonstrated that diastolic dysfunction was frequently present in the investigated subjects and often was not accompanied by recognized heart failure (20.8% with mild and 7.3% with moderate to severe diastolic dysfunction) and appeared as an independent predictor of all-cause mortality (an 8.3- and 10.2-fold increase in the risk of death for mild and for moderate to severe diastolic dysfunction, respectively, compared with patients with normal diastolic function). Taking into consideration the relatively low prognostic value of LVEF in patients with HFPEF, it may well be that an assessment and a proper grading of the magnitude of diastolic dysfunction may soon become a useful tool for risk stratification in HFPEF. However, further studies are needed to establish whether a severity of diastolic dysfunction modulates survival in heart failure patients with preserved LVEF.

Population-Based Studies

There are only a few population-based studies reporting the data on the prognosis for patients with HFPEF.[26] Senni et al. evaluated all patients (n = 216) receiving a first diagnosis of heart failure in Olmsted County, Minnesota, in 1991 (the Rochester Epidemiology Project), most of whom were elderly persons (mean age, 77 years) with moderate to severe symptomatic heart failure (54% in New York Heart Association [NYHA] classes III and IV). Among those who had an EF assessed by echocardiography (n = 137), 43% had preserved LVEF. Survival rates were very poor for the whole heart failure population: 86% ± 2% at 3 months, 76% ± 3% at 1 year, and 35 ± 3% at 5 years, respectively, and did not differ between those with HFPEF and SHF. The authors speculated that the very advanced age of this group (half of the population older than 80 years) could be an important factor explaining no difference in survival between patients with preserved and reduced LVEF. Based on the comprehensive analyses of the Rochester Epidemiology Project, regarding the residents of Olmsted County, Minnesota, 1-, 2-, and 3-year

15. Prognosis in Diastolic Heart Failure

mortality rates were established as 29%, 39%, and 60%, respectively, for those with a new diagnosis of heart failure in 1996–1997 and an LVEF of >45% without any significant valve disease.

In the nested case–control subset of the Framingham Heart Study, the unadjusted annual mortality rate for patients with SHF was higher than for those with HFPEF (18.9% and 8.7%, respectively). The median survival of patients with HFPEF was 7.1 years versus 4.3 years for patients with SHF. However, after an adjustment for covariates, differences in survival remained no longer significant, and both heart failure groups had a risk of death four times higher than their matched controls.

In another population-based project, the Helsinki Aging Study, performed among subjects aged 75–86 with the established diagnosis of heart failure syndrome, 4-year survival rates were 54% and 43% for those with HFPEF and SHF, respectively, and this difference did not reach a statistical significance. However, the results of these three studies should be taken with caution because of the relatively small numbers of studied heart failure patients.

In contrast, the Cardiovascular Health Study was larger and recruited 5,532 community-living participants who were at least 65 years of age, of whom 269 (4.9%) were diagnosed as having heart failure and 63% had normal a LVEF. Forty-five percent of heart failure patients and 16% of those without heart failure died during a 6.4-year follow-up period. All-cause mortality rates were higher for patients with heart failure with decreased versus preserved LVEF; they rose from 87 per 1,000 patient-years for those with heart failure and normal LVEF ($\geq$55%) to 115 for those with borderline LVEF (45%–54%), and reached 154 per 1,000 patient-years for patients with impaired LVEF (<45%). Interestingly, however, the mortality impact of heart failure (the population-attributable risk) calculated in this study was greater in the group with HFPEF, reflecting the combined effect of moderate risk and high prevalence of heart failure in the presence of preserved LVEF.

Also in a large, racially mixed urban heart failure population (comprising data from >3,400 American heart failure patients from the Resource Utilization Among Congestive Heart Failure [REACH] study), the annualized age-, sex-, and race-adjusted mortality rate was significantly lower for patients with HFPEF (11.2%) than for those with SHF (13.0%).

The recently published results of the United Kingdom Heart Failure Evaluation and Assessment of Risk Trial (UK-HEART) have also confirmed that 5-year mortality rates for patients with HFPEF and SHF are high; however, they are lower for the former group (25% and 42%, respectively).

Hospital-Cohort Studies

In a recently published review, Hogg et al. identified 12 hospital cohort studies reporting mortality rates for patients with HFPEF. They concluded that despite different methodologic approaches to survival analyses, these studies seemed to confirm a better survival for patients with preserved LVEF than for those with SHF at all time points from admission. Nevertheless, mortality rates for subjects with HFPEF were still unacceptably high, reaching 15%–20% within first year after discharge and even exceeding 40%–50% after 4–5 years of follow-up.

The results of two relatively large studies by Varadarajan et al.[27] and Lenzen at al.[28] are of particular interest. Varadarajan et al. investigated the survival patterns of 2,258 patients with a primary hospital discharge diagnosis of heart failure. Contrary to the other authors, they reported a significantly lower 5-year survival rate for 963 patients with normal LVEF ($\geq$55%) than for 1,295 subjects with an LVEF of <55% (22% and 28%, respectively). The Euro Heart Failure Survey, designed to evaluate to what extent treatment guidelines are implemented in clinical practice, provided a wealth of information on heart failure patient characteristics and management. In particular, the differences between those with preserved and reduced LVEF could be reliably analyzed. Lenzen et al. demonstrated a slightly better short-term outcome for patients with HFPEF than for those with SHF (12-week mortality rates, 10% and 12%, respectively). After adjustment for age, gender, comorbidities, and pharmacologic treatment, patients with reduced LVEF still had about a 40% risk of death.

Owan et al. recently published an interesting study on secular trends in the prevalence and prognosis of heart failure with preserved and reduced LVEF among patients hospitalized with decompensated heart failure at Mayo Clinic hospitals from 1987 through 2001. Of 6,076 patients with heart failure discharged over this time period, data on LVEF were available for 4,596 (76%), and 47% had been diagnosed as having HFPEF (LVEF ≥50%). The proportion of patients with HFPEF was higher among community patients (55%) than among referral patients (45%). They reported that the epidemiologic features of heart failure were likely to change mainly because of alterations in population demographics, relevant changes in the prevalence of heart failure risk factors, and novel treatments applied for heart failure patients. The authors noticed a significant increase in the prevalence of HFPEF among discharged heart failure patients in the three consecutive 5-year periods: 38% (1987–1991), 47% (1992–1996), and 54% (1997–2001). This trend was seen in both community and referral patients with heart failure. At the same time, the number of admissions for heart failure with reduced LVEF did not change. Owan et al. demonstrated that patients with HFPEF had a slightly more favorable long-term outcome than did subjects with SHF, but the outcomes in both groups were very poor (1- and 5-year all-cause mortality rates were 29% vs. 32% and 65% vs. 68% for HFPEF vs. SHF, respectively). Interestingly, the difference in survival in favor of patients with preserved LVEF was mainly observed in the younger group (those aged <65 years; hazard ratio, 0.87, $p = 0.003$) and become marginal in patients who were ≥65 years of age (hazard ratio, 0.97, $p = 0.06$). The authors emphasized that during a 15-year study period survival improved for patients with SHF but remained constant for those with HFPEF.

Similar to this study, two recently published population-based studies on the epidemiology and prognosis in HFPEF are worth mentioning.[29] Bursi et al. prospectively identified and characterized patients with incident and prevalent heart failure in the period of 2003–2005 living in Olmsted County, Minnesota. All 556 heart failure subjects who were recruited (78% inpatients, 53% incident cases) underwent a detailed echocardiographic assessment, and preserved LVEF (≥50%) was present in 55%. At 6 months follow-up, mortality was high irrespectively of LVEF (16% in heart failure patients with reduced and preserved LVEF, which was four to five times higher than expected). Adjustment for age, sex, comorbidities, and heart failure duration did not influence the results.

Bhatia et al. analyzed the patients hospitalized with a primary diagnosis of heart failure in 103 hospitals in Ontario, Canada, which constituted a subset of the Enhanced Feedback for Effective Cardiac Treatment study. The unadjusted rate in all-cause mortality did not differ between 880 patients with HFPEF (LVEF >50%) and 1,570 patients with SHF (LVEF <40%) at 30 days (5% vs. 7%, $p = 0.08$) and at one year (22% vs. 26%, $p = 0.07$). Even after adjustment for other significant predictors, the risk of death remained similar in both groups.

Among patients hospitalized for acute heart failure decompensation, at least 50% have normal LVEF. In this population, survival may be favorably affected by preserved LVEF, but it still remains very worrisome. Ghali et al.[30] reported that 2-year survival rates significantly differed between HFPEF patients (36%) and those with SHF heart failure (64%). Data from more than 100,000 hospitalizations from the Acute Decompensated Heart Failure National Registry database seem to confirm these findings.[31] In-hospital mortality was lower for patients with HFPEF than for patients with reduced LVEF (2.8% vs. 3.9%; adjusted odds ratio, 0.86; $p = 0.005$), but the duration of intensive care unit stay and the total hospital length of stay were similar for both groups.

Clinical Trial Populations

There are three recently published papers that provide data on the mortality of patients with HFPEF who were enrolled in clinical trials.[14,18,32] Two of the trials, which recruited patients with a wide spectrum of LVEF (DIG and the CHARM Program), uniformly demonstrated that those with preserved LVEF had a more favorable outcome. Additionally, the total mortality reported in all the three trials was still unacceptably high but significantly lower than observed in population-based and hospital-cohort studies.

In the DIG study, 7,788 patients with stable heart failure (mean age, 63 years; 25% women) were recruited to digoxin or to placebo. Of them, 6,800 had impaired LVEF (≤45%) and had 988 preserved LVEF (>45%). During a mean follow-up period of 37 months, the overall crude mortality rate was nearly 34% (23% for patients with preserved LVEF and 35% for those with reduced LVEF). Of interest, a remarkable 28% absolute difference in mortality rates between the lowest and the highest LVEF groups (LVEF ≤15%, 52% vs. LVEF >55%, 24%) was detected.

The CHARM Program enrolled 7,599 heart failure patients with a broad spectrum of heart failure who were randomized to treatment with candesartan or placebo. During the mean follow-up period of 38 months, 24% of patients died (17% among those with LVEF ≥43% and 29% among patients with LVEF <43%).

The Perindopril in Elderly People with Chronic Heart Failure study recruited 850 elderly heart failure patients (aged ≥70 years) with preserved LVEF and echocardiographic evidence of diastolic dysfunction. They were randomized to therapy with either perindopril or placebo. The mortality rate was relatively low; during the first year of the study, there were only 36 (4.5%) deaths, which was much less than expected. The investigators suggested that it might be a result of benign prognosis in subjects with diastolic heart failure or alternatively (which seems to be more likely) this clinical trial selectively enrolled low-risk patients.

The above-mentioned studies also provide information on cause-specific mortality in HFPEF patients versus those with impaired LVEF. In the DIG trial, most deaths (79%) were cardiovascular related. Patients with preserved LVEF had a significantly lower risk of cardiovascular death as compared to those with SHF (hazard ratio = 0.60, 0.48–0.74). Deaths due to arrhythmias, heart failure worsening, and other cardiovascular causes were more frequent among SHF patients. In contrast, noncardiovascular deaths occurred more frequently in those with HFPEF (5.6% vs. 3.8%, respectively, for patients with preserved vs. reduced LVEF).

An interesting analysis of the DIG database was performed by Ahmed al.[33] They used a propensity-score methodology in order to reduce any potential imbalance in baseline covariates between patients with reduced and preserved LVEF and evaluated long-term mortality. In a propensity score–matched cohort of DIG patients, those with preserved LVEF had reduced all-cause mortality, all-cause mortality, and heart failure mortality (hazard ratios: 0.73, 0.60, and 0.58, respectively).

Similarly, in the CHARM Program, 80% of all deaths were cardiovascular related. There was a statistically significant trend toward more cardiovascular deaths, sudden deaths, fatal myocardial infarctions, and deaths due to heart failure in patients with reduced LVEF. The rate of noncardiovascular death was fairly constant across the whole spectrum of LVEF. The Perindopril in Elderly People with Chronic Heart Failure study investigators reported that cardiovascular deaths accounted for 75% of all deaths, but the rate of cardiovascular death was low, reaching 3.2% within the first year of follow-up.

Predictors of Mortality

In patients with heart failure and preserved LVEF, there is a strong association between prognosis and an underlying heart failure etiology, with the worst outcome seen among patients with ischemic heart failure or heart failure in the course of uncorrected valvular heart disease. For patients with HFPEF of nonischemic and nonvalvular origin, the annual mortality rate usually does not exceed 2%–3%, whereas in the whole population it is estimated to be around 5%–10%. In patients with HFPEF from the Coronary Artery Surgery Study registry, the 6-year survival rate was 68% for those with three-vessel coronary artery disease and 92% for those without any coronary artery disease. In the study of McAlister et al.,[34] among patients with ischemic heart failure, 1-, 2-, and 3-year survival rates were almost identical for patients with preserved and reduced LVEF (83% vs. 82%, 66% vs. 66%, and 60% vs. 59%, respectively). Those with nonischemic HFPEF had better outcomes, with 1-, 2-, and 3-year survival rates of 92%, 85% and 70%, respectively.

Age itself constitutes the major independent determinant of mortality in heart failure, and advanced age significantly worsens the prognosis in terms of both mortality and hospital admissions for patients with HFPEF.[35,36] On the basis of several reports, Zile et al. estimated that 5-year mortality rates and 1-year rates of rehospitalization due to heart failure worsening were 15% and 25%, 33% and 50%, and 50% and 50%, for HFPEF patients aged <50, 50–70, and >70 years, respectively. Some studies demonstrated that, for elderly patients, mortality did not significantly differ among subjects with SHF and HFPEF.

Race may be another factor significantly modifying the natural history of HFPEF. Unfortunately, nonwhite patients are usually underrepresented in the epidemiologic studies of heart failure, and definitive conclusions are still not possible. In a group of 2,740 white and 563 African-American patients with HFPEF (LVEF >40%, NYHA classes II to IV), African-American patients had a significantly higher mortality risk than white individuals (hazard ratio = 1.34, 95% CI = 1.13–1.60).[37] Racial differences in survival rate were most prominent in patients with a nonischemic etiology (hazard ratio = 1.6; 95% CI = 1.2–2.0) than in those with ischemic heart failure (hazard ratio = 1.1; 95% CI = 0.9–1.4). On the other hand, in a biracial cohort of patients covered by the Veterans Health Administration health care system, mortality and heart failure readmission rates did not differ by race among patients with HFPEF.[38]

There is growing evidence that prognosticators with an established role in the risk stratification in SHF may also be applicable for heart failure patients with preserved LVEF. In 233 consecutive outpatients with HFPEF (LVEF >50%) who experienced an episode of acute decompensation, Valle et al.[39] demonstrated that plasma brain natriuretic peptide was a strong and independent predictor for cardiovascular mortality and readmission during a 6-month follow-up period.

According to Guazzi et al.,[40] exercise capacity indices derived from cardiopulmonary exercise testing can be reliably used as prognosticators for patients with HFPEF. In particular, augmented ventilatory response to exercise, an index of ominous outcome in SHF, was independently related to unfavorable outcome also in heart failure patients with preserved LVEF.

Only recently has it been shown that anemia coexisting with heart failure is associated with high morbidity and mortality. It should be noted that also for HFPEF patients a reduced hemoglobin level predicts an increased risk of cardiovascular hospitalization and all-cause mortality.[41,42] In the CHARM Program, despite an inverse correlation between hemoglobin level and LVEF, anemia was independently associated with an increased risk of death and hospitalization for patients with reduced and preserved LVEF. Patients with HFPEF and anemia had higher incidences of all-cause mortality, cardiovascular deaths, deaths due to heart failure, fatal myocardial infarctions, and finally noncardiovascular deaths than did subjects with a normal hemoglobin level.

Analogously, there is some evidence suggesting that impaired renal function expressed as increased serum creatinine level, high blood urea nitrogen level[43] or reduced estimated glomerular filtration rate[44] is a strong and independent predictor of poor outcome in patients with HFPEF. The following variables have also been found as independent predictors of mortality in heart failure patients with reduced LVEF: blood pressure, lung disease, diabetes, NYHA class, peripheral vascular disease, cancer, dementia, dialysis, respiratory rate, and serum sodium.

Hospital Admissions

Based on the available epidemiologic studies, one can conclude that for patients with HFPEF morbidity is alarmingly high, as evidenced by frequent consultations in outpatient clinics, high rate of rehospitalizations, and subsequent increased health care costs.[45–47] In a population of community-dwelling elderly persons, Liao et al. compared the long-term health care costs of heart failure patients with preserved and reduced LVEF. The costs remained similar for both groups and also after adjustment for comorbid conditions. For the prevalent and incident cases, the relative 5-year costs were respectively 3% higher or 4% lower for patients with reduced versus those with preserved LVEF (nonsignificant difference for both). Philbin et al.[48] previously reported that among hospitalized heart failure patients the length of stay and hospital charges were similar for heart failure patients with reduced and preserved LVEF. Hogg et al. estimated that approximately 40% of overall health care system costs of heart failure are accounted for by patients with HFPEF.

Several studies have demonstrated similar rates of hospital admissions due to cardiovascular and noncardiovascular causes for heart failure patients with preserved and reduced LVEF, particularly if the hospital cohort populations were studied. Zile et al. estimated that the 1-year rehospitalization rate approached 50% for HFPEF patients aged 50 years and more, which was almost identical to that for subjects with SHF. In a population-based study of hospitalized heart failure patients, Bhatia et al. reported no significant differences in inhospital care and complications between 880 patients with HFPEF (LVEF >50%) and 1,570 patients with SHF (LVEF <40%). The rates of renal failure, cardiac arrest, acute coronary syndrome (myocardial infarction or unstable angina), and admission to a coronary care unit and/or an intensive care unit were comparable (patients with SHF demonstrated higher rates of only hypotension and cardiogenic shock). Moreover, the rates of 30-day and 1-year readmissions for heart failure were similar for patients with preserved and reduced LVEF (4.5% vs. 4.9%, $p = 0.66$; 13.5% vs. 16.1%, $p = 0.09$). In the recent study by Berry et al.[49] of 528 acutely hospitalized heart failure patients, those with preserved LVEF tended to have a slightly lower risk of hospital readmissions due to heart failure but a similar rate of subsequent readmissions for any reason when compared with SHF patients. The high rate of hospitalization for both groups should be noted: during the median follow-up of 814 days, 73% of patients were readmitted to the hospital at least once.

Population-based studies of nonhospitalized subjects usually report a lower risk of hospital admissions for patients with HFPEF. In the Olmsted County heart failure incident case study, the proportions of patients never hospitalized or hospitalized more than times for heart failure over 5 years among those with preserved or reduced LVEF were 24% versus 10% and 25% versus 49%, respectively. Dauterman et al. show, after adjustment for covariates, a 1-year heart failure–related readmission rate 22% higher for patients with SHF than for those with HFPEF. In the CHARM Program, the rate of hospitalization because of heart failure deterioration declined with an increasing EF up to 45%. The same relationship was observed for combined fatal and nonfatal myocardial infarction. According to McDermott et al.,[50] 55% of patients with reduced versus 41% of patients with preserved LVEF were either readmitted or had an emergency room visit within 6 months after discharge. For patients hospitalized with heart failure aged 70 years or more, readmission rates during the following 3 months were higher for SHF patients than for HFPEF patients (42% vs. 29%). In a group of 916 diastolic heart failure and 6,701 SHF patients without valvular heart disease in the DIG trial, during a median 38 months of follow-up, patients with heart failure and preserved LVEF had a similar risk, compared with SHF, of all-cause hospitalization (67% vs. 64%), but a significantly reduced risk of cardiovascular hospitalization (hazard ratio = 0.84, 0.73–0.96) and heart failure-related hospitalization (hazard ratio = 0.63, 0.51–0.77).

Remaining Questions and Conclusion

The available evidence does not allow us to conclude definitely whether the natural history of heart failure with preserved or reduced LVEF is different, and this still needs to be established. The existing data cannot simply be compared mainly because of inconsistent methodologies (such as a small number of patients, inclusion of outpatients and/or hospitalized patients, post hoc analyses of trial-derived databases of heart failure populations undergoing specific selections, age and/or racial differences of studied groups, heterogenous criteria for the definition of HFPEF, various cut-off values for normal and impaired systolic LV function, imaging modalities, to name but a few). Undoubtedly, all of these issues significantly hamper the proper interpretation of available epidemiologic data. On the other hand, however, they reveal an urgent need for properly designed prospective studies that will uncover the unique features of HFPEF to discriminate this pathology from SHF.

Based on the most recent epidemiologic data demonstrating an increasing prevalence of HFPEF in modern communities, together with high morbidity and mortality rates, it is presumed that this clinical syndrome may soon become responsible for a substantial amount of heart failure. In the context of comprehensive management of patients with HFPEF, studies focusing on precise risk stratification in this population of heart failure patients are needed.

References

1. Redfield MM, Jacobsen SJ, Burnett JC Jr, Mahoney DW, Bailey KR, Rodeheffer RJ. Burden of systolic and diastolic ventricular dysfunction in the community: appreciating the scope of the heart failure epidemic. JAMA 2003;289:194–202.
2. Bursi F, Weston SA, Redfield MM, Jacobsen SJ, Pakhomov S, Nkomo VT, Meverden RA, Roger VL. Systolic and diastolic heart failure in the community. JAMA 2006;296:2209–2216.
3. Hogg K, Swedberg K, McMurray J. Heart failure with preserved left ventricular systolic function: epidemiology, clinical characteristics, and prognosis J Am Coll Cardiol 2004;43:317–327.
4. Zile MR, Brutsaert DL. New concepts in diastolic dysfunction and diastolic heart failure. Part I: diagnosis, prognosis, and measurements of diastolic function. Circulation 2002;105:1387–1393.
5. Thomas MD, Fox KF, Coats AJ, Sutton GC. The epidemiological enigma of heart failure with preserved systolic function. Eur J Heart Fail 2004;6:125–136.
6. Franklin KM, Aurigemma GP. Prognosis in diastolic heart failure. Prog Cardiovasc Dis 2005;47:333–339.
7. Senni M, Redfield MM. Heart failure with preserved systolic function. A different natural history? J Am Coll Cardiol 2001;38:1277–1282.
8. Swedberg K, Cleland J, Dargie H, Drexler H, Follath F, Komajda M, Tavazzi L, Smiseth OA, Gavazzi A, Haverich A, Hoes A, Jaarsma T, Korewicki J, Levy S, Linde C, Lopez-Sendon JL, Nieminen MS, Pierard L, Remme WJ; Task Force for the Diagnosis and Treatment of Chronic Heart Failure of the European Society of Cardiology. Guidelines for the Diagnosis and Treatment of Chronic Heart Failure: Executive Summary (update 2005): The Task Force for the Diagnosis and Treatment of Chronic Heart Failure of the European Society of Cardiology. Eur Heart J 2005;26:1115–1140.
9. Hunt SA; American College of Cardiology; American Heart Association Task Force on Practice Guidelines (Writing Committee to Update the 2001 Guidelines for the Evaluation and Management of Heart Failure). ACC/AHA 2005 Guideline Update for the Diagnosis and Management of Chronic Heart Failure in the Adult: a report of the American College of Cardiology/American Heart Association Task Force on Practice Guidelines (Writing Committee to Update the 2001 Guidelines for the Evaluation and Management of Heart Failure). J Am Coll Cardiol 2005;46:e1–e82.
10. Brogan WC, 3rdHillis LD, Flores ED, Lange RA. The natural history of isolated left ventricular diastolic dysfunction. Am J Med 1992;92:627–630.
11. Setaro JF, Soufer R, Remetz MS, Perlmutter RA, Zaret BL. Long-term outcome in patients with congestive heart failure and intact systolic left ventricular performance. Am J Cardiol 1992;69:1212–1216.
12. Judge KW, Pawitan Y, Caldwell J, Gersh BJ, Kennedy JW. Congestive heart failure symptoms in patients with preserved left ventricular systolic function: analysis of the CASS registry. J Am Coll Cardiol 1991;18:377–382.
13. Gottdiener JS, McClelland RL, Marshall R, Shemanski L, Furberg CD, Kitzman DW, Cushman M, Polak J, Gardin JM, Gersh BJ, Aurigemma GP, Manolio TA. Outcome of congestive heart failure in elderly persons: influence of left ventricular systolic function. The Cardiovascular Health Study. Ann Intern Med 2002;137:631–639.
14. Curtis JP, Sokol SI, Wang Y, Rathore SS, Ko DT, Jadbabaie F, Portnay EL, Marshalko SJ, Radford MJ, Krumholz HM. The association of left ventricular ejection fraction, mortality, and cause of death in stable outpatients with heart failure. J Am Coll Cardiol 2003;42:736–742.
15. Aronow WS, Ahn C, Kronzon I. Prognosis of congestive heart failure in elderly patients with normal versus abnormal left ventricular systolic function associated with coronary artery disease. Am J Cardiol 1990;66:1257–1259.
16. Aronow WS, Ahn C, Kronzon I. Prognosis of congestive heart failure after prior myocardial infarction in older men and women with abnormal versus normal left ventricular ejection fraction. Am J Cardiol. 2000;85:1382–1384.
17. Pfeffer MA, Swedberg K, Granger CB, Held P, McMurray JJ, Michelson EL, Olofsson B, Ostergren J, Yusuf S, Pocock S; CHARM Investigators and Committees. Effects of candesartan on mortality and morbidity in patients with chronic heart failure: the CHARM-Overall programme. Lancet 2003;362:759–766.
18. Solomon SD, Anavekar N, Skali H, McMurray JJ, Swedberg K, Yusuf S, Granger CB, Michelson EL, Wang D, Pocock S, Pfeffer MA; Candesartan in Heart Failure Reduction in Mortality (CHARM) Investigators. Influence of ejection fraction on cardiovascular outcomes in a broad spectrum of heart failure patients. Circulation 2005;112:3738–3744.
19. Owan TE, Hodge DO, Herges RM, Jacobsen SJ, Roger VL, Redfield MM. Trends in prevalence and outcome of heart failure with preserved ejection fraction. N Engl J Med 2006;355:251–259.

20. Cohn JN, Johnson G. Heart failure with normal ejection fraction. The V-HeFT Study. Veterans Administration Cooperative Study Group. Circulation. 1990;81(2 Suppl):III48–II53.

21. Senni M, Tribouilloy CM, Rodeheffer RJ, Jacobsen SJ, Evans JM, Bailey KR, Redfield MM. Congestive heart failure in the community: a study of all incident cases in Olmsted County, Minnesota, in 1991. Circulation 1998;98:2282–2289.

22. Vasan RS, Larson MG, Benjamin EJ, Evans JC, Reiss CK, Levy D. Congestive heart failure in subjects with normal versus reduced left ventricular ejection fraction: prevalence and mortality in a population-based cohort. J Am Coll Cardiol 1999;33:1948–1955.

23. Kupari M, Lindroos M, Iivanainen AM, Heikkila J, Tilvis R. Congestive heart failure in old age: prevalence, mechanisms and 4-year prognosis in the Helsinki Ageing Study. J Intern Med 1997;241:387–394.

24. Chen HH, Lainchbury JG, Senni M, Bailey KR, Redfield MM. Diastolic heart failure in the community: clinical profile, natural history, therapy, and impact of proposed diagnostic criteria. J Card Fail 2002;8:279–287.

25. McCullough PA, Khandelwal AK, McKinnon JE, Shenkman HJ, Pampati V, Nori D, Sullivan RA, Sandberg KR, Kaatz S. Outcomes and prognostic factors of systolic as compared with diastolic heart failure in urban America. Congest Heart Fail 2005;11:6–11.

26. MacCarthy PA, Kearney MT, Nolan J, Lee AJ, Prescott RJ, Shah AM, Brooksby WP, Fox KA. Prognosis in heart failure with preserved left ventricular systolic function: prospective cohort study. BMJ 2003;327:78–79.

27. Varadarajan P, Pai RG. Prognosis of congestive heart failure in patients with normal versus reduced ejection fractions: results from a cohort of 2, 258 hospitalized patients. J Card Fail 2003;9:107–112.

28. Lenzen MJ, Scholte op Reimer WJ, Boersma E, Vantrimpont PJ, Follath F, Swedberg K, Cleland J, Komajda M. Differences between patients with a preserved and a depressed left ventricular function: a report from the Euro Heart Failure Survey. Eur Heart J 2004;25:1214–1220.

29. Bhatia RS, Tu JV, Lee DS, Austin PC, Fang J, Haouzi A, Gong Y, Liu PP. Outcome of heart failure with preserved ejection fraction in a population-based study. N Engl J Med 2006;355:260–269.

30. Ghali JK, Kadakia S, Bhatt A, Cooper R, Liao Y. Survival of heart failure patients with preserved versus impaired systolic function: the prognostic implication of blood pressure. Am Heart J 1992;123:993–997.

31. Yancy CW, Lopatin M, Stevenson LW, De Marco T, Fonarow GC; ADHERE Scientific Advisory Committee and Investigators. Clinical presentation, management, and in-hospital outcomes of patients admitted with acute decompensated heart failure with preserved systolic function: a report from the Acute Decompensated Heart Failure National Registry (ADHERE) Database. J Am Coll Cardiol 2006;47:76–84.

32. Cleland JG, Tendera M, Adamus J, Freemantle N, Polonski L, Taylor J; PEP-CHF Investigators. The Perindopril in Elderly People With Chronic Heart Failure (PEP-CHF) study. Eur Heart J 2006;27:2338–2345.

33. Ahmed A, Perry GJ, Fleg JL, Love TE, Goff DC Jr, Kitzman DW. Outcomes in ambulatory chronic systolic and diastolic heart failure: a propensity score analysis. Am Heart J 2006;152:956–966.

34. McAlister FA, Teo KK, Taher M, Montague TJ, Humen D, Cheung L, Kiaii M, Yim R, Armstrong PW. Insights into the contemporary epidemiology and outpatient management of congestive heart failure. Am Heart J 1999;138:87–94.

35. Jones RC, Francis GS, Lauer MS. Predictors of mortality in patients with heart failure and preserved systolic function in the Digitalis Investigation Group trial. J Am Coll Cardiol 2004;44:1025–1029.

36. O'Connor CM, Gattis WA, Shaw L, Cuffe MS, Califf RM. Clinical characteristics and long-term outcomes of patients with heart failure and preserved systolic function. Am J Cardiol 2000;86:863–867.

37. East MA, Peterson ED, Shaw LK, Gattis WA, O'Connor CM. Racial differences in the outcomes of patients with diastolic heart failure. Am Heart J 2004;148:151–156.

38. Agoston I, Cameron CS, Yao D, Dela Rosa A, Mann DL, Deswal A. Comparison of outcomes of white versus black patients hospitalized with heart failure and preserved ejection fraction. Am J Cardiol 2004;94:1003–1007.

39. Valle R, Aspromonte N, Feola M, Milli M, Canali C, Giovinazzo P, Carbonieri E, Ceci V, Cerisano S, Barro S, Milani L. B-type natriuretic peptide can predict the medium-term risk in patients with acute heart failure and preserved systolic function. J Gerontol A Biol Sci Med Sci 2005;60:1339–1344.

40. Guazzi M, Myers J, Arena R. Cardiopulmonary exercise testing in the clinical and prognostic assessment of diastolic heart failure. J Am Coll Cardiol 2005;46:1883–1890.

41. Brucks S, Little WC, Chao T, Rideman RL, Upadhya B, Wesley-Farrington D, Sane DC. Relation of

TABLE 16.1. Diastolic heart failure trials with clinical end points.

Trial	Drug studied	Inclusion criteria	Primary end piont	Results
PEP-CHF (n = 850)	Perindopril	Age ≥ 70, HF, LVEF ≥ 40%	Total mortality and HF-related hospitalization	$p = 0.5$ for primary end point, $p = 0.033$ for HF-related hospitalization at 1 year
CHARM-Preserved (n = 3,025)	Candesartan	HF, LVEF ≥ 40%	Cardiovascular death and HF-related hospitalization	$p = 0.1$ for primary endpoint
I-PRESERVE (n = 4,100)	Irbesartan	Age ≥ 60, HF, LVEF ≥ 45%	Time to all-cause death or cardiovascular hospitalization	Ongoing study
SENIORS (n = 2,128)	Nebivolol	Age ≥ 70, HF (1/3 patients had LVEF > 35%)	All-cause mortality and cardiovascular hospitalization	$p = 0.03$ for primary end point
TOPCAT (n = 4,500)	Spironolactone	Age ≥ 50, HF, LVEF ≥ 45%	Cardiovascular mortality, cardiac arrest, HF-related hospitalization	Ongoing study
DIG ancillary (n = 988)	Digitalis	HF, LVEF ≥ 45%	HF-related hospitalization or HF mortality	$p = 0.136$ for primary outcome, $p = 0.09$ for HF-related hospitalizations

Note: HF, heart failure; LVEF, left ventricular ejection fraction; TOPCAT, Trial of Aldosterone Antagonist Therapy in Adults With Preserved Ejection Fraction Congestive Heart Failure study.

thickness of interventricular septum or posterior wall ≥13 mm, and abnormal Doppler indexes of diastolic flow (E/A ratio <0.5 or deceleration time >280 ms or isovolumic relaxation time >105 ms).

The primary end point of the study was a composite of total mortality and unplanned heart failure–related hospitalization. Secondary end points included each component of the primary end point, cardiovascular mortality, and heart failure symptomatic status assessed by New York Heart Association (NYHA) classification. In most patients a 6-min corridor walk test was performed, and in a substantial proportion of patients N-terminal prohormone brain natriuretic peptide was measured.

Eight hundred fifty patients were randomized.[5] Their mean age was 76 years, and 55% were women. The median follow-up period was 2.1 years. Recruitment and event rates were lower than expected, reducing the power of the study to show the difference in primary end point to 35%. A significant proportion of patients withdrew from perindopril (28%) and placebo (26%) after 1 year. Overall, the primary end point occurred in 107 patients assigned to placebo and in 100 of those assigned to perindopril (hazard ratio = 0.919; 95% CI, 0.700–1.208; $p = 0.545$). Analysis performed at 1 year, when compliance was 90%, showed an almost significant reduction in the primary outcome (hazard ratio = 0.692; 95% CI, 0.474–1.010; $p = 0.055$) and a significant reduction

in hospitalization for heart failure (hazard ratio = 0.628; 95% CI, 0.408–0.966; $p = 0.033$) with perindopril compared with placebo (Figures 16.1 and 16.2).[5] The NYHA functional class ($p < 0.001$) and the distance of the 6-min corridor walk test ($p = 0.02$) improved in patients assigned to perindopril.[5]

Thus, although the PEP-CHF study lacked the power to show an effect on its primary end point, the symptomatic improvement, better exercise capacity, and reduced number of heart failure–related hospitalizations observed with perindopril at 1 year, when most patients were on assigned therapy, suggest that perindopril may be of benefit for elderly patients with heart failure and LV diastolic dysfunction.

Two other studies showed a positive effect of enalapril on the symptomatic improvement of patients with diastolic dysfunction. One was conducted with a group of elderly patients with prior myocardial infarction,[6] and one was a subanalysis of the Vasodilator in Heart Failure Trials.[7] On the contrary, no positive effect of enalapril was shown in the subanalysis of 50 patients in the CONSENSUS trial.[8]

Angiotensin Receptor Blockers

The rationale for implementation of an angiotensin receptor blocker (ARB) is based on an assumption that this drug class proved effective in the

16. Treatment of Diastolic Heart Failure

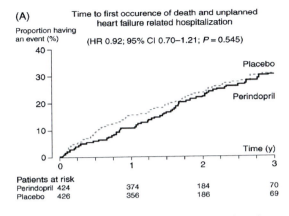

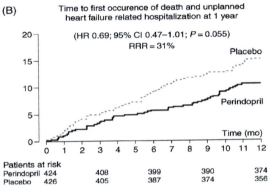

FIGURE 16.1. Results of the PEP-CHF study with respect to the combined primary outcome assessed **(A)** and after 1 year of observation **(B)**.

treatment of arterial hypertension and caused regression of LV hypertrophy, thus counteracting two major predictors of heart failure with preserved systolic function.[9] Furthermore, it is presumed that blockade of only one of the angiotensin receptors, AT1, renders the AT2 receptor available for its agonist. Advantages of the angiotensin binding to the AT2 receptor include activation of collagenases and induction of fibroblast apoptosis leading to reversal of myocardial fibrosis.[10,11] Finally, there is evidence from animal studies that angiotensin receptor blockade prevents development of fibrosis, hypertrophy, and heart failure in a rat model of heart failure with preserved LV systolic function.[12]

In patients with heart failure and impaired systolic function ARBs were shown to improve mortality and morbidity when used in addition to[13] or instead of[14] ACE inhibitors. Most data pertaining to this topic come from the Candesartan in Heart Failure — Assessment of Reduction in Mortality and Morbidity (CHARM) study.[15]

There are no studies of ARBs given to patients with proven diastolic dysfunction. However, one of the components of the CHARM study, CHARM-Preserved, provided important data on patients with relatively preserved LV systolic function.[16]

CHARM-Preserved was a multicenter, randomized, placebo-controlled study in which 3,025 patients were randomized[16] to receive candesartan in a dose of up to 32 mg per day or placebo. Patients aged 18 years or older, with symptoms of heart failure (NYHA classes II to IV) of at least 4 weeks' duration, with a history of hospitalization for a cardiac reason, and an LVEF >40% were

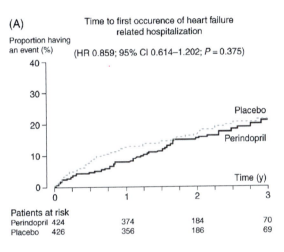

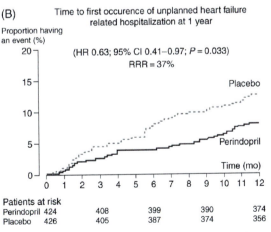

FIGURE 16.2. Results of the PEP-CHF study with respect to heart failure hospitalization outcome assessed **(A)** and after 1 year of observation **(B)**.

eligible for the study. Assessment of LV diastolic function was not required. Physicians were free to prescribe all treatments other than ARBs. It should be emphasized that approximately 30% of patients in this arm had an LVEF of 60% or more.

The primary outcome measure was a composite of cardiovascular death and hospitalization for heart failure. Median follow-up was 36.6 months. The primary end point occurred in 333 patients (22%) in the candesartan arm and in 336 patients (24%) in the placebo arm (unadjusted hazard ratio = 0.89; 95% CI, 0.77–1.03; $p = 0.118$). The number of cardiovascular deaths in the active treatment group was identical to that in the placebo group (170 and 170, respectively), but fewer patients in the candesartan group were admitted to a hospital for heart failure (230 vs. 279; $p = 0.017$). Thus, candesartan proved to have a moderate impact on preventing hospitalization for heart failure in patients with preserved LV systolic function.

The results of the CHARM-Preserved study must be interpreted in the context of the entire CHARM study, which was one of the largest trials performed with subjects with heart failure, with more than 7,600 patients included.[15] In addition to CHARM-Preserved, the overall program included two other components — CHARM-Added and CHARM-Alternative. CHARM-Added included 2,548 patients with depressed LVEF (≤40 %) who were receiving an ACE inhibitor.[13]

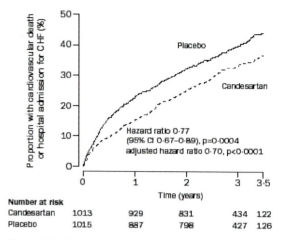

FIGURE 16.4. Primary outcome results of the CHARM-Alternative trial. (Reprinted from Granger et al.,[14] with permission of Elsevier.)

CHARM-Alternative also included patients (2,028 subjects) with an EF ≤40% but who were not treated with an ACE inhibitor because of intolerance or contraindication.[14]

The effect of candesartan on all-cause mortality was analyzed for the overall program, and a composite of cardiovascular death and hospital admission for heart failure was the primary end point in all three component studies.

In CHARM-Overall, candesartan induced a 1.6% absolute reduction in all-cause mortality (unadjusted hazard ratio = 0.91; 95% CI, 0.83–1.00), which did not quite reach the level of statistical significance ($p = 0.055$). However, a significant reduction in the combined incidence of cardiovascular death and hospital admission for heart failure (hazard ratio = 0.84; 95% CI, 0.77–0.91; $p < 0.0001$) was observed.[15] The composite of cardiovascular death and congestive heart failure hospitalization was reduced significantly by 15% ($p = 0.011$) in CHARM-Added[13] and by 23% ($p = 0.0004$) in CHARM-Alternative[14] (Figures 16.3 and 16.4).

In CHARM-Preserved, the trend was similar but driven solely by the decrease in congestive heart failure–related hospital admissions. It should be noted that, compared with patients with impaired systolic function enrolled in the CHARM study, those included in the CHARM-Preserved were older and more likely to be in NYHA class II, and there was a higher proportion of women.[16]

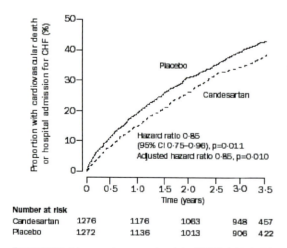

FIGURE 16.3. Primary outcome results of the CHARM-Added trial. (Reprinted from McMurray et al.,[13] with permission of Elsevier.)

There was no indication that these patients had DHF, because diastolic function was not assessed. The objective diagnostic data available at study entry are convincing enough to state that an overwhelming majority of patients included in CHARM-Preserved had heart failure.

Kasama et al.[17] recently examined a new, potentially advantageous mechanism of angiotensin receptor blockade by candesartan specifically in patients with heart failure and preserved LV function. The authors used a radiolabeled analog of guanethidine, the adrenergic neuron-blocking agent that utilizes the same myocardial pathways as norepinephrine, to show in radionuclide studies that myocardial adrenergic uptake and release of neurotransmitters was improved after 6 months of treatment with candesartan. This effect was attributed to inhibition of β-adrenergic receptor–mediated signaling by an ARB.

The ongoing I-PRESERVE study (Irbesartan in Heart Failure with Preserved Systolic Function)[18] is likely to provide additional relevant data on the effect of ARBs in this group of patients. This study is examining the effect of the ARB irbesartan at a dose of 300 mg per day in patients with heart failure and preserved LV function. The study is enrolling 4,100 subjects aged ≥60 years with heart failure symptoms corresponding to NYHA classes II to IV, LVEF ≥45%, and either hospitalization for heart failure within 6 months or corroborative evidence of heart failure, or the substrate for DHF. In patients with no recent hospitalization for heart failure, current NYHA class III or IV is required, together with chest x-ray evidence of pulmonary congestion, presence of LV hypertrophy, or left bundle branch block on the electrocardiogram or the echo evidence for LV hypertrophy or enlarged left atrium in the absence of atrial fibrillation.

Thus, although the diagnosis of diastolic dysfunction is not required, the presence of its substrate will be recorded in a substantial proportion of patients. Stringent criteria used in this study to diagnose heart failure will likely prevent patients without this condition from being entered into the trial.

The primary end point is the time from randomization to first occurrence of the composite outcome of all-cause death or cardiovascular hospitalization. The minimum follow-up period will be 2 years.

Secondary end points include cardiovascular death; all-cause mortality; combined cardiovascular death, nonfatal myocardial infarction, nonfatal stroke; combined heart failure mortality or heart failure hospitalization; changes in quality of life as measured by the Minnesota Living with Heart Failure questionnaire; changes in NYHA class; and changes in brain natriuretic peptide level. The study was launched in 2002, and its results are expected soon.

The Hong-Kong Diastolic Heart Failure study[19] planned to randomize patients with heart failure symptoms and echocardiographically proven diastolic abnormalities in the absence of a significant systolic dysfunction (EF >45%). There were three treatment arms: the ACE inhibitor ramipril, the ARB irbesartan combined with diuretics, and diuretics alone. Recruitment was abandoned due to the low number of patients recruited (only 40 out of almost 1,400 screened).[20] The main reasons for rejections were current treatment with ACE inhibitors, low LVEF (below 45%), valvular heart disease, and hematologic abnormalities. Although the study was not completed, it did provide the important information that patients with isolated diastolic LV dysfunction may have many comorbidities, making them ineligible for inclusion in clinical trials and/or represent a smaller than expected proportion of patients with heart failure. Importantly, however, only fewer than 2% of patients were excluded because they were thought to have no evidence of heart failure.

β-Adrenergic Receptor Blockers

The rationale for the use of β-adrenergic receptor blockers in DHF comes from their ability to prolong the diastole, thus promoting diastolic filling and improving myocardial perfusion.[21] β-Receptor blockade with metoprolol,[21] carvedilol,[22] and atenolol and nebivolol[23] was shown to improve echocardiographic indices of diastolic function in small groups of patients with heart failure and depressed or preserved LV function. Some less well-known mechanisms of β-blockers' action were claimed to play a role in this improvement: normalization of calcium handling in sarcoplasmic reticulum, influence on sympathetic nerve activity, and optimization of myocardial energy production with reduction in fatty acid oxidation.[24]

The effect of carvedilol was examined in the Swedish Evaluation of Diastolic Dysfunction Treated with Carvedilol study,[25] which included 113 patients. Patients had symptomatic heart failure with an LVEF of >45% and compromised diastolic function: abnormal early to atrial diastolic flow velocity ratio (84% of patients), prolonged isovolumic relaxation time (14%), or pathologic pulmonary venous inflow profile (2%). Echocardiographic examination was performed at baseline and after 6 months of treatment. The objective was to compare the effect of carvedilol versus placebo on diastolic function as assessed by Doppler echocardiography. The primary end point was defined as regression of diastolic dysfunction determined by changes in mitral Doppler flow profile, isovolumic relaxation time, early to atrial diastolic flow velocity ratio, and pulmonary flow velocities.

Follow-up was completed with 93 patients. Differences in the primary end point between the placebo and carvedilol groups were not significant. Among patients treated with carvedilol the composite primary end point showed improvement in diastolic function in 51% of patients, remained unchanged in 19%, and showed deterioration in 30%. In the placebo group the composite primary end point improved in 40% of patients, was unchanged in 22%, and worsened in 38%.

One parameter improved significantly in the carvedilol group compared with placebo: early to atrial diastolic flow velocity ratio ($p = 0.046$). No significant changes in the deceleration time, isovolumic relaxation time, or pulmonary systolic to diastolic velocity ratio were observed.

In the carvedilol group, the mean heart rate decreased from 74/min at baseline to 60/min after follow-up ($p < 0.0001$), and there was a trend toward a better effect of treatment on diastolic function parameters in patients with a higher baseline heart rate.

The change in the mitral early to atrial flow velocity ratio was interpreted as an indication of improvement in LV diastolic dysfunction. No clinical outcomes were assessed in this study.

The influence of carvedilol on echocardiographic measures of abnormal diastolic mitral inflow was examined in a study by Palazouli et al.[26] This study included 23 patients with ischemic or dilated cardiomyopathy and severe heart failure (NYHA class III or IV) with an EF of <35%. All patients had a restrictive mitral inflow pattern with an E/A wave ratio of >1, a deceleration time of the E wave of <130 ms, and an isovolumic relaxation time of <60 ms. Patients were randomized to receive carvedilol in a dose up to 50 mg/day or placebo. Echocardiographic assessment performed at 12 months showed, in comparison with the baseline study, a significant decrease in E wave velocity from 76.8 ± 7 cm/s to 70.4 ± 5 cm/s ($p < 0.03$), an increase in A wave velocity from 27.4 ± 4 cm/s to 39.3 ± 4 cm/s ($p < 0.01$), an increase in deceleration time from 113 ± 6 ms to 139.5 ± 16 ms ($p < 0,02$), and an increase in isovolumic relaxation time increase from 49.4 ± 7 to 74.2 ± 8 ms ($p < 0.01$). The recovery of diastolic function parameters was accompanied by an increase in EF and reversed chamber remodeling. The authors attributed the influence of carvedilol on diastolic function to a decrease in heart rate and blood pressure as well as to its ancillary effects, such as antiinflammatory and antifibrotic actions, vascular peripheral dilatation with resulting wall rigidity amelioration, reduction of parietal tension, a decrease in wall thickness, and recovery of coronary blood flow.

The Study of the Effects of Nebivolol Intervention on Outcomes and Rehospitalization in Seniors with Heart Failure (SENIORS) trial[27] included 2,128 heart failure patients 70 years old or older. The study was designed as a parallel group, double-blind, randomized, multicenter international trial comparing nebivolol, titrated from 1.25 to 10 mg once daily, with placebo. Most patients were in NYHA class II or III (56% and 38%, respectively).

The majority of enrolled patients (64% in the nebivolol group and 65% in the placebo group) had significantly impaired LV systolic function (an EF of 35% or less), but the population with a higher EF (>35%) constituted more than one third of the study group: 36% in the nebivolol and 35% in the placebo group.

The primary outcome of the SENIORS trial was a composite of all-cause mortality and cardiovascular hospital admission. Secondary end points included all-cause mortality, all-cause hospitalizations, cardiovascular mortality, cardiovascular hospitalization, and functional capacity assessed by NYHA classification and a 6-min walk test result.

Mean follow-up was 21 months. The primary outcome occurred in 31.1% in the nebivolol group and in 35.3% of placebo group (hazard ratio = 0.86; 95% CI, 0.74–0.99; $p = 0.039$), with the absolute risk reduction of 4.2%.

The risk reduction for patients with preserved LV function was almost identical to that for patients with a low EF regardless of the cut-off point used for EF (35% or 40%). Among patients with an LVEF of ≤35%, the primary outcome occurred in 21.7% in the nebivolol group and in 25.1% in the placebo group and among those with an EF >35% in 17.6% and 21.9%, respectively (the p value for interaction with an EF of 0.42.).

Among the secondary outcomes, a statistical difference in favor of nebivolol occurred in the composite of cardiovascular mortality and cardiovascular hospitalization (28.6% vs. 33%; $p = 0.027$).

The postulated mechanisms of the beneficial action of nebivolol include a reduction in LV wall stress, attenuation of adverse neurohormonal activation, and reduction in the incidence of acute coronary syndromes. On the basis of the SENIORS study, nebivolol has been recommended for elderly heart failure patients irrespective of LVEF.

It is interesting to note that in a recently published echocardiographic substudy of SENIORS, no significant changes in either systolic or diastolic function parameters were observed in patients with an EF of >35%. In patients with a low EF, systolic function improved, but no changes in diastolic function were recorded. It is therefore unlikely that improvement in diastolic performance was responsible for the clinical benefit in either of the two groups.[28]

Calcium Channel Blockers

Experimental data indicate that nonhydropyridine calcium channel blockers can prevent diastolic failure, at least in animals with hypertrophic cardiomyopathy. In mice with a troponin T mutation, prone to develop severe primary DHF, administration of diltiazem can prevent the occurrence of pathologic changes.[29]

For patients with hypertrophic cardiomyopathy, verapamil had a beneficial effect attributed to improvement in LV diastolic function. Verapamil was shown to favorably shift the pressure–volume relations in diastole, increase the peak filling rate, and decrease the time from the beginning of rapid diastolic filling to the peak filling.[29–31]

There is some evidence that a similar beneficial effect may be expected for patients with diastolic dysfunction with an etiology other than hypertrophic cardiomyopathy. For example, in a small group of 20 patients with heart failure and an EF of >45%, 5 weeks of treatment with verapamil significantly improved exercise capacity and LV diastolic filling parameters.[32] Although it is speculated that improved calcium handling is responsible for these effects, the heart rate reduction seen after verapamil or diltiazem administration can also be regarded as a contributing factor.

Aldosterone Antagonists

Aldosterone antagonists are useful for patients with SHF.[2,3] Because they have been found to prevent structural and functional changes in the circulatory system, such as myocardial fibrosis with increased collagen turnover, altered autonomic balance, and decreased arterial compliance,[32,33] they may also be expected to have a beneficial effect for patients with diastolic dysfunction. Objective data regarding the effect of aldosterone antagonists in diastolic dysfunction are, however, scarce.

In an echocardiographic study conducted with 30 patients with hypertension, heart failure, and evidence of abnormal diastolic function with an EF exceeding 50%, administration of spironolactone for 6 months resulted in a significant improvement in sensitive quantitative tissue Doppler measures of myocardial function: strain rate and peak systolic strain. Posterior wall thickness and left atrial area were also reduced.[34]

In a prospective randomized study conducted with 34 patients with essential hypertension, LV hypertrophy, and abnormal diastolic LV function, treatment with the aldosterone antagonist canrenone in a dose of 50 mg/day caused a significant improvement in diastolic parameters (peak lengthening rate of LV diameter and peak thinning rate of the LV posterior wall) obtained from digitized M-mode echocardiography, as well as an improvement in Doppler indices of mitral inflow. This improvement was not accounted for by blood pressure or LV mass changes and was attributed to an opposition of the profibrotic effect of aldosterone.[35]

The Trial of Aldosterone Antagonist Therapy in Adults With Preserved Ejection Fraction Congestive Heart Failure study began in September 2006. The purpose of this trial is to evaluate the effectiveness of spironolactone in reducing all-cause mortality in patients with heart failure with preserved systolic function. Patients 50 years old or older with clinical signs and symptoms of heart failure (dyspnea, rales, edema, jugular vein distension) or chest x-ray evidence of pleural effusion, pulmonary congestion, or cardiomegaly and an LVEF of ≥45% who have been hospitalized for heart failure are randomized into two groups: one receiving spironolactone 15–45 mg/day and the other receiving placebo. Primary outcomes include cardiovascular mortality, aborted cardiac arrest, and hospitalization for the management of heart failure. It is planned to enroll 4,500 patients in 150 medical centers. The study is to be completed in 2011.

Digitalis

The DIG ancillary trial[36] enrolled 988 patients with symptoms of heart failure and an LVEF above 45%. As in the main DIG trial, there was no effect on mortality, but hospitalization related to heart failure was significantly reduced in the digitalis group compared with the placebo group.

In the ancillary trial 492 patients were treated with digoxin and 496 received placebo. The numbers of deaths in these groups were 115 (23.4%) and 116 (23.4%), respectively, with a risk ratio of 0.99 and a 95% CI of 0.76–2.28. The results for the combined end point of death and hospitalization because of worsening heart failure were risk ratio = 0.82 and a 95% CI of 0.63–1.07. Again, in the DIG trial, assessment of LV diastolic function was not required.

It was found in a post hoc analysis of the DIG trial by Ahmed et al.[37] that the clinical drug effects depend on its serum concentration. A DIG study subgroup of 1,687 patients, in whom digoxin serum concentration was measured, was analyzed

and compared with 3,861 patients receiving placebo. In a studied subgroup, 24% of patients were women and 12% had an EF of >45%, 982 patients had a low serum digoxin concentration (0.5–0.9 ng/mL), and 705 had a high serum digoxin concentration (≥1 ng/mL). During follow-up there were 29% deaths among the low serum digoxin concentration patients and 42% of deaths among the high serum digoxin concentration patients compared with 33% deaths in the placebo group. Figure 16.5 shows the respective reduction and increase in all-cause mortality in the low and high serum digoxin concentration groups compared with placebo. A low serum digoxin concentration was associated with a 22% mortality reduction (unadjusted hazard ratio = 0.81; 95% CI, 0.67–0.97; $p = 0.025$) and a high serum digoxin concentration with a 23% relative increase in total mortality (unadjusted hazard ratio = 1.19; 95% CI, 0.98–1.45, $p = 0.08$). Furthermore, a low serum digoxin concentration was associated with a 38% reduction in the risk for all-cause, cardiovascular, and heart failure hospitalizations (hazard ratio = 0.62; 95% CI, 0.51–0.76, $p < 0.0001$); a high serum digoxin concentration was associated with a reduction in heart failure hospitalization (hazard ratio = 0.61; 95% CI, 0.49–0.76; $p < 0.0001$). Taking into account the beneficial effect of a low serum digoxin concentration in all heart failure patients, including those with preserved LV function, the

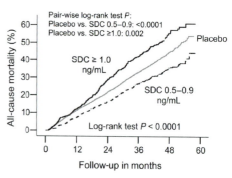

FIGURE 16.5. Kaplan-Meier plots for cumulative risk of death due to all causes based on serum digitalis concentration (SCD). (Reprinted from Ahmed et al.,[37] with permission of Oxford University Press.)

authors emphasized the need for serum digoxin concentration monitoring to achieve levels of 0.5–0.9 ng/mL. Based on the study results, the authors identified patient groups at greater risk for high serum digoxin concentration: elderly, women, and those with pulmonary congestion or renal impairment treated with diuretics; for these patients, digoxin should be started at a dose of 0.0625 mg/day and its concentration measured during therapy.

Diuretics

There are no specific studies related to the use of diuretics for patients with diastolic dysfunction. Because pulmonary congestion is one of the most important features of this condition, it may be expected that use of diuretics may be equally important for patients with DHF as it is for those with SHF.

Medical Treatment for Patients with Heart Failure and Preserved Left Ventricular Function Enrolled in the Euro Heart Survey

The Euro Heart Survey on heart failure was carried out between 2000 and 2001 and analyzed the case notes of 10,701 consecutive discharge or death patients diagnosed with heart failure.[38] Analysis showed that treatment with ACE-inhibitors, β-blockers, statins, digitalis or spironolactone did not cause a significant difference in all-cause mortality between patients with LV systolic dysfunction and those with preserved LV systolic function. The former three drug classes influenced mortality positively and glycosides influenced mortality adversely; however, statistical significance was not achieved (Figure 16.6).

Treatment of the Underlying Disease

Identification of factors responsible for diastolic dysfunction is crucial for the therapeutic process as only a small proportion of patients with symptoms of heart failure and preserved LV function have no identifiable underlying cardiac pathology.[3] Diseases that are known to impair diastolic function include hypertension, coronary artery disease, diabetes, obesity, aortic stenosis, atrial fibrillation, hypertrophic obstructive and non-

obstructive cardiomyopathy, and restrictive cardiomyopathies (e.g., amyloidosis, sarcoidosis, and hemochromatosis).[39]

Although no initial patient evaluation flowchart dedicated specifically to DHF exists, it seems prudent to consider the above-mentioned conditions in the differential diagnosis of patients with heart failure and preserved LV function. The American Heart Association/American College of Cardiology guidelines[3] include certain elements in the initial evaluation of a patient with heart failure (echocardiography, blood glucose measurement, and, in defined cases, coronary arteriography, screening for amyloidosis or hemochromatosis), that may reveal pathologies leading to diastolic dysfunction.

From a practical point of view, it should be mentioned that most often patients with heart failure and normal systolic function are elderly women with arterial hypertension complicated by LV wall hypertrophy.[40] It was found almost 10 years ago that treatment of hypertension in the elderly leads to a substantial reduction in the incidence of heart failure. Administration of a thiazide diuretic was shown to reduce blood pressure significantly and to reduce the incidence of heart failure by 50%.[41]

An alteration in LV diastolic performance, reflected by the prolongation of isovolumic relaxation time, decreased rate of early filling, and increased passive stiffness, is one of the earliest functional abnormalities in arterial hypertension.[42] Arterial hypertension with LV hypertrophy is characterized by diastolic dysfunction with unchanged EF, unchanged or decreased end-diastolic volume, and increased filling pressure, which in turn leads to pulmonary venous congestion and dyspnea.[43] It was shown in a metaanalysis of randomized studies that in patients with arterial hypertension regression of LV wall hypertrophy can be best achieved with ACE inhibitors compared with diuretics, β-adrenergic receptor blockers, and calcium antagonists.[44]

Ischemia due to coronary heart disease or as a consequence of hypertension with LV wall hypertrophy is another leading cause of diastolic dysfunction. It was shown in an experimental model that diastolic dysfunction becomes evident within a few heart beats after sudden coronary artery occlusion.[45] There is some evidence that in patients

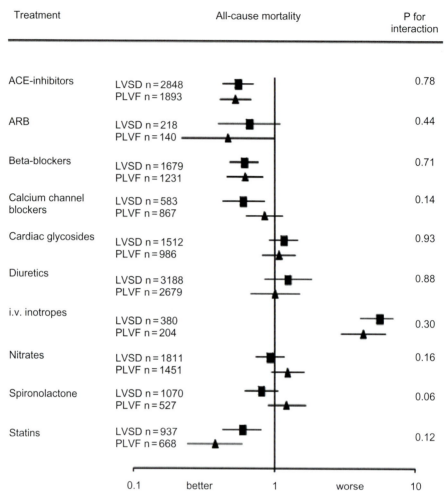

FIGURE 16.6. All-cause mortality rates in the Euro Heart Failure Survey population with respect to pharmacologic treatment of patients with left ventricular systolic dysfunction (LVSD) and preserved left ventricular function (PLVF). (Reprinted from Lenzen et al.,[38] with permission of Oxford University Press.)

with ischemic heart disease coronary revascularization improves diastolic function.

For a group of 53 patients who underwent coronary artery bypass grafting, an echocardiographic examination was performed before the operation and repeated 3 and 12 months after the procedure. An improvement in diastolic function occurred both at rest and during dobutamine infusion. Because conventional Doppler transmitral velocity measurement did not show significant changes, diastolic function assessment was done by mitral annular velocity measurement with tissue Doppler implementation. Improvement was seen only in patients who did not have signs of reversible ischemia on postoperative myocardial scintigraphy. Improvement occurred at 3 months after an operation in most cases but in some was delayed to 1 year.[46] In another study, improvement in diastolic function was also seen after coronary artery bypass grafting and was more pronounced in patients who underwent an on-pump operation than in those who underwent an off-pump procedure.[47]

Diastolic dysfunction in diabetes may result from increased myocardial stiffness, a hallmark of diabetic cardiomyopathy, or may be caused by common comorbidities such as hypertension and coronary artery disease. Strict metabolic control may improve myocardial function in diabetes.[48] Treatment of hypertension is essential; blood pressure values of 130/80 mm Hg should be achieved. Angiotensin-converting enzyme inhibitors are the preferred drugs for hypertensive patients, but adequate blood pressure control can usually be achieved only with two or more drugs.[49] Coronary revascularization, percutaneous or surgical, should be accompanied by precise glycemic control.[50] It should be mentioned that for patients with diabetes who have symptomatic heart failure, thiazolidinediones must be avoided because of the risk of fluid retention and edema aggravation, especially patients also treated with insulin.[51]

Treatment of cardiomyopathies is symptomatic.[52] For patients with amyloidosis and heart failure, diuretics should be given with caution because of the risk of hypotension; digitalis is contraindicated because of the increased risk of arrhythmias. Pacemaker implantation is performed in cases of conduction disturbances; warfarin is administered in atrial standstill (lack of mechanical contraction even in the absence of atrial fibrillation). Results of heart transplantation are poor; in familial hemochromatosis, attempts to transplant heart and liver have been made. Chelation therapy with desferrioxamine administered in hemochromatosis may reverse myocyte damage.[53] Heart involvement in sarcoidosis is treated with corticosteroids, methotrexate, cyclophosphamide, or hydroxychloroquine. Heart and heart–lung transplantation have been used in selected patients. The implantable cardioverter defibrillator should be implanted in patients who have a high risk of sudden death due to arrhythmias.[54]

Medical treatment of hypertrophic cardiomyopathy comprises β-adrenergic receptor blockers, calcium antagonists, disopyramide, and amiodarone. Septal ablation, surgical myo/myectomy, mitral valve repair, and heart transplantation are also implemented.[55]

Other Forms of Treatment

Nonpharmacologic Treatment

There have been attempts to implement nonpharmacologic methods of treatment for patients with diastolic dysfunction. These include coronary revascularization (as in the Euro Heart Survey, discussed earlier) and exercise training. The effect of intracoronary bone marrow cell transfer on LV diastolic function was also investigated.

Exercise training proved effective for a group of women with NYHA class II and III heart failure and an EF above 45%. Implementation of a 12-week low to moderate exercise and education program resulted in significant improvement in the 6-min walk test compared with controls, who participated in the education program only.[56] Similarly, the efficiency of a cardiac rehabilitation program was reported for a group of elderly patients.[57] There is no proof, however, that the effect on diastolic function was the underlying mechanism for exercise tolerance improvement.

Recently the effect of intracoronary bone marrow cell transfer in patients with myocardial infarction on LV diastolic function was investigated. In the randomized Bone Marrow Transfer to Enhance ST Elevation Infarct Regeneration trial,[58] transmitral flow velocities (E/A ratio), diastolic myocardial velocities (Ea/Aa ratio), isovolumic relaxation time, and deceleration time were measured 4.5 ± 1.5 days after percutaneous coronary intervention and repeated after 6 and 18 months of follow-up. Intracoronary cell transfer resulted in improved echocardiographic parameters of diastolic function. An overall effect of cell transfer on the E/A ratio (0.33 ± 0.12; 95% CI, 0.09–0.57; $p = 0.008$) and the Ea/Aa ratio (0.29 ± 0.14; 95% CI, 0.01–0.57; $p = 0.04$) was observed, whereas isovolumic relaxation time and deceleration time were not affected by the treatment.

Other Existing and Developing Treatment Options

Several small studies addressed the efficacy of other agents in diastolic dysfunction. It was found that statins may improve survival of patients with DHF.[59] In an observational study of 137 patients with heart failure and an EF of ≥50%, it was found that patients receiving statins had significantly higher survival rates than those not receiving statins: their relative risk of death was 0.22 with a 95% CI of 0.07–0.64 and $p = 0.006$. During the mean follow-up period of 21 months, 20 deaths and 43 cardiovascular hospitalizations occurred. The latter were not affected significantly by statin treatment. These results should be interpreted with caution, because the numbers were small and the study was not randomized, with treatment ordered at the physician's discretion.

The use of statins should be further explored because of their abilities to prevent myocardial fibrosis and hypertrophy and to increase arterial distensibility through improved endothelial function, which may indirectly lead to improved diastolic function. It was also postulated[60] that the inherent, lipid-dependent effects of statins on vascular atherosclerosis may play a role. As mortality of patients with DHF is related only partly to the heart failure itself, with other causes such as myocardial infarction, stroke, and peripheral vascular disease accounting for 20%–30% of deaths,[61] treatment strategies that prevent progression of atherosclerosis may influence mortality.[60]

Alagebrium chloride (ALT-711), a compound that breaks glucose cross-links, was shown, in a group of 23 patients diagnosed with DHF, to improve indices of LV diastolic filling and decrease LV mass after 16 weeks of treatment. The authors also reported improvement in quality of life as assessed by the Minnesota Living with Heart Failure score.[62]

5-Methyl-2-(1-piperazinyl) benzenesulfonic acid (MCC-135) is a new compound that acts on the sarcoplasmic reticulum by enhancing calcium uptake and reducing its leakage from the reticulum. It exerts a lusitropic effect as confirmed in animal studies.[63] The compound is now being studied in humans. The MCC-135 trial[64] enrolled 511 patients with heart failure who were randomized to one of the dosage regimens: 5 mg, 25 mg, or 50 mg twice daily or placebo given for 24 weeks.

In each subgroup a cohort with an EF of >40% on echocardiographic examination was identified; altogether 230 such patients were included. The study completed recruitment and the results are pending.

Other approaches are being tested in animal models. N-Methylethanolamine was studied in a rat model of DHF. This compound prevented myocardial stiffening through inhibition of phospholipase D activity, leading to decreased collagen synthesis.[65] Adenoviral gene transfer of sarcoplasmic reticulum Ca^{2+}-ATPase in senescent rats resulted in improved hemodynamic parameters of diastolic function: time constant of isovolumic relaxation and maximal rate of pressure fall.[66]

Recommendations from Major Treatment Guidelines

The most recent editions of both the European Society of Cardiology[2] and the American Heart Association/American College of Cardiology[3] guidelines on the diagnosis and treatment of chronic heart failure include a section on patients with preserved LV function. Both documents make a distinction between heart failure with preserved systolic function and DHF, emphasizing that, at present, there is no clear evidence that patients with primary DHF benefit from any specific drug regimen. Specific comments and recommendations from both groups are shown in Tables 16.2 and 16.3.

TABLE 16.2. European Society of Cardiology recommendations on treatment of heart failure with preserved left ventricular function.*

General recommendations	Possible beneficial effect
Identification and treatment of	Prevention of tachyarrhythmias, restoration of sinus rhythm if possible, ventricular rate control
Myocardial ischemia	
Hypertension and hypertrophy	
Myocardial or pericardial constriction	
Drug therapy	
β-Adrenergic receptor blocking agents	Lower heart rate and prolong diastolic period
Verapamil-type calcium antagonists	Lower heart rate and prolong diastolic period; benefit proved in selected cases of hypertrophic cardiomyopathy
Angiotensin-converting enzyme inhibitors	Improve relaxation and cardiac distensibility; regression of hypertrophy and fibrosis; antihypertensive effect
Angiotensin II receptors blockers	Antihypertensive effect; abolish the deleterious effects of angiotensin II
Diuretics	Effective on fluid overload episodes; caution necessary not to lower preload excessively to avoid stroke volume reduction
Digitalis	Symptomatic improvement

*Class of recommendation IIa, level of evidence C.[2]

16. Treatment of Diastolic Heart Failure

TABLE 16.3. Recommendations for treatment of patients with heart failure and normal left ventricular ejection fraction.

Recommendation	Class	Level of evidence
Physicians should control systolic and diastolic hypertension, in accordance with published guidelines	I	A
Physicians should control ventricular rate in patients with atrial fibrillation	I	C
Physicians should use diuretics to control pulmonary congestion and peripheral edema	I	C
Coronary revascularization is reasonable for patients with coronary artery disease in whom symptomatic or demonstrable myocardial ischemia is judged to be having an adverse effect on cardiac function	IIa	C
Restoration and maintenance of sinus rhythm in patients with atrial fibrillation might be useful to improve symptoms	IIb	C
The use of β-adrenergic blocking agents, angiotensin-converting enzyme inhibitors, angiotensin II receptor blockers, or calcium antagonists in patients with controlled hypertension might be effective to minimize symptoms of heart failure	IIb	C
The use of digitalis to minimize symptoms of heart failure is not well established	IIb	C

Source: Reprinted with permission, ACC/AHA 2005 guideline update.[3]

Acute Heart Failure

Diastolic heart failure may, at least in some patients, be an "intermittent disease," with the acute symptoms precipitated by an increase in blood pressure, aggravation of ischemia, or the onset of atrial fibrillation.

That acute heart failure due to diastolic dysfunction really exists has been clearly shown by Gandhi et al.[67] They examined a group of 38 patients hospitalized for acute pulmonary edema whose systolic blood pressure at admission exceeded 160 mm Hg. Pulmonary congestion rapidly cleared when blood pressure was reduced with nitroglycerin and diuretics. Left ventricular ejection fraction was measured during the acute phase and 24–72 hours after treatment. It was found that a significant reduction of blood pressure was accompanied by no changes in LVEF. In one half of patients, the EF values exceeded 50% during pulmonary edema and did not change after treatment. These findings emphasize the role of hypertension in causing diastolic dysfunction.

In patients with acute heart failure, treatment should be aimed at reduction of hypoxia and pulmonary venous pressure and congestion.[68] Oxygen, morphine, nitroglycerin, and parenteral diuretics may be used. Diuretics should be administered cautiously, as hypovolemia may result in hypotension and reduction in stroke volume. Sodium nitroprusside may be administered in cases of hypertension not responding to treatment.[69] Atrial fibrillation with a rapid ventricular response requires urgent cardioversion, as fast heart rates increase myocardial oxygen demand and decrease coronary perfusion time, leading to myocardial ischemia.[70]

Guidelines on the diagnosis and treatment of acute heart failure issued by the Task Force on Acute Heart Failure of the European Society of Cardiology[71] distinguish six clinical conditions of acute heart failure, among them "hypertensive acute heart failure." This entity is defined as signs and symptoms of heart failure accompanied by high blood pressure and relatively preserved LV function with radiographic evidence of acute pulmonary edema. It is stated that patients presenting with pulmonary edema and hypertension usually have preserved LV systolic function with an EF of >45%. Recommended therapies include oxygen, implementation of continuous positive airway pressure or noninvasive ventilation, or alternatively invasive ventilation for short period of time. Antihypertensive agents should initially lower blood pressure by 30 mm Hg within minutes, followed by a further reduction within hours to values obtained before pulmonary edema. Blood pressure should not be lowered to normal values to avoid organ hypoperfusion. Intravenous loop diuretics, intravenous nitroglycerin, nitroprusside or the calcium channel blocker nicardipine are recommended to combat fluid overload, decrease venous preload and arterial afterload, and increase coronary blood flow. ß-Blockers are not advised in cases of hypertensive crisis with pulmonary edema with the exception of pheochromocytoma for which labetalol may be given.

Conclusion

An effective treatment for DHF has not been established. Most of the treatment principles pertaining to this poorly clinically defined condition are based on one of the following assumptions:

1. Isolated DHF is a relatively rare condition. It often coexists with some degree of systolic dysfunction. Thus, both forms of heart failure should be treated similarly, and management principles worked out for the SHF might also be applicable to patients with predominantly diastolic dysfunction.

2. In most patients with clinical heart failure and preserved LV systolic function, a diastolic dysfunction is the underlying cause.

3. All patient populations designated as having preserved systolic function studied thus far constitute a mixture of those with mild systolic, diastolic, and no heart failure. Therefore, no conclusions on treatment of patients with DHF can be derived from them.

These assumptions are, at least in part, mutually exclusive. To establish an effective therapeutic approach for patients with DHF, the following three fundamental steps seem to be necessary. First, a common definition of DHF should be proposed and accepted. Second, the prevalence and incidence of DHF based on this definition could then be established. Finally, therapies proven to be effective for patients with SHF, as well as any specific measures aimed at improvement of diastolic function, could be tested for patients with primarily DHF, as well as those in whom the systolic and diastolic dysfunction coexist.

Currently, six drug classes are given to patients with heart failure thought to be due to diastolic dysfunction: β-adrenergic receptors blockers, calcium channel blockers, ACE inhibitors, ARBs, diuretics, and aldosterone antagonists. The rationale for their administration includes elimination of ischemia, slowing heart rate, regression of myocardial hypertrophy and fibrosis, and their proven effect on patients with systolic dysfunction. Other treatments likely to favorably affect diastolic function are being developed.

The most solid recommendations for treatment that are in our possession include the following:

1. Treat the underlying condition, with special focus on adequate control of blood pressure in patients with arterial hypertension.
2. Use diuretics for patients with signs and symptoms of congestion.
3. Avoid heart rate acceleration.

In practice, all approaches for which there is evidence of efficacy and safety for patients with SHF need to be used also for patients with DHF as long as the necessary evidence specific to DHF is accumulated.

References

1. Vasan R. Diastolic heart failure. The condition exists and needs to be recognised, prevented and treated. BMJ 2003;327:1181–1182.
2. The Task Force for the Diagnosis and Treatment of Chronic Heart Failure of the European Society of Cardiology. Guidelines for the diagnosis and treatment of chronic heart failure: executive summary (update 2005). Eur Heart J 2005;26:1115–1140.
3. Hunt S, Abraham W, Chin M, et al. ACC/AHA 2005 Guideline Update for the Diagnosis and Management of Chronic Heart Failure in the Adult — Summary Article: A Report of the American College of Cardiology/American Heart Association Task Force on Practice Guidelines (Writing Committee to Update the 2001 Guidelines for the Evaluation and Management of Heart Failure): Developed in Collaboration With the American College of Chest Physicians and the International Society for Heart and Lung Transplantation: Endorsed by the Heart Rhythm Society. Circulation 2005;112: 1825–1852.
4. Cleland J, Tendera M, Adamus J, et al. Perindopril for elderly people with chronic heart failure: the PEP-CHF study. The PEP investigators. Eur J Heart Fail 1999;1:211–217.
5. Cleland JGF, Tendera M, Adamus J, et al. The Perindopril in Elderly People with Chronic Heart Failure (PEP-CHF) Study. Eur Heart J 2006;27: 2338–2345.
6. Aronow W, Kronzon I. Effect of enalapril on congestive heart failure treated with diuretics in elderly patients with prior myocardial infarction and normal left ventricular ejection fraction. Am J Cardiol 1993;71:602–604.
7. Carson P, Johnson G, Fletcher R, et al. Mild systolic dysfunction in heart failure (left ventricular ejection fraction >35%): baseline characteristics, prognosis and response to therapy in the Vasodilator in

16. Treatment of Diastolic Heart Failure

Heart Failure Trials (V-HeFT) J Am Coll Cardiol 1996;27:642–649.

8. The CONSENSUS Trial Study Group. Effects of enalapril on mortality in severe congestive heart failure. Results of the Cooperative North Scandinavian Enalapril Survival Study (CONSENSUS). N Engl J Med 1987;316:1429–1435.

9. Mitsunami K, Inoue S, Maeda K, et al. Three months effects of candesartan cilexetil, an angiotensin II type 1 (AT1) receptor antagonist, on left ventricular mass and hemodynamics in patients with essential hypertension. Cardiovasc Drugs Ther 1998;12:469–474.

10. Unger T. Neurohormonal modulation in cardiovascular disease. Am Heart J 2000;139:S2–S8.

11. De Mello W, Danser A. Angiotensin II and the heart. On the intracrine renin-angiotensin system. Hypertension 2000;33:613–621.

12. Yamamoto K, Masuyama T, Sakata Y, et al. Roles of renin-angiotensin and endothelin systems in development of diastolic hart failure in hypertensive hearts. Cardiovasc Res 2000;47:274–283.

13. McMurray J, Oestergren J, Swedberg K, et al. Effects of candesartan in patients with chronic heart failure and reduced left ventricular systolic function treated with an ACE inhibitor: the CHARM-Added Trial. Lancet 2003;362:767–771.

14. Granger C, McMurray J, Yusuf S, et al. Effect of candesartan in patients with chronic heart failure and reduced left ventricular systolic function and intolerant to ACE inhibitors: the CHARM Alternative Trial. Lancet 2003;362:772–776.

15. Pfeffer M, Swedberg K, Granger C, et al. Effects of candesartan on mortality and morbidity in patients with chronic heart failure: the CHARM-Overall programme. Lancet 2003;362:759–766.

16. Yusuf S, Pfeffer M, Swedberg K, et al. Effects of candesartan in patients with chronic heart failure and preserved left-ventricular ejection fraction: the CHARM-Preserved trial. Lancet 2003;362:777–781.

17. Kasama S, Toyama T, Kumakura H, et al. Effects of candesartan on cardiac sympathetic nerve activity in patients with congestive heart failure and preserved left ventricular ejection fraction. J Am Coll Cardiol 2005;45:661–667.

18. Carson P, Massie B, McKelvie R, et al. The Irbesartan in Heart Failure With Preserved Systolic Function (I-PRESERVE) Trial: rationale and design. J Cardiac Failure 2005;11:576–585.

19. Sanderson J. Re: PEP-CHF study [letter]. Eur J Heart Fail 2000;2:117.

20. Sanderson J. Hong Kong Study Recruitment. European Society of Cardiology Congress, 2002:2327.

21. Andersson B, Sveälv B, Tang M, et al. Longitudinal myocardial contraction improves early during titration with metoprolol CR/XL in patients with heart failure. Heart 2002;87:23–28.

22. Capomolla S, Febo O, Gnemmi M, et al. Beta-blockade therapy in chronic heart failure: diastolic function and mitral regurgitation improvement by carvedilol. Am Heart J 2000;139:596–608.

23. Nodari S, Metra M, Dei L, et al. Beta-blocker treatment of patients with diastolic heart failure and arterial hypertension. A prospective, randomized, comparison of the long- term effects of atenolol vs. nebivolol. Eur J Heart Fail 2003;5:621–627.

24. Wallhaus T, Taylor M, DeGrado T, et al. Myocardial free fatty acid and glucose use after carvedilol treatment in patients with congestive heart failure. Circulation 2001;103:2441–2446.

25. Bergstrom A, Andersson B, Edner M, et al. Carvedilol improves diastolic function in patients with diastolic heart failure. Circulation 2001;104(Suppl II):II7.

26. Palazzuoli A, Carrera A, Calabria P, et al. Effects of carvedilol therapy on restrictive diastolic filling pattern in chronic heart failure. Am Heart J 2004;147:e2–e7.

27. Flather M, Shibata M, Coats A, et al. Randomized trial to determine the effect of nebivolol on mortality and cardiovascular hospital admission in elderly patients with heart failure (SENIORS). Eur Heart J 2005;26: 215–225.

28. Ghio S, Magrini G, Serio A, et al. Effect of nebivolol in elderly heart failure patients with or without systolic left ventricular dysfunction: results of the SENIORS echocardiographic substudy. Eur Heart J 2006;27:562–568.

29. Westermann D, Knollmann B, Steendijk P, et al. Diltiazem treatment prevents diastolic heart failure in mice with familial hypertrophic cardiomyopathy. Eur J Heart Fail 2006;8:115–121.

30. Tendera M, Poloński L, Kozielska E. Left ventricular end-diastolic pressure–volume relationship in hypertrophic cardiomyopathy. Changes induced by verapamil. Chest 1983;84:54–57.

31. Bonow R, Ostrow H, Rosing D, et al. effects of verapamil on left ventricular systolic and diastolic function in patients with hypertrophic cardiomyopathy: pressure–volume analysis with a nonimaging scintillation probe. Circulation 1983;68:1062–1073.

32. Duprez D, De Buyzere M, Rietrzschel E, et al. Inverse relationship between aldosterone and large artery compliance in chronically treated heart failure patients. Eur Heart J 1998;19:1371–1376.

33. MacFayden R, Barr C, Struthers A, et al. Aldosterone blockade reduces vascular collagen turnover,

17
Coronary Artery Disease and Diastolic Left Ventricular Dysfunction

Jean G.F. Bronzwaer and Walter J. Paulus

Introduction

Myocardial ischemia initially results in reversible regional disturbances of ventricular pump function, whereas most changes in regional function following myocardial infarction are irreversible. After acute reduction in coronary flow, both diastolic and systolic dysfunctions occur. If blood flow is not restored, myocardial necrosis results, and the wall motion abnormality becomes fixed.

There are two phenomena, however, that result in potentially reversible myocardial dysfunction. The first is myocardial stunning, which occurs after a severe acute ischemic insult. In this scenario, flow is restored and there is no myocardial necrosis. The syndrome results in spontaneous recovery of myocardial function after restitution of blood flow.[1] Second, myocardial hibernation is a similar phenomenon seen in chronic situations in which there is no identifiable recent acute event but diffuse myocardial dysfunction in the presence of normal or near-normal resting blood flow. In many instances what has been termed *myocardial hibernation* may actually represent repetitive stunning. The process of hibernation may be seen as downregulation of myocardial function, followed by "downregulation" of structure and, if adaptive processes are insufficient, eventually followed by focal cell death and apoptosis.[2] Early changes may be reversible before significant structural changes occur, but the loss of cardiomyocytes is not reversible; therefore, because long-term hibernation may lead to irreversible loss of myocardial function, ischemia should be abolished in a timely fashion. In this scenario,

functional recovery of the myocardium occurs after successful revascularization. Myocardial ischemia, hypoxemia, stunning, hibernation, and myocardial infarction all cause a change in diastolic properties of the left ventricular (LV) myocardium, reversible or irreversible. This chapter, however, deals with the acute changes in myocardial distensibility following low-flow ischemia and high-flow ischemia or hypoxia.

There is no single definition for diastolic dysfunction; many features can be altered, and any one change or their combination is typically called *diastolic dysfunction*, although the pathophysiology and functional significance vary greatly. Thus, the term is used to describe slowed force (or pressure) decay and cellular relengthening rates, increased (or decreased) early filling rates and deceleration, elevated or steeper diastolic pressure–volume (PV) relations, and filling rate–dependent pressure elevation (viscoelasticity)[3]. Clinically, the most common manifestation is an elevated LV end-diastolic pressure and altered filling patterns, but neither of these identifies specific features of diastolic dysfunction.

Despite these difficulties, it remains widely presumed that diastolic abnormalities are important to heart failure pathophysiology, and this is driving new research to elucidate the biochemical and structural mechanisms that underlie it, clarify its role in clinical heart failure, and develop targeted treatments for it. Clinical epidemiology is fueling interest, because many patients with cardiac failure present with preserved ejection fraction (EF), which has rightly or wrongly focused attention on diastolic dysfunction. This chapter reviews recent insights into diastolic dysfunction with acute ischemia. We divide our discussion into two primary components: relaxation and diastolic stiffness defined by the length–tension or PV relationship. We avoid discussion of diastolic filling patterns and tissue velocities because these are more integrative in nature and are dealt with in Chapters 6 and 7.

Ischemia

Low-flow ischemia, in contrast to high-flow ischemia or hypoxia, is characterized not only by oxygen deprivation but also by inadequate removal of metabolites consequent to reduced perfusion and by loss of vascular turgor. Coronary flow and coronary perfusion pressure augment LV systolic performance (Gregg effect) and reduce LV diastolic distensibility (Salisbury effect). Build-up of tissue metabolites, especially inorganic phosphate, reduces the calcium sensitivity of myofilaments, thereby diminishing contractility. Accordingly, in patients with low-flow ischemia, LV systolic performance is lower and LV diastolic distensibility greater than when the same patients were exposed to high-flow ischemia or hypoxia.

Diastolic distensibility may also be influenced by changes in myocardial energetics. Hypoxia exists when oxygen supply is reduced despite adequate perfusion, which increases isovolumic resting tension in isolated guinea pig hearts and causes an upward shift of the diastolic PV curve in humans, indicating reduced distensibility. Reductions in LV diastolic distensibility have also been observed during demand ischemia. Demand ischemia or high-flow ischemia during exercise, tachycardia, or emotion in the presence of chronic coronary stenoses is caused by an increase in coronary blood flow that is insufficient to meet the rise in myocardial oxygen demand. It is responsible for many episodes of chronic stable angina. In this setting, the idea of reduced diastolic LV distensibility caused by Ca^{2+} overload was recently rebutted by experiments in blood-perfused isovolumic rabbit hearts that demonstrated correction of the ischemia-induced decline in LV diastolic distensibility by quick stretches, which disrupted rigor bounds, and not by a

calcium desensitizer (2,3-butanedionemonoxime). Change in high-energy phosphate metabolism may also contribute. For example, inhibition of creatine kinase activity by low-dose iodoacetamide resulted in an increase in free magnesium adenosine triphosphate without alterations in magnesium adenosine triphosphate, inorganic phosphate, or phosphate isomerase and, in intact hearts, resulted in a threefold increase in ventricular end-diastolic pressure and delayed relaxation. The LV end-diastolic pressure increase correlated with free adenosine diphosphate.[3] Supply ischemia or low-flow ischemia is characterized by an imbalance between myocardial oxygen supply and demand caused by a reduction of blood flow and oxygen supply secondary to increased coronary vascular tone, intracoronary platelet aggregation, or thrombus formation and is responsible for myocardial infarction and most episodes of unstable angina.

Pathophysiology

Different types of ischemia have unequal effects on initial LV mechanical dysfunction because of complex interactions among oxygen deprivation, accumulation of tissue metabolites, and vascular turgor.[4] Initial LV mechanical dysfunction was first compared during different types of ischemia in an isolated, isovolumically beating, and retrogradely perfused rabbit heart[5] and later in an anesthetized open-chest, open pericardium dog heart model.[6,7] In the buffer-perfused rabbit heart,[5,8] hypoxic coronary perfusion induced a rise in resting tension, in contrast to reduced coronary perfusion, which produced a fall in resting tension. Moreover, the decline in developed tension progressed faster during reduced than during hypoxic perfusion. In anesthetized dogs, pacing tachycardia in the presence of coronary stenoses and brief coronary occlusion had opposite effects on global and regional diastolic LV distensibility.[6,7] Pacing tachycardia in the presence of coronary stenoses resulted in an upward shift in the global diastolic LV PV and of the regional diastolic pressure–segment length and pressure wall–thickness relations of the ischemic myocardium. During brief coronary occlusion,

17. Coronary Artery Disease

the ischemic region showed no change or a shift to the right of these relations.[9–11]

In contrast to these experimental findings, clinical studies in patients with coronary disease described the initial LV mechanical dysfunction of only a single type of ischemic insult. During pacing-induced[12–14] or spontaneous[15] angina, an upward shift of the global diastolic LV PV relation and of the regional diastolic pressure–radial length[16] and pressure–wall thickness relations[17] of the ischemic myocardium was observed. Since the advent of coronary angioplasty, the myocardial effects of a brief reduction of coronary blood flow could easily be investigated in humans during angioplasty balloon coronary occlusion. Initial studies appreciated the mechanical LV dysfunction of balloon coronary occlusion by loss of global and regional systolic performance,[18] and subsequently by altered diastolic LV performance,[19–22] which appeared to be an earlier and more sensitive marker of LV mechanical dysfunction during ischemia of balloon coronary occlusion. The mechanical dysfunction resulting from balloon coronary occlusion ischemia was further characterized by studies of pharmacologic pretreatment[23] and by comparing the effects of sequential balloon coronary occlusions.[24,25]

In contrast to the experimental data, no clinical study has directly compared initial LV mechanical dysfunction resulting from different types of ischemia in the same patient. In this chapter, we discuss mechanisms of ischemia-induced changes in LV diastolic function based on human data acquired in the catheterization laboratory.[26,27] In these studies we compared LV performance in patients with single-vessel left anterior descending coronary disease during balloon coronary occlusion, during pacing-induced angina, and during balloon coronary occlusion with maintained hypoxic perfusion distal to the balloon occlusion.

Materials and Methods

Patients

Twelve patients (10 men, 2 women; mean age 54 years; age range 42–77 years) were included in the comparative analysis of pacing-induced and balloon coronary occlusion ischemia.[26] Eleven patients (8 men, 3 women; mean age 57 years; age range 42–71 years) were included in the comparative analysis of balloon coronary occlusion ischemia and hypoxia.[27] All patients suffered from exercise-induced angina. The exercise stress test was both clinically and electrocardiographically positive. There was no history of angina at rest or of previous myocardial infarction. There was no evidence of previous myocardial infarction on the electrocardiogram, and there was normal wall motion on the baseline LV angiogram. Diagnostic left heart catheterization and coronary angiography showed normal global and regional LV function and single-vessel coronary artery disease, consisting of a significant (>80%) proximal left anterior descending stenosis. Contralateral coronary injection before balloon dilatation revealed no visible collaterals to the distal left anterior descending coronary artery. β-Blockers and calcium entry blockers were withheld at least 24 hours prior to the study, except for two patients, who had experienced angina during mild exercise during the 48-hour period preceding hospital admission. Premedication consisted of 10 mg diazepam. All patients gave informed consent, the study protocol was approved by the hospital ethics committee, and there were no complications related to the angioplasty procedure or to the study protocol.

Study Protocol

A 7Fr pigtail Sentron tip-micromanometer catheter (Cordis Europe, Rooden, the Netherlands) was advanced from the left femoral artery to the left ventricle, and an 8Fr angioplasty guiding catheter was advanced from the right femoral artery. The tip-micromanometer catheter was calibrated externally against a mercury reference and matched against luminal pressure. All pressures were referenced to atmospheric pressure at the level of the midchest. The pressure signals, the LV dP/dt signal, which was derived from the LV pressure signal by an electronic differentiator, and leads of the electrocardiogram were recorded on a Gould ES 1000 multichannel recorder. A 7Fr NIH catheter was positioned in the coronary sinus from a left antecubital vein or from the right femoral vein to obtain coronary sinus blood samples during the different interventions. Simplus balloon catheters (USCI) were used to perform the coronary angioplasty, and during angioplasty balloon inflation the coronary wedge pressure was measured through the fluid-filled lumen of the balloon catheter, which was connected to a pressure transducer.

The use of coronary wedge pressure as an index of coronary collateral recruitment was demonstrated in previous studies.[28,29] Mean coronary wedge pressure during balloon inflation was 29 ± 11 mm Hg (range 11–45 mm Hg), and the mean pressure difference between coronary wedge pressure and LV end-diastolic pressure at the end of the balloon coronary occlusion was 8 ± 6 mm Hg (range 3–15 mm Hg). Left ventricular angiograms were performed in 30° right anterior oblique projection and matched with the LV tip-micromanometer pressure recording using an angiographic frame marker.

Comparative Effects of Pacing-Induced and Balloon Coronary Occlusion Ischemia on Left Ventricular Function

Following baseline LV angiography and LV tip-micromanometer pressure recordings, LV filling pressures were allowed to return to control level. Right ventricular pacing was initiated at a rate of 90 beats/min and was stepwise increased every 2 min by 30 beats/min. Pacing was continued until the appearance of angina. Immediately upon cessation of pacing, a second LV angiogram and simultaneous tip-micromanometer LV pressure recordings were obtained. To allow diastolic LV pressures to return to baseline, a 15-min interval separated the end of the pacing run from the start of the angioplasty procedure. A third LV angiogram and simultaneous LV tip-micromanometer pressure recordings were obtained at the end of the fourth (patients 1–9) or second (patients 10–12) angioplasty balloon inflation of 60-s duration. All patients experienced chest pain and ischemic ST-segment changes at the end of the balloon coronary occlusion. Coronary angioplasty was successful in all patients with minimal residual coronary stenosis.

Comparative Effects of Balloon Coronary Occlusion and Balloon Coronary Occlusion with Distal Perfusion on Left Ventricular Function

After baseline angiography and LV pressure recordings, LV filling pressures were allowed to return to baseline value. A second LV angiogram was obtained at the end of the second balloon coronary occlusion. After return of LV filling pressures to baseline value, a third angioplasty balloon inflation of equal duration to the second angioplasty balloon inflation was performed. During this third angioplasty balloon inflation, saline was perfused through the distal lumen of the balloon catheter at a flow rate that equaled the normal left anterior descending flow in humans (1 mL/s).[18,30] At the end of this third balloon inflation, an LV angiogram and simultaneous LV pressure recordings were obtained.

Data Analysis

Hemodynamic Data

All hemodynamic data were averaged over a complete respiratory cycle. The time constant of LV pressure decay was derived from an exponential curve fit with zero asymptote pressure to the digitized LV pressure data points, which were obtained at 3-ms intervals by digitizing the LV pressure signal from the moment of LV dP/dt_{min} to a time at which LV pressure equaled LV end-diastolic pressure plus 5 mm Hg.[31]

Angiographic Data

Left ventricular volumes were calculated from single-plane LV cineangiograms performed in 30° right anterior oblique projection using the area length method and a regression equation. Nonsinus and post-extrasystolic beats were excluded from analysis, which was performed on the third to fourth beat after contrast appearance. Left ventricular PV plots were constructed by matching corresponding points of LV pressure and volume using the cineframe marker. Left ventricular stroke work index was calculated as the product of stroke volume index and mean systolic LV pressure. Regional wall motion was analyzed

17. Coronary Artery Disease

using the end-diastolic center of mass and 28 sectors emerging from the center of mass. Radial length was calculated for each frame as the distance from the center of mass to the endocardial contour of an ischemic and nonischemic sector. Percentage systolic shortening was the ratio of the difference between end-diastolic and end-systolic radial lengths divided by the end-diastolic radial length. Each individual angiographic value was the average of three measurements. Intraobserver variabilities for LV volume and radial length measurements were 1.5% and 1.6%, respectively.

Metabolic Data

Blood samples were repetitively obtained from the coronary sinus and from the femoral artery before pacing; during the last 15 s of each pacing step; and 10, 30, and 120 s after cessation of pacing. The same samples were drawn before balloon inflation; at the end of the balloon inflation period; 10, 30, and 120 s after deflation of the balloon; before balloon inflation with distal perfusion; at the end of the balloon inflation period with distal perfusion; and 10, 30, and 120 s after deflation of the balloon and cessation of the distal perfusion. The timing of sampling was based on the previously reported K^+ concentration measured by catheter electrode in the coronary sinus during and following balloon inflations of coronary angioplasty.[32] On each blood sample, pH, K^+, and lactate concentrations were determined. For determination of lactates, blood was rapidly centrifuged, and the supernatant fluid was stored at $-20°C$. Lactate in the supernatant was analyzed by oxidase-catalyzed conversion of lactate to pyruvate and hydrogen peroxide in the presence of oxygen. Potassium concentration was assessed by indirect potentiometry; pH was determined by an ABL 30 blood gas analyzer.

Statistical Analysis

Results are given as mean ± standard deviation. Statistical significance was set at $p < 0.05$ and was obtained by Student's t test for paired data and by Bonferroni's method for multiple comparisons.

Results

Comparative Effects of Pacing-Induced and Balloon Coronary Occlusion Ischemia on Left Ventricular Function in Humans

Two surface lead electrocardiograms (I and II), one precordial lead electrocardiogram, the LV dP/dt signal, the LV tip-micromanometer pressure recording, and the end-diastolic and end-systolic frames of an LV cineangiogram were obtained at rest, upon cessation of pacing during an episode of pacing-induced angina, and at the end of a balloon coronary occlusion in 12 patients subjected to this study protocol.[26] Left ventricular end-diastolic pressure rose from 14 ± 4 mm Hg at rest to 24 ± 7 mm Hg ($p < 0.01$) during pacing-induced ischemia and to 21 ± 8 mm Hg ($p < 0.01$) at the end of balloon coronary occlusion. Left ventricular end-diastolic volume index rose from 83 ± 19 mL/m² at rest (R) to 88 ± 17 mL/m² (NS) during pacing-induced ischemia (PI), and to 96 ± 16 m/m² ($p < 0.05$ vs. R and PI) at the end of balloon coronary occlusion. The similar rise of LV end-diastolic pressure during pacing-induced ischemia and at the end of balloon coronary occlusion and the significant increase in LV end-diastolic volume index at the end of balloon coronary occlusion were consistent with an upward shift of the LV end-diastolic PV relation during pacing-induced ischemia and an upward and rightward shift of the same relation at the end of balloon coronary occlusion.

Figure 17.1 shows a representative example of diastolic LV PV relations at rest, during pacing-induced ischemia, and at the end of balloon coronary occlusion. The diastolic LV PV relation during pacing-induced ischemia was shifted upward, and the diastolic LV PV relation at the end of balloon coronary occlusion was shifted rightward compared with the relation at rest. Left ventricular EF fell from 77% ± 7% at rest (R) to 71% ± 9% during pacing-induced ischemia (PI; NS) and to 47% ± 11% at the end of balloon coronary occlusion ($p < 0.01$ vs. R and PI). Left ventricular peak systolic pressure rose from 126 ± 28 mm Hg at rest to 137 ± 23 mm Hg during pacing-induced angina ($p < 0.05$) and was unaltered at the end of balloon coronary occlu-

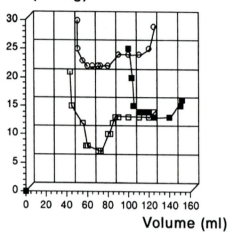

FIGURE 17.1. Diastolic left ventricular pressure–volume relations obtained in a representative patient at rest (□), upon cessation of pacing during an episode of pacing-induced angina (○), and at the end of a balloon coronary occlusion (■). The diastolic left ventricular pressure-volume relation during pacing-induced ischemia was shifted upward and the end-diastolic left ventricular pressure–volume relation at the end of a balloon coronary occlusion was shifted rightward compared with the diastolic left ventricular pressure–volume relation at rest.

sion (127 ± 32 mm Hg). Left ventricular stroke work index was significantly different from rest (R) (75 ± 17 g/m) at the end of balloon coronary occlusion (43 ± 14 g/m; $p < 0.01$ vs. R and PI) but not during pacing-inducing ischemia (PI; 77 ± 15 g/m; Figure 17.2). Heart rate showed a similar increase from 69.1 ± 7.9 beats/min at rest to 82.4 ± 11.8 beats/min during pacing-induced ischemia ($p < 0.01$) and to 82.7 ± 11.4 beats/min at the end of balloon coronary occlusion ($p < 0.01$).

Regional wall motion data of ischemic and nonischemic segments showed a significant drop in percent systolic shortening of the ischemic segment from 40% ± 11% at rest (R) to 25% ± 9% during pacing induced ischemia (PI; $p < 0.01$ vs. R) and to 6% ± 9% at the end of balloon coronary occlusion ($p < 0.01$ vs. R and PI). The nonischemic segment showed no change in percent systolic shortening during pacing-induced ischemia (PI) and a decrease in percent systolic shortening from

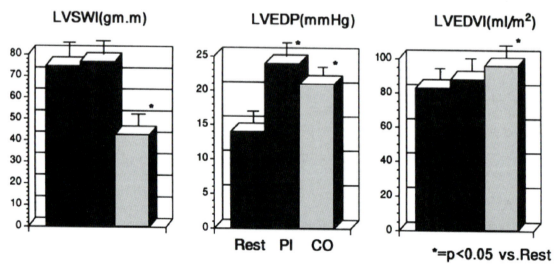

FIGURE 17.2. Bar graphs showing left ventricular stroke work index (LVSWI), left ventricular end-diastolic pressure (LVEDP), and left ventricular end-diastolic volume index (LVEDVI) observed at rest, during pacing-induced ischemia (PI), and at the end of balloon coronary occlusion (CO).

50% ± 8% at rest (R) to 43% ± 8% at the end of balloon coronary occlusion ($p < 0.05$ vs. R and PI). The change in percent systolic shortening of the nonischemic segment was explained by motion of the center of mass toward the area of akinesia, which led to underestimation of systolic shortening of the nonischemic segment at the end of balloon coronary occlusion. The upward shift of the diastolic LV pressure–radial length relation was quantified by Pm, which is a mean pressure value obtained by planimetry of an area enclosed by the two LV pressure–radial length plots and by two lines perpendicular to the radial length axis at the outer borders of a radial length zone for which there was overlap between the two LV pressure–radial length plots and by division of this area by the distance between the two perpendicular lines. The Pm was inversely related to regional LV distensibility.

Comparative Effects of Balloon Coronary Occlusion Ischemia and Hypoxemia on Left Ventricular Function in Humans

Two surface lead electrocardiograms (I and II), one precordial lead electrocardiogram, the LV dP/dt signal, the LV tip-micromanometer pressure recording, and the end-diastolic and end-systolic frames of an LV cineangiogram were obtained at rest, at the end of a balloon coronary occlusion, and at the end of a balloon coronary occlusion with distal perfusion (hypoxemia) in 11 patients subjected to this comparative study protocol.[27] Left ventricular end-diastolic pressure at the end of balloon coronary occlusion with distal perfusion was significantly higher than at rest (34 ± 7 vs. 17 ± 5 mm Hg; $p < 0.001$) and than at the end of the regular balloon coronary occlusion (26 ± 5 mm Hg; $p < 0.01$). Left ventricular minimum diastolic pressure at the end of balloon coronary occlusion with distal perfusion was significantly higher than at rest (26 ± 8 vs. 6 ± 4 mmHg; $p < 0.01$) and than at the end of the regular balloon coronary occlusion (13 ± 4 mm Hg; $p < 0.01$). At the end of balloon coronary occlusion, LV end-diastolic volume index was significantly larger than at rest (79 ± 15 vs. 75 ± 14 mL/m^2; $p < 0.05$), whereas LV end-diastolic volume index at the end of balloon coronary occlusion with distal perfusion was comparable with the value at rest. Because of unaltered LV end-diastolic volume index, the higher LV end-diastolic pressure observed at the end of balloon coronary occlusion with distal perfusion was consistent with a decrease in LV end-diastolic distensibility compared with the resting value and the regular balloon coronary occlusion.

Figure 17.3 shows diastolic LV PV relations at rest, at the end of balloon coronary occlusion, and at the end of balloon coronary occlusion with distal perfusion in a representative patient. The

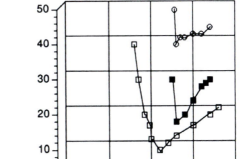

Figure 17.3. Diastolic left ventricular pressure–volume relations obtained in a representative patient at rest (□), at the end of a balloon coronary occlusion (■), and at the end of an equally long balloon coronary occlusion with distal saline perfusion (hypoxemia) (○). The diastolic left ventricular pressure–volume relation during hypoxemia was shifted upward compared with the diastolic left ventricular pressure–volume relation at rest and at the end of balloon coronary occlusion.

Discussion

Left Ventricular Diastolic Dysfunction During Different Types of Ischemia: Experimental Evidence

The complex and often opposite interactions on LV performance of lack of oxygen supply, of accumulation of tissue metabolites, and of vascular turgor have been investigated during the early phase of an ischemic insult in isolated, isovolumically beating, and retrogradely Krebs-perfused rodent hearts. In the guinea pig left ventricle, a switch from aerobic to hypoxic perfusion at constant coronary perfusion pressure induced within a 5-min period a fall in developed tension and a rise in resting tension.[33] Because of the isovolumic contraction mode, this rise in resting tension was consistent with a drop in LV distensibility. Increasing heart rate during the hypoxic perfusion period promoted the rise in resting tension. In a similar type of isolated, buffer-perfused rabbit heart with a constant-volume LV balloon, the acute effects of hypoxia with and without pacing tachycardia were compared with low-flow ischemia with and without pacing tachycardia.[5] Hypoxia caused a faster rise in LV filling pressures and a slower decline in LV developed pressure than low-flow ischemia, which resulted in an initial fall in LV filling pressures. Pacing tachycardia superimposed on hypoxia accelerated the rise in LV filling pressures, whereas pacing tachycardia superimposed on low-flow ischemia resulted in a rise in LV filling pressures in only 2 of the 14 experiments.

Replacement of buffer perfusion by blood perfusion in the same isolated, isovolumically beating, and retrogradely perfused rabbit left ventricle resulted in a consistent elevation of LV filling pressures or a drop in LV distensibility when pacing tachycardia was superimposed on global low-flow ischemia.[34] Hence, in the isovolumic rodent heart the initial LV effects of an ischemic insult can be summarized as follows: (1) Low-flow ischemia results in a loss of LV systolic performance and an increase in LV chamber distensibility; (2) pacing tachycardia superimposed on low-flow ischemia results in a faster loss of LV systolic performance and a decrease in LV diastolic distensibility in blood but not in buffer-perfused preparations; and (3) hypoxia results in a slower loss of LV systolic performance and a decrease in LV chamber distensibility, which is accelerated by superimposition of pacing tachycardia.

In anesthetized or conscious dogs, numerous studies investigated LV performance during brief episodes of single-vessel coronary occlusion and during pacing or exercise stress superimposed on single- or two-vessel coronary stenoses.[9,11,35-40] During brief episodes of single-vessel coronary occlusion (= low-flow ischemia), myocardial shortening of the ischemic segment was replaced by passive bulging, and the diastolic pressure-segment length relation showed a rightward shift, suggestive of increased myocardial distensibility.[6,9,11,40] In conscious dogs with a single-vessel coronary stenosis, exercise (= limited flow-high demand ischemia) resulted in an upward shift of the early portion of the LV diastolic PV relation,[39] and a study in anesthetized pigs,[41] which have less collateral perfusion than dogs, reported an upward shift in the entire LV diastolic pressure-segment length relation after pacing in the presence of a single-vessel coronary stenosis. In anesthetized dogs, a drop in LV systolic performance and an upward shift of the diastolic LV PV relation was observed when pacing tachycardia superimposed on two-vessel coronary stenoses resulted in subendocardial ischemia and a large amount of myocardium at risk.[36-38] When pacing tachycardia superimposed on two-vessel coronary stenoses resulted in transmural myocardial ischemia, there was more profound impairment of LV systolic performance with occasional bulging and unaltered diastolic LV distensibility.[40] In isolated isovolumic dog hearts, global low-flow ischemia resulted in an increase in LV diastolic distensibility,[42] even in the presence of pacing tachycardia,[43] but in the same preparation[44] a hypoxic perfusate of methemoglobin-containing red blood cells resulted in a significant decrease in LV diastolic distensibility.

Comparison of Initial Left Ventricular Dysfunction During Different Types of Ischemia: Clinical Evidence

Previous studies on the initial effects of ischemia on global and regional LV function in humans looked at a single type of ischemic insult: pacing-induced ischemia,[12–14,16,17] exercise-induced ischemia,[45,46] spontaneous coronary spasm,[15] or balloon coronary occlusion ischemia.[18–25] Pacing tachycardia in the presence of triple-vessel coronary disease[12–14] and spontaneous angina[15] resulted in an upward shift of the global diastolic LV PV relation, of the diastolic LV pressure–radial length relation,[16] and of the diastolic LV pressure–wall thickness relation[17] of the ischemic myocardium. Exercise resulted in similar changes, but at end diastole there was a trend for the diastolic LV pressure–radial length relation to converge toward the resting curve.[46] A similar finding was recently reported during exercise after heart transplantation[47] and was explained by a blunted lusitropic LV response to catecholamines because of simultaneous use during exercise of LV preload reserve. At the end of balloon coronary occlusion, all of the previous studies[19,20,22] except one[21] observed an upward shift in the global diastolic LV PV relation and in the regional diastolic LV pressure–radial length relation of the ischemic segment. The present studies[26,27] were the first to compare in the same patient the initial LV effects of different types of ischemia: low-flow ischemia of balloon coronary occlusion, limited flow–high demand ischemia of pacing-induced angina, and/or hypoxemia induced by balloon coronary occlusion with maintained hypoxic perfusion distal to the balloon occlusion.

When comparing pacing-induced ischemia to balloon coronary occlusion ischemia, the following conclusions were reached[26]: (1) During pacing-induced ischemia, LV EF was larger than at the end of balloon coronary occlusion. (2) During both interventions, LV end-diastolic pressure rose but LV end-diastolic volume index was significantly larger than the control value only at the end of balloon coronary occlusion. This was consistent with an upward shift in the end-diastolic pressure volume relation during pacing-induced ischemia and a more rightward shift in the end-diastolic PV relation at the end of balloon coronary occlusion. (3) The upward shift in the diastolic LV pressure–radial length plot of the ischemic segment was larger during pacing-induced ischemia than at the end of balloon coronary occlusion. (4) At the end of balloon coronary occlusion, a correlation was observed for the ischemic segment between systolic shortening and the upward shift in the diastolic LV pressure–radial length plot. This correlation observed at the end of balloon coronary occlusion between systolic shortening of the ischemic segment and the upward shift of the diastolic LV pressure–radial length plot reconciles the contradictory results between the present and some of the previous studies on diastolic LV distensibility changes at the end of balloon coronary occlusion.

The studies by Wijns et al.[19] and by Kass et al.[22] observed a 20% decrease in systolic segmental shortening, a fall in EF from 69% ± 8% to 54% ± 12%, and a decrease in global or regional LV diastolic distensibility, as evident from an upward shift in the diastolic pressure–radial length or PV relations. The present study observed a 34% decrease in systolic segmental shortening and a fall in EF from 77% ± 7% to 47% ± 11 %, which was comparable with the fall in EF observed by Bertrand et al.[21] (from 72% ± 6% to 46% ± 10%). Both the present study and the study by Bertrand et al.[22] observed, respectively, an upward and a rightward shift in the diastolic pressure–radial length relation and no significant change in the radial stiffness modulus. Hence, an interstudy comparison reveals an interaction at the end of balloon coronary occlusion between systolic LV performance and diastolic LV distensibility. This interaction was similar to the correlation observed in the present study[26] at the end of balloon coronary occlusion between individual data on systolic performance and diastolic distensibility.

The variability in depression of systolic performance at the end of balloon coronary occlusion, both individually and among different studies, probably relates to the presence or absence of objective evidence of myocardial ischemia at the end of the balloon occlusion episode, to differences in balloon inflation time, to variable recruitment of collaterals, and to procurement of data during either first or subsequent balloon inflations. In the study of Wijns et al.,[19] balloon inflation time (±30 s) was shorter than in the present study (±60 s), and the balloon inflation used for study of LV performance varied from a third to a tenth balloon inflation, whereas in the present study[26] the balloon inflation varied from a second to a fourth balloon inflation. In the present study all patients had angina and ST-segment changes at the end of balloon coronary occlusion. Moreover, the present study documented the absence of significant coronary collateralization by coronary wedge pressure measurement during balloon coronary occlusion.

Previous studies on the effects of pacing stress on LV performance examined patients with triple-vessel coronary disease and observed an upward shift in the entire diastolic LV PV[12,13] or diastolic pressure–wall thickness relation.[17] The present study[26] examined patients with single-vessel coronary disease, and the smaller amount of myocardium at risk in these patients could explain the occasional limitation of the upward shift of the diastolic LV PV or of the diastolic pressure–radial length relation to early and mid diastole. A similar upward shift limited in the initial portion of the diastolic LV pressure–segment length relation was also recently reported in conscious dogs with a single-vessel coronary stenosis of the left circumflex coronary artery.[39] Despite the presence of single-vessel coronary disease, some patients experienced profound depression of LV systolic performance during pacing-induced ischemia. In these patients the diastolic LV PV and the diastolic pressure–radial length relations failed to change. A similar relation between depressed systolic performance and unaltered diastolic distensibility during pacing-induced ischemia has been reported by other investigators in humans[16] and in anesthetized dogs with two-vessel coronary stenoses.[6] Hence, a drastic reduction of LV systolic performance during either pacing-induced or balloon occlusion ischemia precludes in humans reductions in global or regional diastolic LV distensibility.

The present studies[27] also compared LV diastolic distensibility at the end of a balloon coronary occlusion and at the end of an equally long balloon coronary occlusion during which saline was perfused through the distal lumen of the balloon catheter at a flow rate (= 1 mL/s) that equaled resting left anterior descending flow. The latter intervention resulted in a myocardial oxygen delivery that was 38 times lower than normal and therefore mimicked hypoxemic conditions. During balloon occlusion with distal perfusion, myocardial oxygen delivery was probably comparable with regular balloon occlusion, because the minimal amount of oxygen dissolved in the per-

fusate was offset by reduced oxygen delivery from collateral flow. During balloon inflation with distal perfusion, collateral flow was less than during regular balloon inflation because of higher intravascular pressure created by the perfusion pump in the epicardial coronary arteries distal to the balloon occlusion. Continuous saline perfusion during balloon coronary occlusion caused no change in LV end-diastolic volume at the end of the occlusion episode but a marked elevation in LV minimum and end-diastolic pressures compared with regular balloon coronary occlusion. This profound decrease in LV diastolic distensibility at the end of balloon coronary occlusion with distal perfusion was accompanied by better preservation of LV systolic performance, as evident from the higher LV stroke work index. Hence, the effects of hypoxemia on LV performance in humans resemble the effects of hypoxia in isolated rodent or dog preparations by the smaller depression of LV systolic function and by the larger decrease of LV diastolic distensibility.

Several pathophysiologic mechanisms could contribute to the unequal effect of different types of ischemia on the human myocardium: (1) variable vascular turgor and myocardial stretch during the ischemic episode or during the hyperemic phase following the ischemic episode, (2) build up or washout of tissue metabolites during the ischemic episode, (3) unequal intensity of the ischemic stress episodes, and (4) regional dyssynchrony and biventricular interaction.

Vascular Turgor and Myocardial Stretch During Ischemia and Hyperemia

Coronary perfusion pressure, coronary flow, or both influence LV systolic performance (Gregg phenomenon)[48] and LV diastolic distensibility (Salisbury effect).[49] An increase in coronary perfusion causes transversal stretch of the myocardium, which increases developed force (Gregg effect) through activation of stretch-activated ion channels. Stretch-activated ion channels blockade in isometrically contracting perfused rat papillary muscle completely blunted the increase in developed force and in peak intracellular calcium concentration induced by the Gregg effect.

Salisbury and colleagues[49] were the first to observe in an isovolumic canine left ventricle an increase in LV end-diastolic pressure at increased coronary perfusion pressure. Alterations in LV end-diastolic distensibility follow changes in coronary vascular engorgement and coronary perfusion. The Gregg phenomenon received renewed attention as the initial mediator of the loss of LV systolic function.[50,51] In the isovolumic rodent heart, a Gregg phenomenon was demonstrated during the initial stages of no-flow global myocardial ischemia by the slower decline of LV developed pressure in the microembolized heart without coronary depressurization than after simple interruption of coronary flow.[50] Only in the microembolized heart did the time course of LV pressure decline correspond to the build up of tissue metabolites such as phosphate or H^+, which are known to deactivate cardiac muscle through desensitization of myofilaments. The earlier loss of LV systolic function during interruption of coronary flow was therefore attributed to loss of vascular stretch on adjacent sarcomeres. Vascular turgor could affect muscle sarcomere stretch through mechanical coupling of the vascular network and the myocardium. Recent experiments in pig hearts, however, correlated the initial loss of myocardial function during moderate ischemia of single-vessel coronary stenosis with the fall in high energy phosphates and not with the decrease in muscle preload.[51]

The present observations confirm in humans the importance of coronary vascular turgor as a mediator of the loss in LV systolic performance during low-flow ischemia of balloon coronary occlusion. When coronary vascular turgor was maintained during balloon coronary occlusion by distal perfusion, there was better preservation of LV stroke work at the end of an equally long balloon coronary occlusion. This preservation of LV stroke work could also result from unequal build up of tissue metabolites during regular balloon coronary occlusion and balloon coronary occlusion with distal perfusion. Coronary sinus lactate concentration showed, however, a similar time course in both the regular balloon coronary occlusion and the balloon coronary occlusion with distal perfusion. In both interventions, coronary sinus lactate concentration during the actual balloon inflation period was comparable with arterial lactate concentration, and peak coronary sinus lactate concentration occurred at a comparable moment after release of the angioplasty balloon. This finding suggests the better preservation of systolic performance at the end of balloon coronary occlusion with distal perfusion to be related more to vascular turgor affecting cardiac muscle stretch than to unequal tissue levels of metabolites. Recent insights into how cardiac muscle stretch affects muscle performance suggest an intrinsic molecular property of troponin C to mediate the rising limb of the cardiac muscle length–active tension relation.[52] This implies that vascular turgor affects cardiac muscle performance by a mechanism similar to tissue metabolites, namely, modulation of myofilamentary calcium sensitivity, and that the relative contributions of vascular turgor and of tissue metabolites on the maintenance of systolic function during the initial stages of ischemia are hard to separate.

Moreover, vascular stretch could affect adjacent cardiac muscle sarcomeres not only mechanically but also through release from the coronary endothelium of substances, which have recently been shown to alter cardiac muscle performance also through modulation of myofilamentary calcium sensitivity.[53,54] To measure coronary depressurization during balloon coronary occlusion, we recently obtained high fidelity intracoronary pressure recordings using a 0.018 angioplasty guidewire with a micromanometer pressure transducer mounted on the guidewire tip. Figure 17.6 shows high fidelity recordings of intracoronary pressure distal to the occluded balloon and of LV pressure. During balloon occlusion, there is indeed reduced diastolic intracoronary pressure. During systole, however, there is immediate build up of intracoronary pressure, probably because of squeezing of blood from adjacent normally contracting zones into the balloon occluded epicardial coronary compartment.

This immediate build up of intracoronary pressure during systole argues against the existence of total vascular collapse during balloon occlusion ischemia in humans and confirms the results from recent experiments in pigs, which correlated the initial loss of myocardial function during moderate ischemia of single-vessel coronary stenosis with the fall in high energy phosphates and not

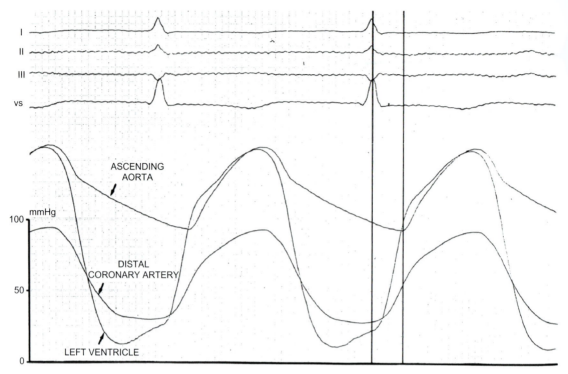

FIGURE 17.6. From top to bottom: Three surface lead electrocardiograms (I, II, III), one precordial lead electrocardiogram, a high fidelity micromanometer aortic pressure recording, a high fidelity micromanometer left ventricular pressure recording, and a high fidelity micromanometer intracoronary pressure recording obtained distal to an inflated angioplasty balloon and derived from a micromanometer pressure transducer mounted on an 0.018 angioplasty guidewire. During balloon occlusion ischemia there is reduced diastolic intracoronary pressure. During systole, however, there is immediate build up of intracoronary pressure, probably because of distention of the balloon occluded epicardial coronary compartment by blood squeezed out of the adjacent and normally contracting left ventricular segments. This build up of systolic intracoronary pressure argues against the existence of total vascular collapse during balloon occlusion ischemia in humans.

with the decrease in muscle preload.[51] Salisbury et al.[49] were the first to observe in an isovolumic canine left ventricle an increase in LV end-diastolic pressure at increased coronary perfusion pressure. Alterations in LV diastolic distensibility after changes in coronary vascular engorgement and coronary perfusion have subsequently been confirmed by other investigators, who observed larger changes in diastolic LV wall stiffness when coronary perfusion pressure was altered in a failing left ventricle than in a normal left ventricle.[55] The relative importance of coronary perfusion pressure versus coronary flow as determinants of myocardial wall stiffness was elucidated by Olsen et al.[56], who observed a significant effect of coronary perfusion pressure and not of coronary flow on LV compliance and who favored direct sarcomere stretching by the coronary vascular tree[57] as the mechanism underlying erectile stiffening of the LV myocardium.

During balloon occlusion ischemia (low-flow ischemia), the drop in coronary perfusion pressure distal to the balloon occlusion could increase diastolic LV distensibility. A rightward and downward shift of the end-diastolic LV PV relation was indeed observed in the present studies in some patients at the end of balloon coronary occlusion (see Figure 17.1). During pacing-induced ischemia (limited flow–high demand ischemia), coronary perfusion pressure distal to the coronary stenosis falls. Based on the Salisbury effect, this drop in coronary perfusion pressure distal to the coronary stenosis would tend to counteract the decrease in LV diastolic distensibility observed during pacing-induced ischemia. On the other hand, during pacing-induced ischemia LV function is assessed during initial relief of the ischemic stress episode in contrast to balloon coronary occlusion ischemia, in which LV function is assessed at the nadir of the ischemic stress episode. Even when a critical coronary stenosis permits no change in total coronary blood flow, a reactive hyperemic response to the ischemic subendocardium following the pacing stress episode could contribute to the observed decrease in diastolic LV distensibility,[58] as previously observed during exercise[59] or isoproterenol infusion[60] in dogs with critical coronary stenosis. During balloon coronary occlusion with distal perfusion (hypoxemia), coronary perfusion pressure was preserved and probably contributed to the larger decrease in diastolic LV distensibility as compared with regular balloon coronary occlusion.

Build Up or Washout of Tissue Metabolites

Low-flow ischemia of balloon coronary occlusion, limited flow–high demand ischemia of pacing-induced angina, and hypoxemia exert different effects on build up of tissue metabolites, such as H^+ and inorganic phosphate. Acidosis as a result of build up of tissue metabolites drives the creatine kinase reaction, which replenishes adenosine triphosphate, depletes creatine phosphate, and produces inorganic phosphate.[7] Despite increased amplitude of the calcium transient and myoplasmic calcium overload, this rise in inorganic phosphate induces contractile failure by reducing the calcium sensitivity of myofilaments.

The present studies measured coronary sinus lactate, H^+, and K^+ concentrations at rest and during and following the pacing-stress episode; during and following the regular balloon coronary occlusion; and during and following an equally long balloon coronary occlusion with distal perfusion (see Figure 17.5). Because no simultaneous coronary sinus flow measurements were performed, the coronary sinus lactate, H^+, and K^+ concentrations provide no quantitative information on myocardial metabolite production rate but allow assessment of the time course of metabolite handling during the different types of ischemic insult. During pacing-induced ischemia, metabolites started to appear in the coronary sinus during the pacing-stress episode before ces-

sation of pacing and continued to be washed out after the pacing-stress episode.

The better preservation of LV systolic performance and the larger decrease in LV diastolic distensibility as compared with balloon occlusion ischemia could well have been influenced by the ongoing washout of tissue metabolites. Partial removal of inorganic phosphate and of H^+ preserved myofilamentary calcium sensitivity and could explain the better preservation of LV systolic performance. Partial removal of metabolites could also explain the larger decrease in diastolic LV distensibility, because preserved myofilamentary calcium sensitivity could allow for diastolic cross-bridge cycling in the presence of a simultaneous myoplasmic calcium overload.

During the low-flow ischemia of balloon coronary occlusion, the time courses of coronary sinus lactate, H^+, and K^+ concentrations were different from the time course during the limited flow–high demand ischemia of pacing-induced ischemia. During the ischemic stress episode of balloon coronary occlusion, there was no rise in coronary sinus lactate concentration (see Figure 17.5), the peak of which was observed after deflation of the angioplasty balloon during the hyperemic phase. At the end of the balloon inflation, when LV function was measured, build up of tissue metabolites and the ensuing decrease in myofilamentary calcium sensitivity could explain the significantly larger decrease in LV stroke work index at the end of balloon coronary ischemia than during pacing-induced ischemia. The time pattern of coronary sinus lactate concentration during balloon occlusion with distal perfusion was comparable with the regular balloon occlusion. Because of the similar time pattern of coronary sinus lactate concentration in both balloon occlusions, the better preservation of LV systolic performance, and the decrease in LV diastolic distensibility observed during balloon inflation with distal perfusion seemed more likely to be related, respectively, to differences in vascular stretch (the Gregg phenomenon) and to differences in vascular engorgement (the Salisbury effect) than to unequal myocardial build up of tissue metabolites. Because of the relative insensitivity of coronary sinus sampling to detect local washout of metabolites and because of the failure to perform great cardiac vein sampling to assess selectively left anterior descending drainage, unequal intracellular accumulation of metabolites during coronary occlusion and during coronary occlusion with distal perfusion was not excluded.

The perfusate used during the balloon inflations with distal perfusion was a mixture of regular saline (pH = 7.0) infused through the distal lumen of the balloon catheter at a constant flow rate of 1 mL/s and blood coming from coronary collaterals (mean coronary wedge pressure = 29 ± 11 mm Hg). Compared with whole blood perfusion, this perfusate was of lower pH, hypokalemic, and hypocalcemic. The higher LV systolic performance observed in the present study during balloon inflation with distal perfusion compared with the regular balloon inflation is, however, unrelated to the altered composition of the perfusate relative to whole blood because in isolated cardiac muscle preparations both acidosis and combined hypokalemia-hypocalcemia exerted a negative inotropic effect.[61] Hypoxic whole blood perfusion could probably have resulted in even better preservation of LV systolic performance and in even larger reductions in LV diastolic distensibility, because the lower pH of the perfusate compared with whole blood perfusion could have resulted in reduced diffusion of hydrogen ions out of the myocardium and because in isovolumic rabbit hearts replacement of buffer perfusion by blood perfusion caused a consistent elevation in LV filling pressures and a consistent fall in LV diastolic distensibility during low-flow–high-demand ischemia.[34] Whole blood perfusion was therefore considered to provide higher mechanical vascular support of surrounding myocardium. Moreover, compared with saline perfusion, whole blood perfusion could modify the release from vascular endothelial cells of factors that influence myofilamentary calcium sensitivity.[53,54]

Patients experienced more severe chest pain during the balloon inflation with distal perfusion, probably consistent with a larger production of bradykinin, which triggers cardiac nociceptors and paracrine secretions from endothelial cells. These factors released from vascular endothelial cells could increase myofilamentary calcium sensitivity and contribute to the better preservation of LV stroke work index observed during the balloon inflation with distal perfusion. Increased cardiac sympathetic stimulation could have resulted from the increased severity of chest pain during the balloon inflation with distal perfusion. At the end of both balloon inflations heart rates were, however, comparable, and, at the end of the balloon inflation with distal perfusion, the prolongation of the time constant of LV pressure decay was larger. The latter cannot be reconciled with a larger lusitropic effect of more intense sympathetic stimulation.

Unequal Intensity of the Ischemic Stress Episodes

Unequal intensity of ischemia could have interfered with global and regional LV functions during the different ischemic stress episodes. In a study of anesthetized dogs, pacing-induced ischemia in the presence of coronary stenoses and coronary occlusion ischemia produced similar changes in systolic and diastolic functions of the ischemic LV region if LV end-diastolic pressure was matched in each experiment during both ischemic stress episodes.[40] In the present clinical studies, comparable levels of LV end-diastolic pressure could not be achieved in each patient, but the pooled patient data comparing pacing-induced and balloon occlusion ischemia revealed similar LV end-diastolic pressures as a result of both ischemic stress episodes. Despite these similar elevations in LV filling pressures, LV EFs and LV end-diastolic volume indices were significantly different.

When comparing balloon occlusion ischemia with hypoxemia, the pooled patient data showed the highest LV end-diastolic pressure during hypoxemia, when the LV stroke work index showed the smallest reduction. These observations cannot be reconciled with the left ventricle operating on a single diastolic LV compliance curve during the different ischemic stress episodes and with unequal severity of ischemia of the different ischemic stress episodes inducing different degrees of LV failure. During balloon occlusion ischemia with distal perfusion, more oxygen could be delivered to the myocardium because of oxygen dissolved in the perfusate. The amount of oxygen dissolved in the perfusate was, however, minimal (±5 mL/L) and approximately 38 times less than in arterial blood. This additional amount of oxygen delivered to the ischemic region during balloon inflation with perfusion was probably

17. Coronary Artery Disease

offset by reduced oxygen delivery to the ischemic region from collateral flow because of the higher intravascular pressure created by the perfusion pump in the epicardial coronary arteries distal to the balloon occlusion. The most accurate assessment of the severity of ischemia in these different types of intervention is measurement of myocardial adenosine triphosphate and creatine phosphate contents in the ischemic myocardium as performed in dogs using a transmural biopsy drill by Momomura et al.[7] during pacing-induced and coronary occlusion ischemia and as performed noninvasively in humans during handgrip-induced angina using nuclear magnetic resonance spectroscopy.[62]

Regional Dyssynchrony and Biventricular Interaction

Slower LV isovolumic relaxation and filling can result from loss of synchronicity of contraction and relaxation of different LV segments.[63,64] As evident from clinical observations in patients with coronary artery disease[65] and from experimental findings in a single-vessel coronary stenosis model in pigs,[41] synchronicity of diastolic wall motion of ischemic and nonischemic LV segments is drastically affected by brief coronary occlusion and only slightly affected by pacing-induced ischemia in the presence of coronary stenoses.

In a patient who had received radiopaque markers in the LV myocardium at the time of coronary bypass surgery, regional wall motion could be accurately followed during balloon occlusion of a saphenous vein bypass graft.[65] During the balloon occlusion, the segmental shortening pattern evolved from systolic shortening to mid systolic bulging and to holosystolic bulging with early diastolic recoil. The dyssynchronous early diastolic recoil slowed isovolumic LV relaxation but did not alter regional diastolic distensibility of the ischemic segment, as evident from the unchanged diastolic pressure–segment length relation of the ischemic segment. This confirmed in humans the findings in numerous animal experiments investigating the regional LV effect of brief coronary artery ligation.[9,11]

A similar loss of synchronous early diastolic filling has also been implicated as the cause of the upward shift of the diastolic LV PV relation in humans during pacing-induced angina.[66] During pacing-induced angina in humans, dyssynchrony between ischemic and nonischemic segments is, however, much smaller than during coronary occlusion, as evident from the ±50 ms reduction in time to peak posterior wall thickness[17] and the ±50 ms reduction in time to peak segment lengthening.[67] Moreover, the decrease in diastolic LV distensibility during pacing-induced angina was larger when the amount of myocardium at risk assessed by a simultaneously performed thallium scan was larger.[68] If dyssynchrony between ischemic and nonischemic LV segments was the mechanism for the decrease in diastolic LV distensibility, an equal magnitude of ischemic and nonischemic areas would tend to cause the largest shifts in diastolic LV distensibility. A similar argument against regional dyssynchrony as the mechanism for the decrease in diastolic LV distensibility during pacing-induced ischemia is provided by patients with aortic stenosis, in whom pacing results in an upward shift in the diastolic LV PV relation despite uniform distribution of subendocardial ischemia.[69] During pacing-induced and balloon coronary occlusion ischemia, LV end-diastolic pressure rose to a similar level. Reactive pulmonary hypertension and right ventricular loading, although not directly measured, were therefore probably comparable in both interventions. Eventual right ventricular interaction through the shared interventricular septum must have been similar and fails to explain the unequal changes in diastolic LV distensibility in both interventions.

Conclusion

Diastolic LV PV and diastolic LV pressure–radial length relations were compared in patients with significant left anterior descending coronary stenosis during pacing-induced ischemia (low-flow–high-demand ischemia), during balloon coronary occlusion (low-flow ischemia), and during balloon coronary occlusion with preserved hypoxic perfusion distal to the balloon occlusion (hypoxemia). During pacing-induced ischemia and at the end of balloon coronary occlusion with distal perfusion, LV systolic performance showed a smaller decrease and LV diastolic distensibility a larger decrease than at the end of balloon coronary occlusion. Better preservation of myofilamentary calcium sensitivity during pacing-induced ischemia as a result of wash-out of tissue metabolites, of mechanical stretch of maintained coronary pressurization, and of endothelial factors released by continuing coronary flow could explain not only the smaller decrease in LV systolic performance but also the larger decrease in LV diastolic distensibility because of diastolic cross-bridge cycling in the presence of a simultaneous myoplasmic calcium overload.

References

1. Kim SJ, Kudej RK, Yatani A, Kim YK, Takagi G, Honda R, Colantonio DA, Van Eyk JE, Vatner DE, Rasmusson RL, Vatner SF. A novel mechanism for myocardial stunning involving impaired Ca(2+) handling. Circ Res 2001;89(9):831–837.
2. Heusch G, Sipido KR. Myocardial hibernation: a double-edged sword. Circ Res 2004;94(8): 1005–1007.
3. Kass DA, Bronzwaer JG, Paulus WJ. What mechanisms underlie diastolic dysfunction in heart failure? Circ Res 2004;94(12):1533–1542.
4. Apstein CS, Grossman W. Opposite initial effects of supply and demand ischemia on left ventricular diastolic compliance: the ischemia-diastolic paradox. J Mol Cell Cardiol 1987;19(1):119–128.
5. Serizawa T, Vogel WM, Apstein CS, Grossman W. Comparison of acute alterations in left ventricular relaxation and diastolic chamber stiffness induced by hypoxia and ischemia. Role of myocardial oxygen supply–demand imbalance. J Clin Invest 1981;68(1):91–102.
6. Paulus WJ, Grossman W, Serizawa T, Bourdillon PD, Pasipoularides A, Mirsky I. Different effects of two types of ischemia on myocardial systolic and diastolic function. Am J Physiol 1985;248(5 Pt 2): H719–H728.
7. Momomura S, Ingwall JS, Parker JA, Sahagian P, Ferguson JJ, Grossman W. The relationships of high energy phosphates, tissue pH, and regional blood flow to diastolic distensibility in the ischemic dog myocardium. Circ Res 1985;57(6):822–835.
8. Wexler LF, Weinberg EO, Ingwall JS, Apstein CS. Acute alterations in diastolic left ventricular chamber distensibility: mechanistic differences between hypoxemia and ischemia in isolated perfused rabbit and rat hearts. Circ Res 1986;59(5):515–528.
9. Tyberg JV, Forrester JS, Wyatt HL, Goldner SJ, Parmley WW, Swan HJ. An analysis of segmental ischemic dysfunction utilizing the pressure-length loop. Circulation 1974;49(4):748–754.
10. Wong BY, Toyama M, Reis RL, Goodyer AV. Sequential changes in left ventricular compliance during acute coronary occlusion in the isovolumic working canine heart. Circ Res 1978;43(2):274–286.
11. Hess OM, Osakada G, Lavelle JF, Gallagher KP, Kemper WS, Ross J Jr. Diastolic myocardial wall stiffness and ventricular relaxation during partial and complete coronary occlusions in the conscious dog. Circ Res 1983;52(4):387–400.
12. Dwyer EM Jr. Left ventricular pressure-volume alterations and regional disorders of contraction during myocardial ischemia induced by atrial pacing. Circulation 1970;42(6):1111–1122.
13. Barry WH, Brooker JZ, Alderman EL, Harrison DC. Changes in diastolic stiffness and tone of the left ventricle during angina pectoris. Circulation 1974; 49(2):255–263.
14. Mann T, Goldberg S, Mudge GH Jr, Grossman W. Factors contributing to altered left ventricular diastolic properties during angina pectoris. Circulation 1979;59(1):14–20.
15. Sharma B, Behrens TW, Erlein D, Hodges M, Asinger RW, Francis GS. Left ventricular diastolic properties and filling characteristics during spontaneous angina pectoris at rest. Am J Cardiol 1983; 52(7):704–709.
16. Sasayama S, Nonogi H, Miyazaki S, Sakurai T, Kawai C, Eiho S, Kuwahara M. Changes in diastolic properties of the regional myocardium during pacing-induced ischemia in human subjects. J Am Coll Cardiol 1985;5(3):599–606.
17. Bourdillon PD, Lorell BH, Mirsky I, Paulus WJ, Wynne J, Grossman W. Increased regional myocardial stiffness of the left ventricle during pacing-induced angina in man. Circulation 1983;67(2): 316–323.
18. Serruys PW, Wijns W, van den BM, Meij S, Slager C, Schuurbiers JC, Hugenholtz PG, Brower RW. Left ventricular performance, regional blood flow, wall motion, and lactate metabolism during transluminal angioplasty. Circulation 1984;70(1):25–36.
19. Wijns W, Serruys PW, Slager CJ, Grimm J, Krayenbuehl HP, Hugenholtz PG, Hess OM. Effect of coronary occlusion during percutaneous transluminal angioplasty in humans on left ventricular chamber stiffness and regional diastolic pressure–radius relations. J Am Coll Cardiol 1986;7(3):455–463.

20. Carlson EB, Hinohara T, Morris KG. Recovery of systolic and diastolic left ventricular function after a 60-second coronary arterial occlusion during percutaneous transluminal coronary angioplasty for angina pectoris. Am J Cardiol 1987;60(7):460–466.
21. Bertrand ME, Lablanche JM, Fourrier JL, Traisnel G, Mirsky I. Left ventricular systolic and diastolic function during acute coronary artery balloon occlusion in humans. J Am Coll Cardiol 1988;12(2):341–347.
22. Kass DA, Midei M, Brinker J, Maughan WL. Influence of coronary occlusion during PTCA on end-systolic and end-diastolic pressure-volume relations in humans. Circulation 1990;81(2):447–460.
23. Kern MJ, Deligonul U, Labovitz A. Influence of drug therapy on the ischemic response to acute coronary occlusion in man: supply-side economics. Am Heart J 1989;118(2):361–380.
24. Deutsch E, Berger M, Kussmaul WG, Hirshfeld JW Jr, Herrmann HC, Laskey WK. Adaptation to ischemia during percutaneous transluminal coronary angioplasty. Clinical, hemodynamic, and metabolic features. Circulation 1990;82(6):2044–2051.
25. Cribier A, Korsatz L, Koning R, Rath P, Gamra H, Stix G, Merchant S, Chan C, Letac B. Improved myocardial ischemic response and enhanced collateral circulation with long repetitive coronary occlusion during angioplasty: a prospective study. J Am Coll Cardiol 1992;20(3):578–586.
26. Bronzwaer JG, De Bruyne B, Ascoop CA, Paulus WJ. Comparative effects of pacing-induced and balloon coronary occlusion ischemia on left ventricular diastolic function in man. Circulation 1991;84(1):211–222.
27. De Bruyne B, Bronzwaer JG, Heyndrickx GR, Paulus WJ. Comparative effects of ischemia and hypoxemia on left ventricular systolic and diastolic function in humans. Circulation 1993;88(2):461–471.
28. Meier B, Luethy P, Finci L, Steffenino GD, Rutishauser W. Coronary wedge pressure in relation to spontaneously visible and recruitable collaterals. Circulation 1987;75(5):906–913.
29. De Bruyne B, Meier B, Finci L, Urban P, Rutishauser W. Potential protective effect of high coronary wedge pressure on left ventricular function after coronary occlusion. Circulation 1988;78(3):566–572.
30. Pepine CJ, Mehta J, Webster WW, Jr., Nichols WW. In vivo validation of a thermodilution method to determine regional left ventricular blood flow in patients with coronary disease. Circulation 1978;58(5):795–802.
31. Paulus WJ, Vantrimpont PJ, Rousseau MF. Diastolic function of the nonfilling human left ventricle. J Am Coll Cardiol 1992;20(7):1524–1532.
32. Webb SC, Rickards AF, Poole-Wilson PA. Coronary sinus potassium concentration recorded during coronary angioplasty. Br Heart J 1983;50(2):146–148.
33. Nayler WG, Yepez CE, Poole-Wilson PA. The effect of beta-adrenoceptor and Ca^{2+} antagonist drugs on the hypoxia-induced increased in resting tension. Cardiovasc Res 1978;12(11):666–674.
34. Isoyama S, Apstein CS, Wexler LF, Grice WN, Lorell BH. Acute decrease in left ventricular diastolic chamber distensibility during simulated angina in isolated hearts. Circ Res 1987;61(6):925–933.
35. Tomoike H, Franklin D, McKown D, Kemper WS, Guberek M, Ross J Jr. Regional myocardial dysfunction and hemodynamic abnormalities during strenuous exercise in dogs with limited coronary flow. Circ Res 1978;42(4):487–496.
36. Serizawa T, Carabello BA, Grossman W. Effect of pacing-induced ischemia on left ventricular diastolic pressure–volume relations in dogs with coronary stenoses. Circ Res 1980;46(3):430–439.
37. Paulus WJ, Serizawa T, Grossman W. Altered left ventricular diastolic properties during pacing-induced ischemia in dogs with coronary stenoses. Potentiation by caffeine. Circ Res 1982;50(2):218–227.
38. Momomura S, Bradley AB, Grossman W. Left ventricular diastolic pressure-segment length relations and end-diastolic distensibility in dogs with coronary stenoses. An angina physiology model. Circ Res 1984;55(2):203–214.
39. Miyazaki S, Guth BD, Miura T, Indolfi C, Schulz R, Ross J Jr. Changes of left ventricular diastolic function in exercising dogs without and with ischemia. Circulation 1990;81(3):1058–1070.
40. Applegate RJ, Walsh RA, O'Rourke RA. Comparative effects of pacing-induced and flow-limited ischemia on left ventricular function. Circulation 1990;81(4):1380–1392.
41. Takahashi T, Levine MJ, Grossman W. Regional diastolic mechanics of ischemic and nonischemic myocardium in the pig heart. J Am Coll Cardiol 1991;17(5):1203–1212.
42. Palacios I, Johnson RA, Newell JB, Powell WJ, Jr. Left ventricular end-diastolic pressure volume relationships with experimental acute global ischemia. Circulation 1976;53(3):428–436.
43. Lorell BH, Palacios I, Daggett WM, Jacobs ML, Fowler BN, Newell JB. Right ventricular distension and left ventricular compliance. Am J Physiol 1981;240(1):H87–H98.

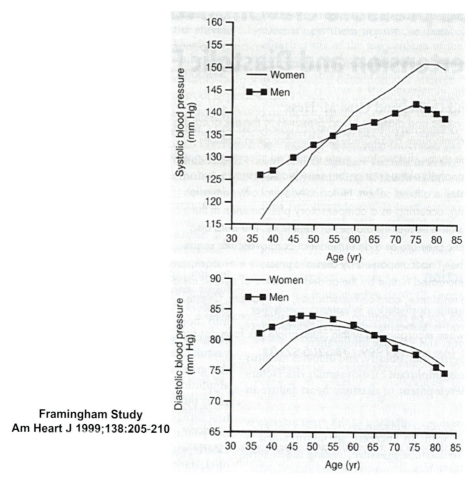

Figure 18.1. Systolic **(top)** and diastolic **(bottom)** blood pressure changes in healthy men and women over time. There is a continuous increase in systolic pressure with age that is more pronounced in females than males. At the age of >75 years, systolic blood pressure decreases due to the losses of patients with the highest blood pressure. In contrast, diastolic pressure increases up to the age of 50 and decreases then in both gender groups from approximately 80 to 75 mm Hg. (From Kannel.[4])

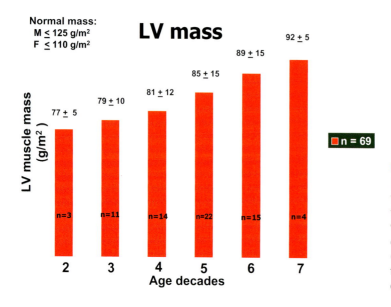

Figure 18.2. Changes in left ventricular (LV) muscle mass in healthy persons over time. Muscle mass increases significantly from 77 g/m^2 at the age of 30 years to 92 g/m^2 at the age of 80 years. These changes are within the normal limits (muscle mass in males, ≤125 g/m^2, in females, ≤110 g/m^2). Thus, there is physiologic LV hypertrophy with aging.

FIGURE 18.3. Changes in transmitral Doppler flow profile (E/A ratio) in healthy persons over time (same population as in Figure 18.2). There is an age-related decrease in E/A ratio from 1.6 at the age of 30 years to 0.88 at the age of 80 years. These changes are parallel with the increase in left ventricular muscle mass (see Figure 18.2). Thus, there is "physiologic diastolic dysfunction" with increasing age parallel with "physiologic left ventricular hypertrophy."

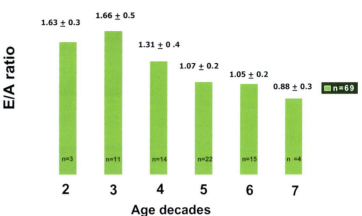

Definition of Diastolic Dysfunction

Diagnosis of diastolic dysfunction is difficult and is mainly based on Doppler-echocardiographic evaluation.[8,9,13] Three different forms of abnormal diastolic filling have been described (Figure 18.4):

1. Delayed relaxation filling pattern
2. Pseudonormalized filling pattern
3. Restrictive filling pattern

These echocardiographic changes characterize different filling patterns of the left ventricle and do not reflect true ventricular stiffness.[6,7,14] From a clinical standpoint, diastolic dysfunction has been differentiated into three forms:

1. **Diastolic filling abnormalities** with delayed relaxation, abnormal filling, or changes in diastolic stiffness
2. **Diastolic dysfunction** with delayed relaxation, abnormal filling, or changes in diastolic stiffness associated with clinical symptoms such as dyspnea on exertion, fatigue, reduced exercise tolerance or atrial fibrillation
3. **Diastolic heart failure** with signs or symptoms of heart failure and preserved systolic function (EF ≥45%) but an abnormal diastolic filling pattern[9,13,15,16]

Clinical symptoms may occur at rest or during exercise and may precipitate during atrial fibrillation or after strenuous exercise.[17] However, echocardiographic abnormalities may occur without clinical symptoms and have no prognostic impact.[12] These echocardiographic findings have been termed "diastolic abnormalities" and are considered to represent "echo findings."[9]

Pathophysiology of Diastolic Dysfunction in Hypertension

The increase in blood pressure is compensated even before left ventricular hypertrophy develops by a change in systolic and diastolic function.[15,18] At the beginning, LV muscle mass is minimally increased (see Figure 18.2), remaining within the normal range but affecting diastolic function (Figure 18.3) without altering systolic performance.[19] The earliest functional changes in hypertension are a prolongation and incoordination of isovolumic relaxation, reduced rate of rapid filling, and increased amplitude of the A wave probably caused by an increase in passive diastolic stiffness (see Figure 18.4).[8,9,13,16]

Parallel to these changes in LV function vascular changes of the large and small arteries occur. These changes are considered at the beginning as "hypertensive" but later become "atherosclerotic."[19] The former are directly caused by the increased blood pressure and can be prevented by lowering the pressure level; however, the latter

Doppler echocardiography

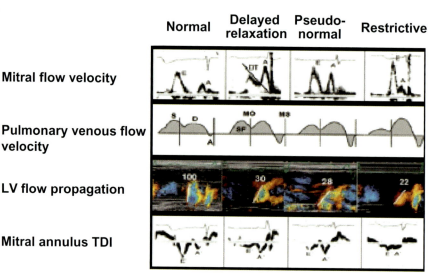

FIGURE 18.4. Doppler echocardiographic findings in healthy people and in patients with diastolic dysfunction. Diastolic dysfunction is separated into delayed relaxation, pseudonormalized, and restrictive filling pattern (top line). Data are shown for mitral flow velocity, pulmonary venous flow velocity, left ventricular (LV) color Doppler flow propagation, and mitral annulus tissue Doppler imaging (TDI). With increasing severity of diastolic dysfunction (from left to right), there is an increase in early diastolic filling with a loss of mitral annulus motion. (From Erbel et al.[14])

form has multiple cardiovascular risk factors such as hyperlipidemia, smoking, aging, and hyperhomocysteinemia.[20] In the pathophysiology of hypertension, vascular changes occur such as endothelial dysfunction and smooth muscle cell hypertrophy.[21,22] Data from the literature (Table 18.1) clearly indicate that, with mild to moderate hypertension, LV hypertrophy develops with changes in diastolic function, whereas systolic function remains normal.

There has been a smooth transition from physiologic diastolic function (see earlier discussion) to **clinically** manifest diastolic dysfunction.[9,15] As a consequence of chronic pressure overload, severe

TABLE 18.1. Studies of patients with hypertension (Hyp) and controls according to different echocardiographic diastolic parameters.

Reference	Year	N	Female (%)	Diastolic dysfunction (%)	BP Hyp (Syst/diast, mm Hg)	BP controls (Syst/diast, mm Hg)	LVMI Hyp (g/m²)	LVMI controls (g/m²)	E/A Hyp (E/A ± SD)	E/A controls (E/A ± SD)	DcT Hyp (ms)	DcT controls (ms)
23	2002	679	41	—	174/95	—	124 ± 26	—	—	—	—	—
12	2003	1779	37	28	—	—	—	—	—	—	—	—
24	2003	99	50	—	134/76	—	119 ± 34	—	0.82 ± 0.33	—	234 ± 48	—
25	2004	113	42	100	150/90	—	—	—	0.72 ± 0.2	—	224 ± 40	—
26	2004	37	38	—	168/96	123/72	145 ± 37	81 ± 9	0.72 ± 0.12	1.03 ± 0.43	—	—
6	2005	85	59	44	148/82	120/68	82 ± 18	79 ± 12	1.2 ± 0.2	1.1 ± 0.2	202 ± 23	197 ± 32
27	2005	30	63	100	142/79	—	117 ± 29	—	0.79 ± 0.15	—	256 ± 52	—
28	2006	60	60	—	166/96	118/74	109 ± 28	87 ± 13	1.1 ± 0.3	0.9 ± 0.4	217 ± 40	189 ± 35
All		2882	49	—	151/87	128/76	116 ± 29	82 ± 11	0.9 ± 0.2	0.9 ± 0.3	227 ± 41	200 ± 36

Note: Data are absolute numbers or mean values ±1 SD. A, peak late diastolic transmitral velocity; BP, blood pressure; DcT, deceleration time; E, peak early diastolic transmitral velocity; LVMI, left ventricular mass index; N, number of patients.

18. Hypertension and Diastolic Function

TABLE 18.2. Cardiovascular risk factors for developing diastolic dysfunction.

Risk factor	Reference
Age ≥ 65 years	3, 10, 12
Female gender	5
Hypertension	12
Coronary artery disease	12
Cardiomyopathies	12, 22
Diabetes	12 22, 29
Glucose intolerance	30
Systolic dysfunction	8, 12, 13, 31
Obesity (body mass index >30 kg/m^2)	12
Dyslipidemia*	27, 30
Renal Doppler parameters†	24
Increased N-terminal prohormone brain natriuretic peptide	17, 28, 31–36

*Low high-density lipoprotein cholesterol and high triglycerides.
†The diastolic to systolic ratio (D/S) and resistance index (RI).

LV concentric hypertrophy may occur.[15,22] Potential cardiovascular risk factors are summarized in Table 18.2. Because women have larger pressure increases than males (see Figure 18.1), the term "little old ladies' heart" has been used mainly to express the clinical picture of elderly females with preserved systolic pump function.

Neurohumoral Adaptation and Diastolic Function in Hypertension

Detection of abnormal diastolic function in the early course of hypertension with the use of a simple screening test is often difficult and not readily accomplished. Although pulsed Doppler and color Doppler echocardiography permit accurate assessment of abnormal diastolic function, a simple screening test may be more helpful.

Neurohumoral adaptation in hypertension is characterized by changes in the renin-angiotensin system, enhanced activity of the sympathetic nervous system, and activation of the natriuretic peptides. In contrast to angiotensin, aldosterone and plasma renin activity as well as natriuretic peptides are elevated independently of the degree of LV hypertrophy and are therefore more suitable for assessing the degree of reduced LV diastolic function. Previous studies have shown that the natriuretic peptides are increased in patients

with systolic heart failure parallel to the increase in diastolic filling pressures.[31,32] In hypertensive patients, natriuretic peptides (free brain natriuretic peptide [BNP] and N-terminal prohormone BNP [NT-pro-BNP]) are increased in those with mildly reduced diastolic function.[30–32] The increase in concentrations of NT-pro-BNP occurred even before the evolution of clinically apparent LV dysfunction and suggests that NT-pro-BNP appears to be a useful marker for detection of early impairment of diastolic function. There was also a close correlation to color Doppler echocardiographic findings suggesting that increased concentrations of NT-pro-BNP increased parallel with LV filling pressures.[26] Another study[33] showed that concentrations of NT-pro-BNP levels are increased in patients with increased filling pressures during exercise and are strongly correlated with the pulmonary capillary wedge pressure at rest and during exercise.

Thus, the neurohumoral system is activated in patients with arterial hypertension even in the presence of mild to moderate hypertension. The most useful laboratory parameters for assessing alterations in neurohumoral activation are the natriuretic peptides, that is, free BNP or NT-pro BNP, the latter seeming more sensitive and specific in hypertensive people than free BNP. These changes in neurohumoral adaptation are associated with increased filling pressures and are correlated with the pulmonary capillary wedge pressure at rest and during exercise, even in the absence of LV systolic dysfunction.

References

1. Peters RM, Flack JM., Diagnosis and treatment of hypertension in children and adolescents. J Am Acad Nurse Pract 2003;15(2):56–63.
2. Chobanian AV, et al. The Seventh Report of the Joint National Committee on Prevention, Detection, Evaluation, and Treatment of High Blood Pressure: the JNC 7 report. JAMA 2003;289(19): 2560–2572.
3. Lye M, Wisniacki N. Heart failure in the elderly: a diastolic problem? Eur J Heart Fail 2000;2(2): 133–166.
4. Kannel WB. Historic perspectives on the relative contributions of diastolic and systolic blood pressure elevation to cardiovascular risk profile. Am Heart J 1999;138(3 Pt 2):205–210.

5. Lim JG, et al. Sex differences in left ventricular function in older persons with mild hypertension. Am Heart J 2005;150(5):934–940.

6. Mottram PM, et al. Relation of arterial stiffness to diastolic dysfunction in hypertensive heart disease. Heart 2005;91(12):1551–1556.

7. Tsioufis C, et al. Left ventricular diastolic dysfunction is accompanied by increased aortic stiffness in the early stages of essential hypertension: a TDI approach. J Hypertens 2005;23(9):1745–1750.

8. Clarkson P, Wheeldon NM, Macdonald TM. Left ventricular diastolic dysfunction. Q J Med 1994; 87(3):143–148.

9. Mandinov L, et al. Diastolic heart failure. Cardiovasc Res 2000;45(4):813–825.

10. Kitzman DW. Diastolic heart failure in the elderly. Heart Fail Rev 2002;7(1):17–27.

11. Arques S, et al. B-type natriuretic peptide and tissue Doppler study findings in elderly patients hospitalized for acute diastolic heart failure. Am J Cardiol 2005;96(1):104–107.

12. Redfield MM, et al. Burden of systolic and diastolic ventricular dysfunction in the community: appreciating the scope of the heart failure epidemic. JAMA 2003;289(2):194–202.

13. Paulus WJ, Vantrimpont PJ, Rousseau MF. Diastolic function of the nonfilling human left ventricle. J Am Coll Cardiol 1992;20(7):1524–1532.

14. Erbel R, Neumann T, Zeidan Z, Bartel T, Buck T. Echocardiography diagnosis of diastolic heart failure. Herz 2002;27(2):99–106. Erratum in Herz 2002;27(4):388.

15. Palmieri V, et al. Relations of diastolic left ventricular filling to systolic chamber and myocardial contractility in hypertensive patients with left ventricular hypertrophy (The PRESERVE study). Am J Cardiol 1999;84(5):558–562.

16. Thomas MD, et al. Echocardiographic features and brain natriuretic peptides in patients presenting with heart failure and preserved systolic function. Heart 2006;92:603–608.

17. Nakae I, et al. Left ventricular systolic/diastolic function evaluated by quantitative ECG-gated SPECT: comparison with echocardiography and plasma BNP analysis. Ann Nucl Med 2005;19(6): 447–454.

18. Kitzman DW, et al. Pathophysiological characterization of isolated diastolic heart failure in comparison to systolic heart failure. JAMA 2002; 288(17):2144–2150.

19. Lukowicz TV, et al. BNP as a marker of diastolic dysfunction in the general population: Importance of left ventricular hypertrophy. Eur J Heart Fail 2005;7(4):525–531.

20. Philbin EF, et al. Systolic versus diastolic heart failure in community practice: clinical features, outcomes, and the use of angiotensin-converting enzyme inhibitors. Am J Med 2000;109(8): 605–613.

21. Brilla CG, Funck RC, Rupp H. Lisinopril-mediated regression of myocardial fibrosis in patients with hypertensive heart disease. Circulation 2000; 102(12):1388–1393.

22. Weber KT, et al. Collagen in the hypertrophied, pressure-overloaded myocardium. Circulation 1987;75(1 Pt 2):I40–I47.

23. Wachtell K, et al. Change in systolic left ventricular performance after 3 years of antihypertensive treatment: the Losartan Intervention for Endpoint (LIFE) study. Circulation 2002;106(2): 227–232.

24. Ogata C, et al. Association between left ventricular diastolic dysfunction and renal hemodynamic change in patients with treated essential hypertension. Hypertens Res 2003;26(12):971–978.

25. Bergstrom A, et al. Effect of carvedilol on diastolic function in patients with diastolic heart failure and preserved systolic function. Results of the Swedish Doppler-echocardiographic study (SWEDIC). Eur J Heart Fail 2004;6(4):453–461.

26. Tanaka H, et al. Losartan improves regional left ventricular systolic and diastolic function in patients with hypertension: accurate evaluation using a newly developed color-coded tissue Doppler imaging technique. J Card Fail 2004;10(5):412–420.

27. Horio T, et al. Pioglitazone improves left ventricular diastolic function in patients with essential hypertension. Am J Hypertens 2005;18(7);949–957.

28. Furumoto T, et al. Increased plasma concentrations of N-terminal pro-brain natriuretic peptide reflect the presence of mildly reduced left ventricular diastolic function in hypertension. Coron Artery Dis 2006;17(1):45–50.

29. Pop-Busui R, et al. Sympathetic dysfunction in type 1 diabetes: association with impaired myocardial blood flow reserve and diastolic dysfunction. J Am Coll Cardiol 2004;44(12):2368–2374.

30. Miyazato J, et al. Fasting plasma glucose is an independent determinant of left ventricular diastolic dysfunction in nondiabetic patients with treated essential hypertension. Hypertens Res 2002;25(3): 403–409.

31. Redfield MM, et al. Plasma brain natriuretic peptide to detect preclinical ventricular systolic or diastolic dysfunction: a community-based study. Circulation 2004;109(25):3176–3181.

18. Hypertension and Diastolic Function

32. Atisha D, et al. A prospective study in search of an optimal B-natriuretic peptide level to screen patients for cardiac dysfunction. Am Heart J 2004;148(3):518–523.
33. Tschöpe C, et al. Elevated NT-proBNP levels in patients with increased left ventricular filling pressure during exercise despite preserved systolic function. J Card Fail 2005;11(5 Suppl):28–33.
34. Celinski R, et al. Relationship between plasma BNP levels and left ventricular diastolic function as measured by radionuclide ventriculography in patients with coronary artery disease. Nucl Med Rev Cent East Eur 2004;7(2):123–128.
35. Dahlstrom U. Can natriuretic peptides be used for the diagnosis of diastolic heart failure? Eur J Heart Fail 2004;6(3):281–287.
36. Wei T, et al. Systolic and diastolic heart failure are associated with different plasma levels of B-type natriuretic peptide. Int J Clin Pract 2005;59(8): 891–894.

19
Diastolic Disturbances in Diabetes Mellitus

Thomas H. Marwick

Introduction

Disturbed glucose metabolism and its sequelae are becoming the most common contributors to the development of cardiovascular disease. Indeed, the relative importance of "diabesity" as a risk factor is greater than ever, reflecting the epidemic of obesity on the one hand and better control of many risk factors, such as smoking and hypercholesterolemia, on the other. However, these adverse cardiovascular effects relate predominantly to the development of atherosclerosis,[1] but in parallel with this (and no less malignant) are the effects of diabetes and abnormal glucose metabolism on myocardial function. The most common initial manifestation of this is diastolic dysfunction.

Manifestations of Myocardial Dysfunction in Diabetes

Diastolic Dysfunction

Diastolic dysfunction is most frequently identified in diabetic patients with normal systolic function as an "incidental" finding at echocardiography. Although some of these patients complain of dyspnea, the impairment in exercise capacity in diabetes,[2] while common, is often ascribed to obesity or deconditioning and not recognized as a symptom.

As in other forms of diastolic dysfunction, delayed or impaired relaxation is the earliest and most common change. Increases in left atrial pressure due to the progressive difficulty in filling the left ventricle may produce pseudonormal filling, but the development of a restrictive filling profile in the absence of systolic dysfunction and other pathology (e.g., myocardial infarction or hypertensive heart disease) is uncommon. The causes for these findings are discussed later, but they likely reflect myocyte abnormalities (the relaxation process being energy intense) as well as structural abnormalities within the interstitium that compromise both systolic and diastolic events. This entity appears to be more associated with type 2 than with type 1 diabetes,[3] perhaps reflecting a contribution from insulin resistance, and the changes are potentiated by the presence of hypertension.[4]

The frequency of such changes alters with the population studied and with how the study is performed (Table 19.1).[5–8] Even among young, well-controlled diabetic subjects with normal blood pressure, impaired relaxation has been reported in 26% of subjects.[6] The detection of abnormal diastolic function is increased to 75% of apparently healthy and asymptomatic diabetic patients with a normal blood pressure and a normal stress echocardiogram by the use of specific techniques and maneuvers to identify pseudonormal flow increases.[5]

The presence of changes in diastolic function due to diabetes is also supported by experiments involving both animal models and human tissue.[9] For example, prolongation of relaxation and reduction of relaxation rate have been reported in

TABLE 19.1. Prevalence of abnormal diastolic characteristics in apparently healthy diabetic subjects.

Reference	Study group	Methodology for identification of pseudonormal filling	Prevalence
5	61 patients with type 2 diabetes and normal systolic function	Transmitral flow, Valsalva maneuver, flow propagation, tissue Doppler echocardiography	75%
6	86 patients with type 2 diabetes, normal systolic function, and negative exercise echocardiogram	Transmitral flow, Valsalva maneuver	47%
7	46 patients with type 2 diabetes, no complications or comorbidity, and negative exercise electrocardiogram	Transmitral flow, Valsalva maneuver, pulmonary venous flow	60%
8	157 asymptomatic patients with type I diabetes	E slope, left atrial emptying, isovolumic relaxation time	27%

muscle preparations.[10] Interestingly, some studies have shown abnormalities to become apparent only after hemodynamic stress,[11,12] and in other animal models only lusitropic function appears to be altered.[13]

Systolic Dysfunction

The most common causes of overt systolic dysfunction in a diabetic subject are coronary artery disease and hypertensive heart disease. Nonetheless, systolic dysfunction in diabetic subjects without coexistent heart disease may be due to a cardiomyopathy caused by the diabetes alone,[14] and this may be symptomatic or asymptomatic. However, although changes in systolic volumes and reduction of ejection fraction (EF) have been reported in diabetic children,[15] overt systolic dysfunction at rest is less common among diabetic subjects than is diastolic dysfunction, although the prevalence of systolic dysfunction is greater in response to exercise.[16]

The presence of a normal EF merely identifies preservation of the volume work of the ventricle and not the time course of ejection. Studies of unselected patients with various etiologies of myocardial dysfunction have shown that diastolic dysfunction is not a purely diastolic entity.[17] This finding is equally true for diabetic subjects, among whom sensitive markers of systolic function have been shown to be impaired in patients both with and without diastolic dysfunction. Indeed, experimental evidence in isolated papillary muscle preparations and animal models also supports the apparent lower prevalence of overt systolic

dysfunction being an artifact of measurement technique.[9]

As disturbances may be identified in both systolic and diastolic functions, a simple and sensitive means of identifying the problem is with the myocardial performance index, which combines isovolumic times in systole and diastole and ejection time. Disturbances of this parameter are similar in patients with hypertension and diabetes, unrelated to age, left ventricular (LV) mass, and EF.[18]

Myocardial Dysfunction

The underlying disease process appears to be a primary disease of the myocardium. Because both overt systolic function (EF) and diastolic dysfunction (abnormal transmitral flow) may be influenced by loading conditions, it seems reasonable to assess the myocardium directly.

Table 19.2 summarizes studies[19–24] that have demonstrated abnormalities in myocardial parameters such as measurement of tissue velocity, strain rate, and strain (Figure 19.1). After exclusion of patients with LV hypertrophy or ischemia, abnormal myocardial characteristics are present in about one fourth of the remaining subjects (Figure 19.2).[25]

These disturbances in longitudinal function appear to be compensated by augmentation of radial function.[22,26] Although the cause of this phenomenon (which seems to be characteristic of early myocardial disease) is unclear, it has been suggested that it reflects reduced subendocardial function. In fact, a number of mechanisms may be responsible (Figure 19.3).

19. Diabetes Mellitus

TABLE 19.2. Abnormalities in myocardial parameters (tissue velocity, strain rate, and strain) in diabetes mellitus.

Reference	N	Criteria	Comments
20	8 type 1 diabetes mellitus (DM) patients and 8 controls	Lower myocardial diastolic velocity in DM patients than in controls (13.8 ± 0.6 vs. 15.6 ± 0.5 cm/s, $p < 0.04$)	Abnormal velocity corresponded with reduced myocardial blood volume (6.6 ± 0.6 vs. 8.2 ± 0.6 units of contrast intensity, $p < 0.04$), but not flow. Short-term therapy with C-peptide improved both resting function and hyperemic response
19	93 DM patients and 93 controls	Patients with DM had lower peak systolic strain and strain rate than controls. Those with DM + left ventricular hypertrophy (LVH) had lower values than patients with DM alone ($p < 0.03$) or LVH alone ($p = 0.01$). Myocardial reflectivity (measured as calibrated integrated backscatter) was greater in all subjects (DM, LVH, both) than in controls ($p < 0.05$)	Exclusion of coronary artery disease with negative ExE is an important step as ischemia/infarction can produce similar changes. The evaluation of subgroups with and without LVH reassures us that this is not simply hypertensive heart disease
21	32 type 2 DM patients and 32 controls	Patients with DM had lower longitudinal myocardial displacement (tracking score 5.8 ± 1.6 vs. 7.7 ± 1.1 mm; $p < 0.001$) and lower peak systolic velocity (4.3 ± 1.5 vs. 5.4 ± 1.0 cm/s; $p < 0.001$) and peak systolic strain rate (−1.2 ± 0.3 vs. −1.6 ± 0.4 s^{-1}; $p < 0.001$)	Carefully selected to minimize comorbidity: normotensive, normal ejection fraction, and no angina, valvular heart disease, or small vessel disease
22	35 type 2 DM patients and 35 controls	Patients with DM had lower longitudinal (basal segment) peak systolic velocities than controls (5.6 ± 1.4 vs. 6.5 ± 1.1 cm/s, $p < 0.01$)	Radial velocity was greater in patients with DM than in controls (5.4 ± 1.3 vs. 4.7 ± 1.4 cm/s; $p < 0.05$), suggesting that radial function compensates for impaired longitudinal function (and hence ejection fraction is preserved)
23	79	27% of patients with DM had Em < 8.5 cm/s or Em/Am < 1	Myocardial Doppler findings were more specific than classic Doppler criteria (abnormal in 41%). Abnormal myocardial velocity associated with exercise intolerance
24	44 DM patients and 33 controls	Reduction of resting myocardial early diastolic velocity (8.5 ± 1.7 vs. 9.6 ± 1.9 cm/s, $p < 0.02$) and systolic velocity (10.7 ± 2.7 vs. 13.6 ± 3.4 cm/s, $p < 0.05$) in DM compared with controls. Impaired increase in myocardial systolic velocity ($p < 0.05$), myocardial early diastolic velocity ($p < 0.0003$), myocardial late diastolic velocity ($p < 0.03$)	Reduction of myocardial stress response

Source: Marwick and Wong.[97]

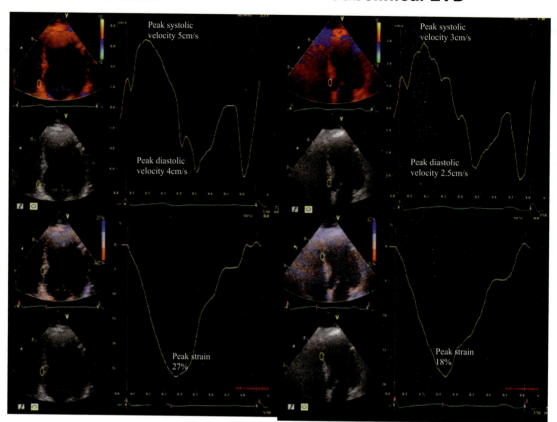

FIGURE 19.1. Typical velocity (top traces) and deformation patterns (bottom traces) in diabetic subjects without and with subclinical left ventricular dysfunction.

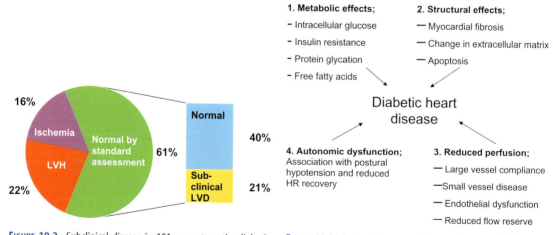

FIGURE 19.2. Subclinical disease in 101 asymptomatic, diabetic subjects with normal ejection fraction. (From Fang et al.[25])

FIGURE 19.3. Potential causes of abnormal myocardial characteristics in diabetes mellitus.

Pathogenesis of Diabetic Heart Disease

Metabolic Disturbances

Abnormalities of glucose supply and utilization and abnormal free fatty acid metabolism may influence contractile function as a consequence of altered nutrient supply. Oxidative stress and toxic molecules including free radicals may alter regulatory and contractile proteins.

Glucose Disturbances

A reduction in glucose supply and utilization may reduce contractile function by reducing the availability of adenosine triphosphate. This phenomenon has been shown in isolated diabetic cardiomyocytes, animal models, and diabetic subjects.[9] The mechanisms of this phenomenon include limitation of glucose transport across the cell membrane by depletion of glucose transporters[27] and inhibition of glucose oxidation by high circulating free fatty acids.[28] This is an important group of mechanisms, as they may be altered by improving glycemic control.

Free Fatty Acid Metabolism

Metabolic disturbances in diabetes lead to enhanced lipolysis, increasing circulating free fatty acids, especially in type 2 diabetes, and their involvement may explain the preponderance of type 2 diabetes in subjects with myocardial dysfunction. This increased supply of fatty acid to myocytes is compounded by hydrolysis of myocardial triglyceride stores, which increases levels of myocardial free fatty acids. The adverse consequences of fatty acids on myocardial structure and performance are due to accumulation of toxic intermediates as well as to inhibition of glucose oxidation.[29] The ability of fatty acids to act as a myocardial energy substrate may be limited by carnitine insufficiency.[30]

Protein Glycation

Although protein glycation occurs with increasing age, this process is accelerated in diabetes, especially with poor glycemic control. The resultant advanced glycation endproducts in turn bind to an advanced glycation endproduct receptor with consequent inflammation and release in cytokines and growth factors. The resultant changes in the extracellular matrix and angiogenesis are responsible for the pathology identified in nephropathy and diastolic dysfunction.[31]

Other Metabolic Changes

In addition to changes in the metabolic milieu, diabetic animals have been shown to have alterations in the coupling of myocardial energetics and mechanical function. For example, in a rat model, slowing of the ventricular relaxation rate has been linked with reduced mitochondrial sarcoplasmic reticulum calcium adenosine triphosphatase (SERCA2).[13] With humans, Diamant et al.[32] have shown diastolic dysfunction in otherwise apparently healthy diabetic subjects to be associated with abnormal high energy phosphate metabolism, as measured by phosphorous spectra with magnetic resonance imaging.

Role of Metabolic Changes

Although the adverse impact of metabolic disturbances would seem to be a plausible explanation for altered myocyte function, the relation between these disturbances and development of structural and echocardiographic changes is time dependent. Unfortunately, although some work has shown an association between LV functional abnormalities and diabetes (especially in the context of diabetic complications),[33] it is difficult to distinguish this from the impact of age, which itself produces alterations in LV function.

For example, alterations in myocardial function but not histologic changes correspond to glucose level in isolated muscle preparations.[34] Disturbances in LV filling[35] and myocardial backscatter[3] are associated with poor glycemic control in humans. Table 19.3 summarizes studies examining the link between glycemic control and LV dysfunction in humans.[36–43] Although the results are far from uniform, the studies showing no association are more commonly small and cross-sectional and use less sensitive techniques for detection of LV dysfunction. Inconsistent responses to therapy probably also reflect the effect of the duration of metabolic disturbance. In rat and canine experimental models, insulin

TABLE 19.3. Relationship between left ventricular dysfunction and glycemic control.

Reference	N	Criteria	Design	Comments
36	20	E/A ratio	Longitudinal	No relationship to glycemic control despite glycosylated hemoglobin reduction from 10% to 7% over 6 months
37	8 type 1 diabetes mellitus (DM) patients and 11 controls	Peak filling rate (RNV)	Cross-sectional	No relationship to glycemic control
38	246 type 2 DM patients	Isovolumic relaxation time increased, E/A reduced	Longitudinal	Diastolic dysfunction worse in those with retinopathy. E/A increased toward normal after insulin therapy only in patients without retinopathy
39	18 type 2 DM patients	Systolic and diastolic parameters	Longitudinal	Improvement with correction of hyperglycemia
40	33 type 2 DM patients	Pre-ejection period (PEP) decreased ($p < 0.05$), left ventricular ejection time (LVET) increased ($p < 0.0025$), and the PEP/LVET ratio decreased ($p < 0.005$)	Longitudinal	3–8 months dietary therapy; changes in those with fasting glucose reduction of 3 mmol/L
41	20 type 1 DM patients, 14 type 2 DM patients, and 12 controls	Peak filling rate lower and time to peak filling increased in type 2 DM vs. type 1 DM and controls ($p < 0.05$)	Cross-sectional	Type 2 patients had worse diastolic dysfunction despite shorter duration and lower glycosylated hemoglobin
42	10 type 2 DM patients and 10 controls	Shorter E duration ($p < 0.01$), higher A ($p < 0.001$) and lower E/A ($p < 0.001$)	Longitudinal	6–12 months better control did not induce changes in abnormal diastolic parameters
43	40 type 1 DM patients and DM 40 controls	DM had higher peak A velocity ($p = 0.002$), lower E/A ratio ($p < 0.001$), and longer isovolumic relaxation time ($p < 0.001$)	Cross-sectional	No relation between diastolic changes and glycemic control

administration has been shown to improve hemodynamic,[44] metabolic,[45] and structural alterations,[46] although delayed treatment did not reverse the interstitial changes in the diabetic heart. It is important to recognize that studies of the efficacy of improved glycemic control have shown improvement in diastolic[47] and systolic[48] functions as well as in myocardial characteristics[49] in humans. The contribution of specific treatments other than glycemic control are discussed in the section on therapeutics.

Myocardial Structural Changes

Structural changes may occur in myocytes (reduction of mitochondria and contractile elements, apoptosis, and, to a lesser degree, fibrosis), vasculature (reduced capillary density), and interstitium (extracellular fibrosis and increased interstitial matrix). All of these structural changes may influence force generation and relaxation and nutrient perfusion. However, although these structural changes have been shown to occur independent of LV hypertrophy and coronary artery disease, they are nevertheless nonspecific and may be due to other causes, including hypertensive heart disease. The association between levels of myocardial backscatter and fibrosis[50] has enabled the use of echocardiography to identify the problem and its response to therapy.

The involvement of fibrosis has been established in experimental models[9] as well as in right ventricular biopsy specimens from humans; these studies have shown fibrotic changes to be perivascular and/or interstitial. Fibrosis may be provoked by protein glycosylation or cell necrosis, although angiotensin production may be an important mediator.[51] Diabetes is associated with increased local production of angiotensin and upregulation of receptor density, which appears to be a sequela of metabolic derangement.[52] This association with the angiotensin/aldosterone pathway may be an important clue to management.

Diabetic Vascular Disease

Apart from the obvious contribution to atherosclerosis, diabetes is associated with abnormalities of small vessel structure and function that are potentiated by the presence of hypertension.[53] The structural changes include thickening of the basement membrane, arterial thickening, perivascular fibrosis, and reduction of capillary density that are analogous to those in the kidney.[54] The importance of vascular changes to subclinical myocardial dysfunction is unresolved. Some studies have shown an association between the two and a common response to therapy.[20,49] However, changes in myocardial blood flow may not be associated with altered myocardial oxygen consumption; diabetic patients do not exhibit lactate production during atrial pacing,[55] and we have found no correlation between vascular and structural changes. The presence of a normal myocardial velocity increment with dobutamine stress (albeit from a lower baseline myocardial velocity)[56] is inconsistent with an ischemic etiology for myocardial dysfunction in diabetes.

Abnormalities of coronary vascular function are well recognized in diabetic subjects,[57] and reduction of coronary flow reserve may potentiate the effects of borderline stenoses. However, the relevance of these findings to diastolic dysfunction and myocardial disease, rather than coronary artery disease, is unclear.

Cardiac Autonomic Neuropathy

Cardiac sympathetic denervation is an important consequence of the autonomic neuropathy associated with diabetes. Simple clinical evidence of this problem includes the lack of heart rate response to postural change, deep breathing, and the Valsalva maneuver as well as more sophisticated measurements, including disturbances of heart rate variability and recovery after exercise. Interestingly, of the various tests of autonomic dysfunction, the best correlate of abnormal filling is orthostatic hypotension.[58]

Apart from influencing vasodilator reserve,[59] autonomic neuropathy is associated with systolic dysfunction during exercise stress[60] as well as diastolic dysfunction.[61] The mechanism of this association in unclear but could be associated with regional variation of sympathetic denervation, with particular apical involvement shown on cardiac single photon emission (SPECT) or positron emission tomography (PET) imaging of ^{123}I-labeled metaiodobenzylguanidine or ^{11}C-labeled hydroxyephedrine,[62–64] as apical untwisting is associated with rapid LV filling.

Clinical Presentation of Diabetic Heart Disease

Subclinical Left Ventricular Dysfunction

Although the most frequent manifestations of diabetic heart disease occur in asymptomatic patients, many of these patients actually have some limitation of exercise capacity.[2,65] The cause of this is likely multifactorial, with contributions from obesity, deconditioning, and diabetic lung disease,[66] among other factors, but some evidence suggests an association between impaired exercise capacity and diastolic dysfunction[67] or preclinical myocardial changes.[68]

The optimum process for identifying patients with diabetic heart disease is unclear. As in other forms of heart failure,[69] it seems likely that early intervention offers the best chance for preventing the progression of this condition. However, as the prevalence of subclinical myocardial changes seems to be 20%–30%,[25] it is unclear how best to screen patients for this problem. The assessment of diastolic dysfunction and tissue characterization are too complicated to be attractive for widespread screening. The reduction in exercise capacity could be a marker of patients who would benefit from sophisticated imaging techniques to identify this condition. Unfortunately, the measurement of brain natriuretic peptide does not seem to be a solution to screening. This marker of overt LV dysfunction[70] is released in response to increased transmural wall stress and appears to have limited efficacy for the detection of subclinical heart disease.[71] Specifically, brain natriuretic peptide does not appear to be a worthwhile marker of diabetic myocardial disease.[25,72]

Overt Heart Failure

The current epidemics of both type 2 diabetes and congestive heart failure mean that the association between the diseases is common. Diabetic subjects represent a disproportionate component of those with diastolic heart failure,[73] and in fact diabetes is more frequent in all heart failure patients,[74] with a 2.4-fold incidence in diabetic men and a 5.1-fold incidence in diabetic women.[75] Conversely, population-based studies in elderly subjects have shown the presence of diabetes to confer a 30% increase in the risk of heart failure.[76] The prognosis of diabetic subjects with heart failure is particularly poor, especially in the setting of coronary artery disease,[77] even after correcting for their worse risk factor profile.[78]

When cardiac damage occurs from one of these known causes, the diabetic heart appears to have a greater propensity to develop heart failure.[79,80] In part, this may be because of the prevalence of other causes of heart failure in diabetes mellitus. For example, hypertension is more common and myocardial infarcts are larger in diabetic subjects. However, another explanation is that this finding is due to subclinical myocardial damage that compromises the ability of the myocardium to deal with an acute insult.

Therapeutic Implications in the Diabetic Heart

There is limited specific evidence about how best to manage myocardial disease in diabetes. For patients who present with reduced exercise capacity, the goal of symptom control is readily understood, but for the majority who do not complain of specific symptoms, the goal of treatment is to prevent the development of overt cardiac failure, for example, after a cardiac event. The efficacy of this strategy remains unproven.

General Measures

The general measures recommended in the guidelines are applicable for diabetic subjects,[81] in particular, the pursuit of optimum blood pressure control and lifestyle interventions. Studies of both conventional transmitral flow parameters and myocardial parameters[19] show that the effect of diabetes is analogous to the effect of hypertension on the myocardium, while the presence of both has a cumulative effect. The benefit of treatment of blood pressure targets in diabetic subjects is widely recognized,[82] and strong arguments have been mounted for treating to below the normal targets.[83] However, preliminary data from a substudy of the CALM II study have shown that enhanced blood pressure control has no benefit on the disturbances of longitudinal ventricular function reported in diabetic subjects.[84]

In diabetic subjects with heart failure, β-blockers, angiotensin-converting enzyme inhibitors or angiotensin receptor blockers are underutilized.[85] This is despite the fact that the latter two have favorable effects in diabetes and some reports, for example, the CHARM-Preserved trial,[86] suggest that they are effective in patients with heart failure and preserved systolic function. Perhaps more importantly, in patients without heart failure in the RENAAL and LIFE trials, losartan reduced new heart failure admissions.[87]

Specific Treatments

Specific treatments for subclinical myocardial disease are directed toward the underlying mechanisms discussed earlier: metabolic interventions to improve glycemic control and insulin resistance, management of fibrosis, and use of cross-link breakers to reduce the impact of protein glycosylation.

Glycemic Control

In the above discussion of the potential metabolic causes of myocardial dysfunction, the severity of disturbances of substrate supply and utilization, free fatty acid metabolism, and oxidative stress all reflect the severity of hyperglycemia. There are limited data to indicate that more aggressive glycemic control has favorable effects on myocardial function. These data include observational data[68,84] and clinical trial data showing that treatment with C-peptide improves both perfusion and function.[20] It is unclear whether glycemic control alone is the effective intervention or whether insulin is a specific requirement for this better control.[49]

As discussed earlier, insulin resistance is another potential contributor to the metabolic effects of diabetes on the heart. Thiazolidinediones reduce insulin resistance, and, despite their association with edema, it does not appear that they increase the likelihood of heart failure (in fact, they seem to reduce it).[88] Although these agents also improve vascular function, their myocardial effects are undefined. The performance of exercise training and lifestyle modification may offer other strategies for improving insulin resistance.

Treatment of Fibrosis

Aldosterone levels are increased in type 2 diabetes and may induce pathologic changes, particularly fibrosis. In registry data, therapy with angiotensin-converting enzyme inhibitors appears to be protective against the development of primary myocardial disturbances.[35] It is unclear whether this effect is indeed anti-fibrotic — angiotensin-converting enzyme inhibitors have also been shown to have important cellular effects as potentiators of insulin action, as well as improving coronary perfusion. Nonetheless, results in non-diabetic populations have shown effects on myocardial structure and function that are incremental to just blood pressure reduction.[89] Although arguments are often made to use angiotensin-converting enzyme inhibitors more widely for diabetic subjects, it is unclear whether this will completely overcome the effects of aldosterone, and direct inhibition of aldosterone might be expected to have an incremental benefit. Indeed, aldosterone inhibition has been shown to have beneficial effects on myocardial function in hypertensive heart disease,[90] although this has not been studied in early diabetic myocardial disease.

Cross-Link Breakers

As described earlier, altered proteins may contribute to increased vascular permeability among other processes — including inflammatory responses via the advanced glycation endproduct receptor — and have been correlated with the severity of diastolic dysfunction. Cross-link breakers may disrupt cross-links between glycosylated proteins.

Experimental studies have shown that the use of the cross-link breaker alagebrium chloride reduced LV hypertrophy and the deposition of type III collagen.[91] Similar studies have shown the cross-link breakers to reduce LV stiffness in aging nondiabetic dogs[92] and reversal of systolic dysfunction, increased aortic stiffness, and increases of myocardial collagen in diabetic animals.[93]

A small study of 23 patients (average age 71 years) with stable diastolic heart failure showed LV mass to decrease with therapy, with an increase in tissue E velocity and a reduction in filling pressure (E/E′). However, despite an improvement in symptom score, there was no change in EF, blood pressure, peak VO_2′ or aortic distensibility. Worryingly, two patients in the treatment arm had events — a myocardial infarction after 12 days therapy and sudden death after 10 weeks. This treatment is, however, worthy of further attention; it appears efficacious, but this may be at the cost of some serious side effects.[94]

Conclusion

Primary myocardial disease in diabetic subjects forms part of a continuum of metabolic disturbances involving the myocardium that include both impaired glucose tolerance and obesity.[95,96] These conditions particularly manifest as diastolic dysfunction, but, as in many other conditions, this abnormality not isolated. Although these patients are commonly "asymptomatic," like many diabetic subjects they may show reduced exercise capacity, which may in part be due to their abnormal LV filling. The main significance of this condition may be its contribution to the development of heart failure in diabetic subjects. Although the general principles for the management of diastolic dysfunction are pertinent, understanding the etiology of the condition will help in the identification of specific therapies for the management of the metabolic milieu, fibrosis, autonomic neuropathy, and possibly myocardial perfusion.

References

1. Fisher M. Diabetes and atherogenesis. Heart 2004; 90:336–340.
2. Regensteiner JG, Sippel J, McFarling ET, Wolfel EE, Hiatt WR. Effects of non-insulin-dependent diabetes on oxygen consumption during treadmill exercise. Med Sci Sports Exerc 1995;27:875–881.
3. Astorri E, Fiorina P, Contini GA, Albertini D, Magnati G, Astorri A, et al. Isolated and preclinical impairment of left ventricular filling in insulin-dependent and non-insulin-dependent diabetic patients. Clin Cardiol 1997;20:536–540.
4. Nicolino A, Longobardi G, Furgi G, Rossi M, Zoccolillo N, Ferrara N, et al. Left ventricular diastolic filling in diabetes mellitus with and without hypertension. Am J Hypertens 1995;8:382–389.
5. Boyer JK, Thanigaraj S, Schechtman KB, Perez JE. Prevalence of ventricular diastolic dysfunction in asymptomatic, normotensive patients with diabetes mellitus. Am J Cardiol 2004;93:870–875.
6. Zabalgoitia M, Ismaeil MF, Anderson L, Maklady FA. Prevalence of diastolic dysfunction in normotensive, asymptomatic patients with well-controlled type 2 diabetes mellitus. Am J Cardiol 2001;87:320–323.
7. Poirier P, Bogaty P, Garneau C, Marois L, Dumesnil JG. Diastolic dysfunction in normotensive men with well-controlled type 2 diabetes: importance of maneuvers in echocardiographic screening for preclinical diabetic cardiomyopathy. Diabetes Care 2001;24:5–10.
8. Raev DC. Which left ventricular function is impaired earlier in the evolution of diabetic cardiomyopathy? An echocardiographic study of young type I diabetic patients. Diabetes Care 1994;17:633–639.
9. Fang ZY, Prins JB, Marwick TH. Diabetic cardiomyopathy: evidence, mechanisms, and therapeutic implications. Endocr Rev 2004;25:543–567.
10. Trost SU, Belke DD, Bluhm WF, Meyer M, Swanson E, Dillmann WH. Overexpression of the sarcoplasmic reticulum Ca(2+)-ATPase improves myocardial contractility in diabetic cardiomyopathy. Diabetes 2002;51:1166–1171.
11. Flarsheim CE, Grupp IL, Matlib MA. Mitochondrial dysfunction accompanies diastolic dysfunction in diabetic rat heart. Am J Physiol 1996;271:H192–H202.
12. Gotzsche O, Darwish A, Hansen LP, Gotzsche L. Abnormal left ventricular diastolic function during cold pressor test in uncomplicated insulin-dependent diabetes mellitus. Clin Sci (Lond) 1995; 89:461–465.
13. Abe T, Ohga Y, Tabayashi N, Kobayashi S, Sakata S, Misawa H, et al. Left ventricular diastolic dysfunction in type 2 diabetes mellitus model rats. Am J Physiol Heart Circ Physiol 2002;282:H138–H148.
14. Rubler S, Dlugash J, Yuceoglu YZ, Kumral T, Branwood AW, Grishman A. New type of cardiomyopathy associated with diabetic glomerulosclerosis. Am J Cardiol 1972;30:595–602.
15. Friedman NE, Levitsky LL, Edidin DV, Vitullo DA, Lacina SJ, Chiemmongkoltip P. Echocardiographic evidence for impaired myocardial performance in children with type I diabetes mellitus. Am J Med 1982;73:846–850.
16. Vered A, Battler A, Segal P, Liberman D, Yerushalmi Y, Berezin M, et al. Exercise-induced left ventricular dysfunction in young men with asymptomatic diabetes mellitus (diabetic cardiomyopathy). Am J Cardiol 1984;54:633–637.
17. Yu CM, Lin H, Yang H, Kong SL, Zhang Q, Lee SW. Progression of systolic abnormalities in patients with "isolated" diastolic heart failure and diastolic dysfunction. Circulation 2002;105:1195–201.
18. Andersen NH, Poulsen SH, Helleberg K, Ivarsen P, Knudsen ST, Mogensen CE. Impact of essential hypertension and diabetes mellitus on left ventricular systolic and diastolic performance. Eur J Echocardiogr 2003;4:306–312.
19. Fang ZY, Yuda S, Anderson V, Short L, Case C, Marwick TH. Echocardiographic detection of early diabetic myocardial disease. J Am Coll Cardiol 2003;41:611–617.
20. Hansen A, Johansson BL, Wahren J, von Bibra H. C-peptide exerts beneficial effects on myocardial blood flow and function in patients with type 1 diabetes. Diabetes 2002;51:3077–3082.
21. Andersen NH, Poulsen SH, Eiskjaer H, Poulsen PL, Mogensen CE. Decreased left ventricular longitudinal contraction in normotensive and normoalbuminuric patients with Type II diabetes mellitus: a Doppler tissue tracking and strain rate echocardiography study. Clin Sci (Lond) 2003;105:59–66.
22. Vinereanu D, Nicolaides E, Tweddel AC, Madler CF, Holst B, Boden LE, et al. Subclinical left ventricular dysfunction in asymptomatic patients with Type II diabetes mellitus, related to serum lipids and glycated haemoglobin. Clin Sci (Lond) 2003; 105:591–599.
23. Saraiva RM, Duarte DM, Duarte MP, Martins AF, Poltronieri AV, Ferreira ME, et al. Tissue Doppler imaging identifies asymptomatic normotensive diabetics with diastolic dysfunction and reduced exercise tolerance. Echocardiography 2005;22:561–570.

24. von Bibra H, Thrainsdottir IS, Hansen A, Dounis V, Malmberg K, Ryden L. Tissue Doppler imaging for the detection and quantitation of myocardial dysfunction in patients with type 2 diabetes mellitus. Diabetes Vasc Dis Res 2005;2:24–30.
25. Fang ZY, Schull-Meade R, Leano R, Mottram PM, Prins JB, Marwick TH. Screening for heart disease in diabetic subjects. Am Heart J 2005;149:349–354.
26. Fang ZY, Leano R, Marwick TH. Relationship between longitudinal and radial contractility in subclinical diabetic heart disease. Clin Sci (Lond) 2004;106:53–60.
27. Garvey WT, Hardin D, Juhaszova M, Dominguez JH. Effects of diabetes on myocardial glucose transport system in rats: implications for diabetic cardiomyopathy. Am J Physiol 1993;264:H837–H844.
28. Rodrigues B, Cam MC, Kong J, Goyal RK, McNeill JH. Strain differences in susceptibility to streptozotocin-induced diabetes: effects on hypertriglyceridemia and cardiomyopathy. Cardiovasc Res 1997;34:199–205.
29. Rodrigues B, Cam MC, McNeill JH. Metabolic disturbances in diabetic cardiomyopathy. Mol Cell Biochem 1998;180:53–57.
30. Malone JI, Schocken DD, Morrison AD, Gilbert-Barness E. Diabetic cardiomyopathy and carnitine deficiency. J Diabetes Complications 1999;13:86–90.
31. Berg TJ, Snorgaard O, Faber J, Torjesen PA, Hildebrandt P, Mehlsen J, et al. Serum levels of advanced glycation end products are associated with left ventricular diastolic function in patients with type 1 diabetes. Diabetes Care 1999;22:1186–1190.
32. Diamant M, Lamb HJ, Groeneveld Y, Endert EL, Smit JW, Bax JJ, et al. Diastolic dysfunction is associated with altered myocardial metabolism in asymptomatic normotensive patients with well-controlled type 2 diabetes mellitus. J Am Coll Cardiol 2003;42:328–335.
33. Annonu AK, Fattah AA, Mokhtar MS, Ghareeb S, Elhendy A. Left ventricular systolic and diastolic functional abnormalities in asymptomatic patients with non-insulin-dependent diabetes mellitus. J Am Soc Echocardiogr 2001;14:885–891.
34. Kita Y, Shimizu M, Sugihara N, Shimizu K, Yoshio H, Shibayama S, et al. Correlation between histopathological changes and mechanical dysfunction in diabetic rat hearts. Diabetes Res Clin Pract 1991;11:177–188.
35. Fang ZY, Schull-Meade R, Downey M, Prins J, Marwick TH. Determinants of subclinical diabetic heart disease. Diabetologia 2005;48:394–402.
36. Gough SC, Smyllie J, Barker M, Berkin KE, Rice PJ, Grant PJ. Diastolic dysfunction is not related to changes in glycaemic control over 6 months in type 2 (non-insulin-dependent) diabetes mellitus. A cross-sectional study. Acta Diabetol 1995;32:110–115.
37. Ruddy TD, Shumak SL, Liu PP, Barnie A, Seawright SJ, McLaughlin PR, et al. The relationship of cardiac diastolic dysfunction to concurrent hormonal and metabolic status in type I diabetes mellitus. J Clin Endocrinol Metab 1988;66:113–118.
38. Hiramatsu K, Ohara N, Shigematsu S, Aizawa T, Ishihara F, Niwa A, et al. Left ventricular filling abnormalities in non-insulin-dependent diabetes mellitus and improvement by a short-term glycemic control. Am J Cardiol 1992;70:1185–1189.
39. Hirai J, Ueda K, Takegoshi T, Mabuchi H. Effects of metabolic control on ventricular function in type 2 diabetic patients. Intern Med 1992;31:725–730.
40. Uusitupa M, Siitonen O, Aro A, Korhonen T, Pyorala K. Effect of correction of hyperglycemia on left ventricular function in non-insulin-dependent (type 2) diabetics. Acta Med Scand 1983;213:363–368.
41. Astorri E, Fiorina P, Gavaruzzi G, Astorri A, Magnati G. Left ventricular function in insulin-dependent and in non-insulin-dependent diabetic patients: radionuclide assessment. Cardiology 1997;88:152–155.
42. Beljic T, Miric M. Improved metabolic control does not reverse left ventricular filling abnormalities in newly diagnosed non-insulin-dependent diabetes patients. Acta Diabetol 1994;31:147–150.
43. Lo SS, Leslie RD, Sutton MS. Effects of type 1 diabetes mellitus on cardiac function: a study of monozygotic twins. Br Heart J 1995;73:450–455.
44. Litwin SE, Raya TE, Anderson PG, Daugherty S, Goldman S. Abnormal cardiac function in the streptozotocin-diabetic rat. Changes in active and passive properties of the left ventricle. J Clin Invest 1990;86:481–488.
45. Stroedter D, Schmidt T, Bretzel RG, Federlin K. Glucose metabolism and left ventricular dysfunction are normalized by insulin and islet transplantation in mild diabetes in the rat. Acta Diabetol 1995;32:235–243.
46. Thompson EW. Structural manifestations of diabetic cardiomyopathy in the rat and its reversal by insulin treatment. Am J Anat 1988;182:270–282.
47. Sykes CA, Wright AD, Malins JM, Pentecost BL. Changes in systolic time intervals during treatment of diabetes mellitus. Br Heart J 1977;39:255–259.
48. Shapiro LM, Leatherdale BA, Coyne ME, Fletcher RF, Mackinnon J. Prospective study of heart disease in untreated maturity onset diabetics. Br Heart J 1980;44:342–348.

49. von Bibra H, Hansen A, Dounis V, Bystedt T, Malmberg K, Ryden L. Augmented metabolic control improves myocardial diastolic function and perfusion in patients with non-insulin dependent diabetes. Heart 2004;90:1483–1484.

50. Picano E, Pelosi G, Marzilli M, Lattanzi F, Benassi A, Landini L, et al. In vivo quantitative ultrasonic evaluation of myocardial fibrosis in humans. Circulation 1990;81:58–64.

51. Fiordaliso F, Li B, Latini R, Sonnenblick EH, Anversa P, Leri A, et al. Myocyte death in streptozotocin-induced diabetes in rats in angiotensin II-dependent. Lab Invest 2000;80:513–527.

52. Kajstura J, Fiordaliso F, Andreoli AM, Li B, Chimenti S, Medow MS, et al. IGF-1 overexpression inhibits the development of diabetic cardiomyopathy and angiotensin II-mediated oxidative stress. Diabetes 2001;50:1414–1424.

53. Kawaguchi M, Techigawara M, Ishihata T, Asakura T, Saito F, Maehara K, et al. A comparison of ultrastructural changes on endomyocardial biopsy specimens obtained from patients with diabetes mellitus with and without hypertension. Heart Vessels 1997;12:267–274.

54. Fischer VW, Barner HB, Leskiw ML. Capillary basal laminar thickness in diabetic human myocardium. Diabetes 1979;28:713–719.

55. Sakamoto K, Yamasaki Y, Nanto S, Shimonagata T, Morozumi T, Ohara T, et al. Mechanism of impaired left ventricular wall motion in the diabetic heart without coronary artery disease. Diabetes Care 1998;21:2123–2128.

56. Fang ZY, Najos-Valencia O, Leano R, Marwick TH. Patients with early diabetic heart disease demonstrate a normal myocardial response to dobutamine. J Am Coll Cardiol 2003;42:446–453.

57. Strauer BE, Motz W, Vogt M, Schwartzkopff B. Impaired coronary flow reserve in NIDDM: a possible role for diabetic cardiopathy in humans. Diabetes 1997;46(Suppl 2):S119–S124.

58. Kahn JK, Zola B, Juni JE, Vinik AI. Radionuclide assessment of left ventricular diastolic filling in diabetes mellitus with and without cardiac autonomic neuropathy. J Am Coll Cardiol 1986;7:1303–1309.

59. Scognamiglio R, Avogaro A, Casara D, Crepaldi C, Marin M, Palisi M, et al. Myocardial dysfunction and adrenergic cardiac innervation in patients with insulin-dependent diabetes mellitus. J Am Coll Cardiol 1998;31:404–412.

60. Scognamiglio R, Fasoli G, Ferri M, Nistri S, Miorelli M, Egloff C, et al. Myocardial dysfunction and abnormal left ventricular exercise response in autonomic diabetic patients. Clin.Cardiol 1995;18:276–282.

61. Erbas T, Erbas B, Kabakci G, Aksoyek S, Koray Z, Gedik O. Plasma big-endothelin levels, cardiac autonomic neuropathy, and cardiac functions in patients with insulin-dependent diabetes mellitus. Clin Cardiol 2000;23:259–263.

62. Mantysaari M, Kuikka J, Mustonen J, Tahvanainen K, Vanninen E, Lansimies E, et al. Measurement of myocardial accumulation of 123I-metaiodobenzylguanidine for studying cardiac autonomic neuropathy in diabetes mellitus. Clin Auton Res 1996;6:163–169.

63. Hartmann F, Ziegler S, Nekolla S, Hadamitzky M, Seyfarth M, Richardt G, et al. Regional patterns of myocardial sympathetic denervation in dilated cardiomyopathy: an analysis using carbon-11 hydroxyephedrine and positron emission tomography. Heart 1999;81:262–270.

64. Allman KC, Stevens MJ, Wieland DM, Hutchins GD, Wolfe ER Jr, Greene DA, et al. Noninvasive assessment of cardiac diabetic neuropathy by carbon-11 hydroxyephedrine and positron emission tomography. J Am Coll Cardiol 1993;22:1425–1432.

65. Regensteiner JG. Type 2 diabetes mellitus and cardiovascular exercise performance. Rev Endocr Metab Disord 2004;5:269–276.

66. Ford ES, Mannino DM. Prospective association between lung function and the incidence of diabetes: findings from the National Health and Nutrition Examination Survey Epidemiologic Follow-up Study. Diabetes Care 2004;27:2966–2970.

67. Poirier P, Garneau C, Bogaty P, Nadeau A, Marois L, Brochu C, et al. Impact of left ventricular diastolic dysfunction on maximal treadmill performance in normotensive subjects with well-controlled type 2 diabetes mellitus. Am J Cardiol 2000;85:473–477.

68. Fang ZY, Sharman J, Prins JB, Marwick TH. Determinants of exercise capacity in patients with type 2 diabetes. Diabetes Care 2005;28:1643–1648.

69. Hunt SA, Abraham WT, Chin MHea, et al. ACC/AHA 2005 Guideline Update for the Diagnosis and Management of Chronic Heart Failure in the Adult. J Am Coll Cardiol 2005;46.

70. McCullough PA, Nowak RM, McCord J, Hollander JE, Herrmann HC, Steg PG, et al. B-type natriuretic peptide and clinical judgment in emergency diagnosis of heart failure: analysis from Breathing Not Properly (BNP) Multinational Study. Circulation 2002;106:416–422.

71. Rodeheffer RJ. Measuring plasma B-type natriuretic peptide in heart failure: good to go in 2004? J Am Coll Cardiol 2004;44:740–749.

72. Valle R, Bagolin E, Canali C, Giovinazzo P, Barro S, Aspromonte N, et al. The BNP assay does not identify mild left ventricular diastolic dysfunction in asymptomatic diabetic patients. Eur J Echocardiogr 2006;7:40–44.

73. Redfield MM, Jacobsen SJ, Burnett JC Jr, Mahoney DW, Bailey KR, Rodeheffer RJ. Burden of systolic and diastolic ventricular dysfunction in the community: appreciating the scope of the heart failure epidemic. JAMA 2003;289:194–202.

74. Coughlin SS, Pearle DL, Baughman KL, Wasserman A, Tefft MC. Diabetes mellitus and risk of idiopathic dilated cardiomyopathy. The Washington, DC, Dilated Cardiomyopathy Study. Ann Epidemiol 1994;4:67–74.

75. Kannel WB, McGee D. Diabetes and cardiovascular disease: the Framingham study. JAMA 1979;241:2035.

76. Aronow WS, Ahn C. Incidence of heart failure in 2,737 older persons with and without diabetes mellitus. Chest 1999;115:867–868.

77. de Groote P, Lamblin N, Mouquet F, Plichon D, McFadden E, Van Belle E, et al. Impact of diabetes mellitus on long-term survival in patients with congestive heart failure. Eur Heart J 2004;25:656–662.

78. Stone PH, Muller JE, Hartwell T, York BJ, Rutherford JD, Parker CB, et al. The effect of diabetes mellitus on prognosis and serial left ventricular function after acute myocardial infarction: contribution of both coronary disease and diastolic left ventricular dysfunction to the adverse prognosis. The MILIS Study Group. J Am Coll Cardiol 1989;14:49–57.

79. Bell DS. Heart failure: the frequent, forgotten, and often fatal complication of diabetes. Diabetes Care 2003;26:2433–2441.

80. Stone PH, Muller JE, Hartwell T, York BJ, Rutherford JD, Parker CB, et al. The effect of diabetes mellitus on prognosis and serial left ventricular function after acute myocardial infarction: contribution of both coronary disease and diastolic left ventricular dysfunction to the adverse prognosis. The MILIS Study Group. J Am Coll Cardiol 1989;14:49–57.

81. Hunt SA, Baker DW, Chin MH, Cinquegrani MP, Feldman AM, Francis GS, et al. ACC/AHA guidelines for the evaluation and management of chronic heart failure in the adult: executive summary. J Heart Lung Transplant 2002;21:189–203.

82. Tight blood pressure control and risk of macrovascular and microvascular complications in type 2 diabetes: UKPDS 38. UK Prospective Diabetes Study Group. BMJ 1998;317:703–713.

83. Tuomilehto J, Rastenyte D, Birkenhager WH, Thijs L, Antikainen R, Bulpitt CJ, et al. Effects of calcium-channel blockade in older patients with diabetes and systolic hypertension. Systolic Hypertension in Europe Trial Investigators. N Engl J Med 1999;340:677–684.

84. Andersen NH, Poulsen SH, Poulsen PL, Knudsen ST, Mogensen CE. Effects of blood pressure lowering and metabolic control on systolic left ventricular long axis function in type 2 diabetes mellitus. Eur J Echo 2005;6:S47.

85. Fonarow GC. An approach to heart failure and diabetes mellitus. Am J Cardiol 2005;96:47E–52E.

86. Yusuf S, Pfeffer MA, Swedberg K, Granger CB, Held P, McMurray JJ, et al. Effects of candesartan in patients with chronic heart failure and preserved left-ventricular ejection fraction: the CHARM-Preserved trial. Lancet 2003;362:777–781.

87. Carr AA, Kowey PR, Devereux RB, Brenner BM, Dahlof B, Ibsen H, et al. Hospitalizations for new heart failure among subjects with diabetes mellitus in the RENAAL and LIFE Studies. Am J Cardiol 2005;96:1530–1536.

88. Rajagopalan R, Rosenson RS, Fernandes AW, Khan M, Murray FT. Association between congestive heart failure and hospitalization in patients with type 2 diabetes mellitus receiving treatment with insulin or pioglitazone: a retrospective data analysis. Clin Ther 2004;26:1400–1410.

89. Brilla CG, Funck RC, Rupp H. Lisinopril-mediated regression of myocardial fibrosis in patients with hypertensive heart disease. Circulation 2000;102:1388–1393.

90. Mottram PM, Haluska B, Leano R, Cowley D, Stowasser M, Marwick TH. Effect of aldosterone antagonism on myocardial dysfunction in hypertensive patients with diastolic heart failure. Circulation 2004;110:558–565.

91. Candido R, Forbes JM, Thomas MC, Thallas V, Dean RG, Burns WC, Tikellis C, Ritchie RH, Twigg SM, Cooper ME, Burrell LM. A breaker of advanced glycation end products attenuates diabetes-induced myocardial structural changes. Circ Res 2003;92:785–792.

92. Asif M, Egan J, Vasan S, Jyothirmayi GN, Masurekar MR, Lopez S, et al. An advanced glycation end product cross-link breaker can reverse age-related increases in myocardial stiffness. Proc Natl Acad Sci USA 2000;97:2809–2813.

93. Liu J, Masurekar MR, Vatner DE, Jyothirmayi GN, Regan TJ, Vatner SF, et al. Glycation end-product cross-link breaker reduces collagen and improves cardiac function in aging diabetic heart. Am J Physiol Heart Circ Physiol 2003;285:H2587–H2591.

94. Little WC, Zile MR, Kitzman DW, Hundley WG, O'Brien TX, Degroof RC. The effect of alagebrium chloride (ALT-711), a novel glucose cross-link breaker, in the treatment of elderly patients with diastolic heart failure. J Card Fail 2005;11;191–195.

95. Rutter MK, Parise H, Benjamin EJ, Levy D, Larson MG, Meigs JB, et al. Impact of glucose intolerance and insulin resistance on cardiac structure and function: sex-related differences in the Framingham Heart Study. Circulation 2003;107:448–454.

96. Wong CY, O'Moore-Sullivan T, Leano R, Byrne N, Beller E, Marwick TH. Alterations of left ventricular myocardial characteristics associated with obesity. Circulation 2004;110:3081–3087.

97. Marwick TH, Wong CY. Role of exercise and metabolism in heart failure with normal ejection fraction. Prog Cardiovasc Dis 2007;49:263–274.

20
Hypertrophic Cardiomyopathy

Saidi A. Mohiddin and William J. McKenna

Introduction

Abnormalities of ventricular and atrial function that result in suboptimal left ventricular (LV) filling in diastole are thought to be important causes of symptoms and functional limitation in patients with hypertrophic cardiomyopathy (HCM). Indeed, many of the pathophysiologic mechanisms believed to account for "diastolic" heart failure are floridly expressed in HCM, and HCM may prove a useful "supermodel" for the study of diastolic heart disease and its treatment.

Hypertrophic cardiomyopathy is a genetically determined condition defined by apparently unexplained LV hypertrophy associated with symptoms of myocardial ischemia and heart failure and with increased risk of arrhythmic sudden death.[1,2] Clinical practice is largely based on an understanding of disease process; in an almost complete absence of randomized trial data, dynamic outflow obstruction is often managed invasively, defibrillators are used when sudden death risk is deemed relatively high, and symptoms of heart failure are treated with negative inotropes and diuretics. While many of these strategies are based on an understanding of the pathophysiologic processes in HCM and there is clinical evidence that they are effective treatments, the mechanisms underlying the heart failure–related symptomatology in HCM are less well understood and affected patients can be difficult to treat effectively.

Most of the research and clinical studies into HCM have been directed by debate over the importance of LV outflow tract obstruction (LVOTO), the relative merits of alternative methods of LVOTO reduction, and the need to identify and treat patients at high risk of sudden death. More modern cross-sectional and prospective studies confirm that most patients with HCM do not have LVOTO, and the risks of sudden death are lower than originally thought.[3–6] In fact, symptoms of heart failure and atrial arrhythmia often dominate the clinical course of many patients, with these complications often responsible for late-presenting disease.[5,7–9] Abnormalities of LV filling are thought to be a major cause of dyspnea and exercise intolerance in many patients, particularly those without LVOTO. Because adequate LV filling depends on elevated LV filling pressures for augmenting systolic function at rest and/or in response to exercise (or increased afterload), symptoms and exercise limitation may result from elevated pulmonary venous pressures or from reduced maximum cardiac output as preload reserve is limited.

Congestive heart failure is the most common diagnosis in hospitalized patients over the age of 65 years.[10–14] Recent evidence from the National Heart, Lung and Blood Institute–sponsored Cardiovascular Health Study and elsewhere has suggested that as many as half of elderly patients presenting with overt congestive heart failure have normal LV systolic function as documented by a normal LV ejection fraction.[10,11,13–15] This disease, often termed *diastolic heart failure*, thus presents in epidemic proportions. Dyspnea on exertion and exercise limitation resulting from more moderate abnormalities of LV filling must be considerably more common.

This chapter begins with a description and discussion of the hypertrophic cardiomyopathies. We then briefly discuss the critical events in LV filling, a process also referred to as *atrioventricular coupling,* to emphasize the importance of appropriate interaction of both constant and variable atrial and ventricular cardiac chamber properties. Molecular and histopathologic evidence of abnormalities affecting LV relaxation, LV compliance, and atrial function is presented, following which we examine evidence from patient studies for the clinical importance of abnormal diastolic performance. Finally, we comment on limitations in the methods available for assessing LV filling and the need for refined measurement tools in the development of intervention strategies tailored to specific abnormalities of LV filling.

We end this introduction with a disclaimer. In the HCM patient, several other pathophysiologic processes (e.g., LV obstruction, myocardial ischemia, arrhythmia, chronotropic incompetence, inappropriate vasodilatation) may be present concurrently with filling abnormalities and contribute to symptoms and/or exercise limitation. Arterial compliance and expansion of the circulating volume may be important in the development of diastolic heart failure in some hypertensive patients[12,16] and may contribute to symptoms in an elderly or hypertensive HCM patient. Extracardiac expression of the disease-causing gene in certain forms of HCM may also complicate symptomatology.[17-21] We consider only the contributions that ventricular and atrial disease may make to abnormal diastole.

The Hypertrophic Cardiomyopathies

Hypertrophic cardiomyopathy is a primary myocardial disease defined by LV hypertrophy and associated with small LV cavities and a supranormal ejection fraction.[1,2,22] It has a prevalence of approximately 1 in 500[23,24] and is typically inherited in an autosomal dominant fashion.[25,26] Left ventricular hypertrophy develops in the absence of increased loading conditions; although resting outflow obstruction may develop as a consequence of LV hypertrophy in about one fourth of patients,

an elevated ventricular pressure load is not the primary mechanism underlying myocyte hypertrophy. In fact, the magnitude of LV hypertrophy found in HCM is often far greater than that associated with load-related forms of LV hypertrophy. In most HCM patients, LV hypertrophy develops during puberty, following which further increases in LV wall thickness are uncommon.[27,28]

Treatment of disabling symptoms, risks of sudden death, risks of thromboembolic disease, and provision of appropriate genetic counseling dominate the clinical approach to the HCM patient. The development of clinical complications is often not clearly related to readily assessed disease characteristics, but classification into "types" of HCM is useful in patient management. For the purposes of this section, we consider types of HCM on the basis of (1) morphology, (2) molecular cause, (3) sudden death risk, and (4) symptom status.

Morphologic Variants

Hypertrophic cardiomyopathy was originally identified and is still diagnosed on the basis of morphologic LV abnormalities. The diagnosis is conventionally made after the demonstration, by cardiac imaging, of a criterion severity of LV hypertrophy. By definition, the LV hypertrophy has developed in the absence of another cause for the hypertrophy such as increased afterload, metabolic abnormalities, and infiltrative disease, although other conditions such as hypertension can clearly coexist and interact. Premolecular era definitions of HCM also specify an idiopathic etiology; in clinical practice, the majority of diagnoses of HCM are made without genetic information, and the "idiopathic" criterion remains relevant in that it refers to the exclusion of valve disease, hypertension, systemic metabolic disease, and myocardial infiltration.

The distribution or pattern of the hypertrophy within the LV has lead to morphologic subclassifications such as asymmetric septal hypertrophy, reversed asymmetric septal hypertrophy, apical, midcavity, or Maron-type obstructive HCM, apical (Japanese) HCM (Figure 20.1). A "burned-out" HCM with septal wall thinning, LV dilation, and systolic impairment develops in about 10% of patients and can develop into a dilated cardiomy-

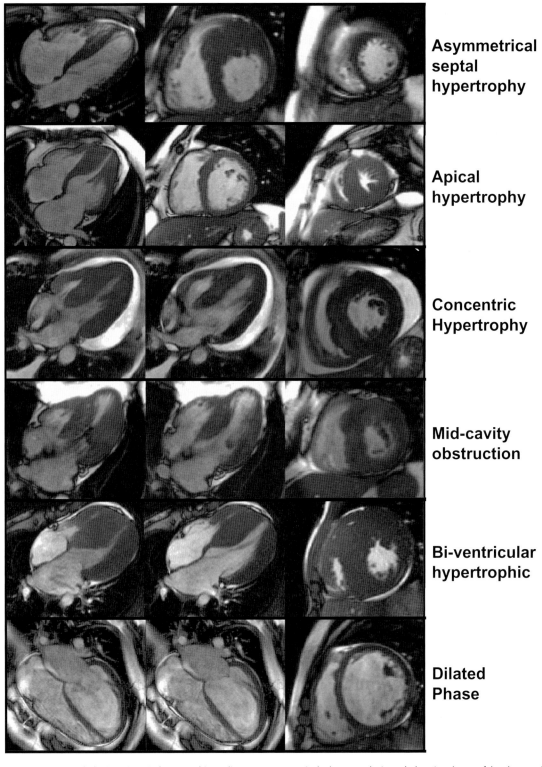

FIGURE 20.1. Morphologic variants in hypertrophic cardiomyopathy. A single genetic abnormality may be associated with "classic" asymmetric septal hypertrophy, other patterns of left ventricular hypertrophy, an apparently normal cardiac phenotype, and progressive left ventricular dilatation and systolic impairment. Left ventricular hypertrophy/morphology is only one of the phenotypic features of hypertrophic cardiomyopathy, and as yet undefined genetic and/or environmental factors contribute to the variable phenotypic consequences of the fundamental cellular defect. (Images courtesy of Dr. James Moon.)

opathy.[27,29-32] Progressive dilatation of the left atrium is common and is associated with increased risks of thromboembolic disease and atrial fibrillation; our practice is to anticoagulate patients with a left atrial dimension of greater than 50 mm, even in the absence of atrial fibrillation.[33-35] Many studies have shown that there is a great variation in morphologic patterns of disease resulting from an identical disease-causing gene mutation in both the same and in different pedigrees. Additionally, cases of HCM with no or mild hypertrophy (normal phenotype or mild LV hypertrophy despite positive genotype) suggest that genetic or molecular perspectives on HCM may offer a more comprehensive classification system.

The pattern of LV hypertrophy poorly predicts clinical manifestations and has little relevance to therapy. However, in some individuals, the pattern of LV hypertrophy in concert with other characteristics of the heart may result in dynamic obstruction during systole. This obstruction is most frequently of the LV outflow tract (i.e., LVOTO) but may alternatively (or also) be in the mid-LV or the right ventricular outflow tract. A dynamic, often labile degree of LVOTO is found in approximately one fourth of at-rest patients in relatively unselected cohorts.[36,37] and the division into obstructive and nonobstructive disease has robust *clinical* utility (Figure 20.2). The precise determinants of LVOTO have been debated for decades;[38-41] regardless, the consequences of LVOTO on afterload, wall tension, preload, and so on undoubtedly make major contributions to symptoms. These include those suggestive of heart failure, myocardial ischemia, and impaired consciousness, all of which will often improve after abolition or reduction of LVOTO. Persisting symptoms, and those in individuals without obstruction (the majority of patients), can be much more difficult to treat.

Molecular Variants

The identification of β-myosin heavy chain mutations as a cause of some cases of HCM was rapidly followed by descriptions of more than 200 disease-causing mutations in more than 10 other genes encoding components of the basic contractile unit the sarcomere.[25,26] Mutations in nonsarcomeric genes, including mitochondrial and "energy-homeostasis" genes may also cause a phenotype clinically indistinguishable from sarcomeric gene HCM.[19,42] Mutations affecting other cellular processes are also likely to be causes of some cases of HCM, and transgenic studies have implicated calcium-signaling genes as likely suspects.[43,44] A classification into distinct HCM entities on the basis of cause promises a rational basis for prognostication and targeted therapy and has the attraction of etiologic clarity. Such a classification could, for example, be defined by the specific causative molecular lesion (e.g., mutation of arginine to histidine at residue 403 of β-myosin), by the gene affected (e.g. troponin T), or by the (putative) effect on cellular function (e.g., sarcomeric function, calcium handling, or energy utilization).

There are several limitations to a molecular classification. There is a striking degree of genetic heterogeneity where several hundred mutations in 10 or more genes have been identified as causes, with several families having apparently private or unique mutants. This clearly condemns a simple mutation-based classification to tremendous complexity and limited applicability.[25,26] A feature of most genetic studies is the striking infidelity between individual mutation and resulting disease phenotype. This is of sufficient magnitude to limit the clinical/prognostic utility of almost any classification scheme based on molecular/genetic considerations. Currently, only 50%–60% of patients have a mutation in the coding sequences of one of the identified genes, but as many as 10% may have mutations in more than one gene.[45-47] This, and the multiplicity of mutations, makes genetic testing cumbersome, expensive, and of relatively low yield. As such, routine genetic testing is difficult to justify, with results contributing significantly only to the detection of family members at risk of developing the disease. Finally, our understanding of how any of the inherited molecular abnormalities initiates the hypertrophic response remains very limited, and available data suggest other, undefined, modifying factors are of great importance.[48-51] There are notable exceptions, including some mutants associated with high risks of early mortality,[52-55] atrial fibrillation,[56] midcavity hypertrophy and obstruction,[21] and severe disease despite minimal or no hypertrophy.[54,55]

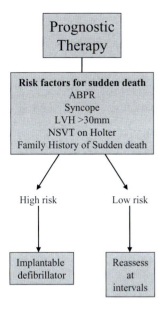
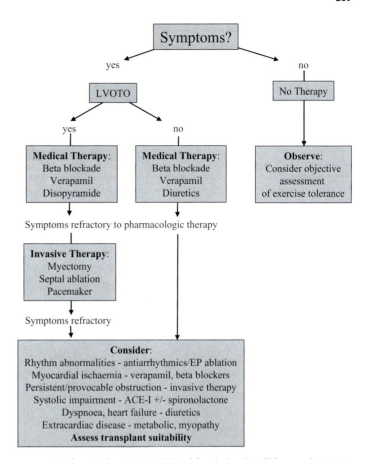

FIGURE 20.2. A contemporary approach to the management of prognostic and symptomatic concerns in hypertrophic cardiomyopathy patients. In most medical centers, an assessment of sudden death risk relies on the summation of individual risk factors that are given equal weight. The 6-year survival rate for patients with no, one, or two risk factors is 95%, 93%, and 82%, respectively,[71] and defibrillator implantation is often advised if two or more risk factors are present. There is little evidence to guide the frequency at which assessments should be made, but as the highest risks of death are in the third and fourth decades of life, annual review in this age group is reasonable. β-Blockers, verapamil, diuretics, and disopyramide are the mainstay of medical therapy for patients with obstructive physiology with symptoms refractory to pharmacologic therapy. ABPR, abnormal blood pressure response to exercise; ACE-I, angiotensin-converting enzyme inhibitor; LVH, left ventricular hypertrophy; LVOTO, left ventricular outflow tract obstruction; NSVT, nonsustained ventricular tachycardia.

To date, most mutations identified as causes of HCM are in genes that code for components of the sarcomere; alterations in contractility, in sensitivities to changes in calcium concentration, in the efficiency of adenosine triphosphate utilization, and cell injury have all been suggested as potential mechanisms by which these mutated proteins initiate LV hypertrophy.[26,44,51,57–59] An interaction between the basic molecular defect and other variables leads to multiple pathologic processes in the myocardium, and the concept of a hypertrophic cellular circuit has been developed. (Figure 20.3)

The sum effect of circuit activity is a group of diseases that are diverse etiologically but share myocyte hypertrophy, cell death, myocardial ischemia, myocyte disarray, interstitial fibrosis, and chamber remodeling, albeit to variable degrees. In the absence of an identifiable "primary" cause of LV hypertrophy such as hypertension, we currently identify the resulting phenotypes as a single clinical entity on the basis of LV wall thickness alone. Several of these processes and/or their secondary effects continue contributing to cardiac dysfunction long after hypertrophy has

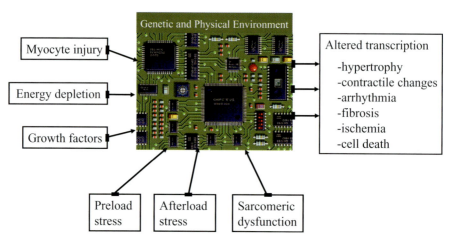

FIGURE 20.3. A conceptual model of the hypertrophic circuit in the cardiomyocyte and other cardiac cells. Quite dissimilar conditions result in cardiac hypertrophy phenotypes that share similar elements, presumably as a result of activating shared pathways altering nuclear expression. This view of hypertrophy emphasizes the potential value of hypertrophic cardiomyopathy as a model system for the investigation of factors that determine severity of cardiac hypertrophy, as an identical genetic abnormality often results in a variable hypertrophic phenotype.

developed.[27,29,30,60] These aspects of the phenotype may be independent of the magnitude of LV wall thickness, may make major contributions to diastolic dysfunction and to other manifestations of the disease, and are likely to be progressive.[27,28,33–35,61–67]

Risk of Arrhythmic Sudden Death

Identifying individuals at high risk of sudden death remains a major clinical challenge. Ventricular tachycardia and fibrillation are the most common final modes of sudden death, and implantable cardioverter defibrillator devices (ICDs) are effective for secondary prevention and for primary prevention in selected high-risk individuals.[68–71] Therapy with ICDs carries significant risks and costs that currently obviate more indiscriminate use.

The arrhythmic substrate has been attributed to a variety of mechanisms that are not mutually exclusive and include abnormal calcium handling (enhanced automaticity, delayed after depolarization), myocyte disarray and fibrosis (reentrant circuits), myocardial ischemia, altered hemodynamic/autonomic reflexes, and intolerance of tachyarrhythmia due to ischemia, LVOTO, or diastolic dysfunction.[36,54,71–76] Given these several plausible mechanisms, perhaps it is not surprising that all individual risk factors identified to date have poor predictive value. Currently, risk stratification is accomplished by scoring for the presence or absence of the following; a family history of sudden death, a history of syncope, severe magnitude of LV hypertrophy, abnormal (hypotensive) blood pressure responses to exercise, and non-sustained VT on Holter monitoring.[69,71,76] Risks of sudden death and the use of ICD implantation in adolescents are higher, but the predictive value of these risk factors are not as well established in this age group.[77] Our strategy is to combine risk factors and recommend primary ICD therapy if two or more risk factors are present in a patient over 30 years of age or for a single risk factor in adult patients younger than 30 years of age.[71] Newer risk factors and quantitative or synergistic combinations of risk factors may enhance the predictive power.

Diastolic abnormalities have not been adequately assessed as risk factors for sudden death in HCM. However, altered myocellular calcium handling, myocardial ischemia, and interstitial fibrosis/scarring are mechanisms shared by both arrhythmogenesis and stiff myocardium, and diastolic heart failure without systolic dysfunction is associated with reduced prognosis.[10,11] Addition-

Symptomatic and Asymptomatic Hypertrophic Cardiomyopathy

Currently, there are few indications for treatment of the asymptomatic patient, other than ICD therapy in those thought to be at high risk of ventricular arrhythmia (see Figure 20.2) and anticoagulation when thromboembolic risks are considered sufficiently elevated. Patients may present with symptoms, or symptoms may develop years after initial diagnosis. Symptoms include those associated with heart failure, myocardial ischemia, atrial/ventricular arrhythmia, and dynamic/provocable LVOTO.

The management approach to the symptomatic HCM patient with LVOTO assumes that obstruction makes a significant contribution to the development of symptoms. Reduction of LVOTO is often very successful in symptom improvement, but patients may have residual symptoms.[78,79] For the symptomatic HCM patient without LVOTO, therapeutic options are few and often unsatisfactory.

Clinical investigations in the symptomatic or limited nonobstructive patient often detect evidence of ischemia; abnormal diastolic measurements with echocardiography, nuclear imaging, or catheterization; systolic abnormalities; atrial enlargement; myocardial scarring with magnetic resonance imaging; and atrial/ventricular arrhythmias. No individual or profile of abnormality reliably distinguishes symptomatic from asymptomatic patients or correlates sufficiently well with measured exercise limitation. Therapy is therefore often targeted at the prominent symptom or abnormality, for example, arrhythmia suppression, preload reduction with diuretics, angiotensin-converting enzyme inhibitors for LV dilatation, verapamil or β-blockers for ischemia, and so on.

Abnormal LV filling, encompassing abnormal LV relaxation, atrial dysfunction, LV compliance, and ventricular interaction, is thought to make major contributions to heart failure symptoms and exercise intolerance in such patients. Left ventricular filling is a complex and interactive process determined by preload, afterload, systolic events, and the passive and active properties of the cardiac chambers and vascular structures. Not surprisingly, even though it has been relatively easy to demonstrate alterations in LV filling, the specific determinants of abnormal filling and their clinical importance have been more difficult to accurately identify and quantify. Given that LV filling depends on the appropriate interaction of several cardiac properties, a comprehensive description of diastole will include several parameters.

The development of "diastolic profiling" has also been limited by the absence of specific therapies and therefore clinical importance. Recent developments in cardiac resynchronization therapy and a better understanding of myocyte and matrix metabolism have suggested potential interventions. Clinical trials will require rational patient selection and will be limited by difficulties in identification and quantification of LV filling abnormalities, for example, in LV chamber compliance and atrial function.

Summary

Hypertrophic cardiomyopathy has proved remarkably heterogeneous at every level of investigation, and there is no single useful classification framework for the disease. A useful clinical approach begins with assessments of both risk and symptom status (see Figure 20.2). Diastolic abnormalities are likely to play an important role in the development of symptoms and are difficult to treat. No single pathologic mechanism is solely responsible for abnormal LV filling. The development of assessment tools for diastole is essential for the development and testing of rational therapies.

Left Ventricular Filling and Preload Reserve

Preload reserve refers to the capacity to modulate the stroke volume by virtue of the relationship between the magnitude of LV filling and the Starling relationship. As discussed later, the size and geometry of the HCM heart mean that preload reserve is particularly dependent on optimal LV filling. As a consequence of myocyte and myocardial abnormalities, it is also prone to the development of LV filling abnormalities. Optimal LV filling in diastole requires the appropriate coupling of passive and active properties of the left atrium and the LV.

Components of Diastole

The definition and temporal limits of diastole can be described in both cellular and hemodynamic terms as outlined in other reviews and conceptual models.[80-84] For our purposes, a simple description encompassing major cellular and hemodynamic events may be helpful.

Following peak LV force generation during the systolic phase of the cardiac cycle, energy-dependent sequestration of calcium into the sarcoplasmic reticulum leads to rapid dissociation of actin-myosin fibril cross-linking and marks the beginning of "cellular" diastole. As a result, the rapid decline in LV pressure results in aortic valve closure, and thus "hemodynamic" diastole begins shortly after "cellular" diastole. A period of isovolumic relaxation follows until atrial pressure exceeds that in the LV, and the mitral valve opens and early rapid filling occurs until atrioventricular chamber pressure equilibration again ensues (diastasis) and there is little or no flow across the valve. The passive capacitance and intracavitary pressure in the left atrium and pulmonary veins as well as LV relaxation velocity, LV restoring forces (a suction effect as the LV "springs" from and systolic toward equilibrium volume), and compliance all influence early LV filling. If sinus rhythm is present, late diastolic atrial contraction causes a second LV filling phase, providing the final stretch to myocardial fibers and thereby increasing LV stroke volume via the Frank-Starling mechanism. This phase of LV filling is dependent on the interaction of atrial systolic force (itself dependent on atrial preload and atrial inotropy) and the LV's passive pressure–volume (PV) characteristics (compliance). Cellular diastole is terminated by energy-dependent actin-myosin cross-linking and cycling after intracellular calcium is again increased, effecting excitation-contraction coupling. The mitral valve closes as LV pressure rises to exceed left atrial pressure and

diastole, as defined hemodynamically, comes to an end.

From this brief description, it can be appreciated that many constant and variable (or active and passive) properties will influence LV filling. Systolic LV performance and afterload, LV relaxation, atrial chamber inotropy, and compliance all determine LV filling volumes. Thus, a decreased LV end-systolic volume as a result of reduced afterload or from enhanced inotropy will increase restoring forces and enhance filling (and vice versa). Uncoordinated LV systolic contraction resulting from ischemia or conduction abnormalities/pacing might not only directly impair ejection volume but also prolong isovolumetric relaxation time by delaying regional LV relaxation and also increase LV end-systolic volumes and reduce restoring forces. A compliant left atrium and adequate atrial inotropy maintain an atrio-ventricular pressure gradient in early and late diastole, respectively, and minimize mean atrial pressure.[85]

Preload Reserve

Left ventricular end-diastolic volume, representing fiber stretch, influences LV contractile function and stroke volume via the Frank-Starling mechanism. Left ventricular end-diastolic volume is determined by end-diastolic pressure and the passive material properties of the ventricular myocardium (compliance or elasticity). The final filling pressure is generated by atrial ejection and thus LV end-diastolic volume is partly dependent on atrial systolic function. This atrial booster-pump activity is itself responsive to inotropic effects and to Frank-Starling potentiation (atrial fiber stretch by atrial preload).[86-88] The coupling of pulmonary venous/left atrial pressure and compliance and LV relaxation/suction kinetics in early diastole and of atrial systole and LV passive compliance in late diastole are responsible for the augmentation of cardiac output related to Frank-Starling enhancement of final LV volumes and preload reserve.

Increases in cardiac output are mediated through increases in stroke volume (reduction of LV end-systolic volume and/or increases in end-diastolic volume) and heart rate (reducing diastolic filling time). In the resting HCM heart, LV volumes are typically small, frequently with near obliteration of end-systolic cavity volume, suggesting further decreases in end-systolic volume can make only minimal contributions to an increased stroke volume. As such, augmented ventricular end diastolic volume and preload reserve are probably much more important for increasing cardiac output in an HCM heart than in a normal heart. Apparently "normal" age-related decreases in LV compliance and atrial impairment are described in normal hearts[89-95] and may have much greater consequences in an aging HCM heart more dependent on preload reserve.

Diastolic Abnormalities in Hypertrophic Cardiomyopathy

Small LV volumes, abnormal relaxation kinetics, reduced chamber compliance, atrial systolic abnormalities, and myocellular dysfunction are features of HCM. These abnormalities may restrict preload reserve, resulting in elevated pulmonary venous pressures and/or inadequate cardiac output. Tolerance of exertion, particularly as diastole is abbreviated by increased heart rates, may be severely compromised by restrictions in LV filling.

Left ventricular filling abnormalities demonstrated in HCM can be primary consequences of the myopathic disease process or manifestations of compensatory mechanisms. Several cellular, histologic, and anatomic/chamber abnormalities have been well described and can all, theoretically, affect atrioventricular coupling. We consider some of these abnormalities here and how they might be relevant in diastole.

Myocellular Abnormalities

Early LV pressure decline (relaxation) results from deactivation of actin-myosin cross-linking following the reduction in cytoplasmic Ca^{2+} concentration. Passive restoring forces result in a sucking effect as the ventricular chamber recoils toward its equilibrium volume. Cytoplasmic Ca^{2+} removal is an energy-dependent process during which Ca^{2+} is sequestered into the sarcoplasmic reticulum through the smooth endoplasmic reticulum Ca^{2+} ATPase (SERCA) and is also extruded into the extracellular space via the Na^+/Ca^{2+} exchange.[96,97] Extracellular and sarcoplasmic reticulum Ca^{2+} are available in the subsequent cardiac cycle for release through the L-type Ca^{2+} and ryanodine receptor channels, respectively, to effect excitation-contraction coupling. Adenosine triphosphate availability, β-adrenergic activity, and a host of other factors modulate channel and contractile kinetics.

In HCM, abnormalities that are either primary or secondary consequences of mutant expression and that may affect relaxation at the cellular level include abnormalities in the expression or regulation of SERCA, Na^+/Ca^{2+}, ryanodine receptor, and L-type channels; the availability of adenosine triphosphate and other energy substrates; as well as direct mutant effects on contractile protein properties such as actin-myosin uncoupling, Ca^{2+} responsiveness, and kinetics of Ca^{2+} association/dissociation from contractile proteins.[98-106] These myocellular abnormalities may affect the function of both ventricular and atrial myocytes. As they may be either a direct or a secondary consequence of the causative molecular abnormality, their profile may be very different in cardiomyopathies resulting from different genetic causes.

Histological Abnormalities

In most pathologic states, LV hypertrophy is the result of myocyte hypertrophy, hyperplasia of smooth muscle cells and fibroblasts, and the accumulation of extracellular matrix. In HCM, additional histologic features can include myofibrillar disarray, replacement and interstitial fibrosis, microvascular abnormalities, and inflammation.[67,107] Although none of these abnormalities is always present or pathognomonic, myofibrillar disarray is common in HCM and an uncommon finding in "secondary" LV hypertrophy in which myocyte hypertrophy is characterized by an increase in actin and myosin fibers in parallel arrangement.[106,108,109] Left ventricular hypertrophy in HCM is frequently more severe than in pressure overload states, and the accumulation of fibrillar collagen and other matrix components is more profound.[67] The fibrillar component of the normal myocardium has several functions, including (1) maintenance of alignment between myocytes, (2) acting as a protective restraint to prevent damage from excessive mechanical loads, (3) transmission of contractile force, and (4) storage of mechanical energy in coiled fibers to contribute to diastolic recoil (restitution forces).

Excessive myocardial fibrosis, documented histologically[66,110-114] and inferred by delayed gadolinium enhancement on cardiac magnetic resonance imaging[115,116] is a prominent feature in HCM, hypertensive heart disease, and dilated cardiomyopathy (Figure 20.4). The extracellular matrix in HCM hearts has been estimated to comprise between 9% and 22% of total volume, in contrast to 2.6%–20% in hypertensive hearts and 1.1%–3.8% in normal hearts.[111,112,117] Collagens I (85%) and III (11%) are the major fibrillar collagens of the myocardial extracellular matrix.[118,119] Collagen I has the tensile strength of steel, and small increases in this substance substantially add to myocardial stiffness. The total collagen content in HCM hearts has been reported as up to 72% higher than hypertrophied non-HCM hearts.[113,120] Fibrotic changes are found throughout the myocardium but appear to be most prominent in areas of marked myofibrillar disarray.[112,114] Excessive myocardial fibrosis and myofibrillar disarray are likely to increase passive LV chamber stiffness, and consequent reductions in preload reserve may contribute to heart failure symptoms in HCM and other forms of LV hypertrophy.

Chamber Function and Geometry

Left Ventricular Shape, Size, Wall Thickness, and Compliance

Differences in the material properties of the myocardium among different subjects may obscure relationships between LV size and wall thickness and LV filling properties. Nonetheless, the magnitude of hypertrophy and patterns of its distribution as well as chamber size have been correlated with measures of diastolic dysfunction in other forms of LV hypertrophy and less clearly in HCM.[121-124]

Left ventricular remodeling to reduce wall tension has been thought a compensatory mechanism to accommodate the basic contractile abnormality resulting from a sarcomeric mutation. The smaller LV cavity size and increased wall thickness in HCM reduce LV wall tension according to Laplace's law (wall tension = [intracavitary pressure × chamber radius]/[2 × wall thickness]). Assuming invariant myocardial material properties, a given pressure increase will result in a smaller increase in wall stress and therefore a smaller volume increase in a smaller chamber or in a chamber with thicker walls. Thus, increasing LV wall thickness or reducing LV cavity volume will reduce compliance (compliance = change in volume/change in pressure) above and beyond the altered myocardial properties discussed earlier. Adverse effects of reduced LV volume on diastolic function are described after LV volume reduction surgery for dilated cardiomyopathies.[125]

Atrial Function

The atria have reservoir, conduit, and pump functions, but interest in the left atrial contribution to LV filling has largely been limited to a view that altered left atrial properties are compensatory for LV abnormalities and culminate in increased risks of atrial fibrillation. Indeed, left atrial enlargement developing secondary to chronically elevated LV filling pressures has been proposed as a barometer of diastolic dysfunction.[126,127] Left atrial enlargement is very prominent in HCM, and left atrial dysfunction may be particularly important.

FIGURE 20.4. Myocardial fibrosis viewed in three ways. (A) Gadolinium delayed hyperenhancement on in-vivo cardiac MRI. The persistence within myocardial segments of the magnetic resonance contrast agent gadolinium is interpreted as demonstrating the replacement of normal myocardial tissue with scar tissue/matrix material on a macroscopic scale (as in B). Microscopic or diffuse myocardial scarring (as in B) will not be detected as delayed hyperenhancement. Delayed hyperenhancement (pale areas) is shown in consecutive short axis slices through the left ventricle. (Images courtesy of Dr. James Moon.) (B) Confluent myocardial scarring ex-vivo. This cross section of an explanted hypertrophic cardiomyopathy heart shows confluent myocardial fibrosis. The epicardial coronary arteries were unobstructed. The patient underwent cardiac transplantation for symptoms of severe heart failure. (C) Microscopic myocardial scarring histologically. Microscopic areas of scarring are seen in these biopsy samples of the interventricular septum obtained from the right ventricle.

20. Hypertrophic Cardiomyopathy

A

B

C

provide information on the major phases of LV filling, relaxation, and compliance and left atrial systolic function and compliance. Less invasive assessment methods with echocardiography and pulmonary artery catheters have been used to estimate LV compliance[137] and can be adapted to assess left atrial function.

Clinical Significance of Diastolic Abnormalities in Hypertrophic Cardiomyopathy

By virtue of chamber size and hypertrophy, the left ventricle of an HCM heart is particularly dependent on optimum atrioventricular coupling to maintain an adequate LV end-diastolic volume with acceptable filling pressures. Abnormalities expressed in the HCM heart, many of which are progressive, are likely to degrade atrial and ventricular diastolic performance and progressively impair LV filling. This section looks at the available evidence that filling abnormalities actually result in functional abnormalities and/or clinical manifestations in patients.

Limitations of Clinical Studies

Symptoms of heart failure and exercise intolerance are common in HCM. Several and coexisting pathophysiologies are likely to contribute, and abnormal LV filling is a major suspect. Resting abnormalities in LV diastolic filling parameters were documented decades ago in HCM.[37,61,110,138–149] Much of the earlier work, while documenting perturbations in LV relaxation and compensatory augmentation of atrial emptying, failed to either analyze or to demonstrate a strong relationship (or any relationship) between diastolic filling parameters and functional capacity.

More recent studies have compared symptoms or exercise performance to various estimates or measures of diastolic performance. Most investigators used echocardiographic, nuclear, or catheter data to assess diastole. Several limitations are evident in these studies: (1) there is no gold standard measure that assesses all major components of LV filling in diastole; (2) the demonstration of elevated filling pressures does not necessarily identify the failing component(s) of diastole; (3) it is unclear which pressure measurement best represents LV filling (e.g., mean pulmonary artery wedge pressure, mean left atrial pressure, post-A/pre-A LV end-diastolic pressure); (4) pressure measurements are (pre- and post-) load dependent; (5) resting measurements of LV filling cannot assess nonconstant (e.g., inotrope/load-dependent LV relaxation and atrial contractility) and nonlinear (e.g. LV compliance) variables; (6) inclusion of obstructed and nonobstructed patients may confound the results as symptoms may have several causes; and (7) inclusion of a high percentage of asymptomatic and young patients limits the power of a study to associate the measured diastolic parameter with functional impairment.

Invasive Hemodynamic Studies

Chan et al.[150] compared pulmonary artery wedge pressure, cardiac index, and blood pressure after diuresis and infusion of fluid volume in 13 HCM patients. Similar to responses from normal controls, all three indices were higher in the resting upright state after fluid infusion. At peak upright exercise testing, pulmonary artery wedge pressure was also significantly higher in patients when fluid replete than in the same patients after diuresis, but cardiac index and blood pressure were similar. Thus, as a higher pulmonary artery wedge pressure in the volume replete was not associated with greater cardiac index, the authors concluded that stroke volume was insensitive to preload; hearts were operating near the Starling plateau. In this study, the mean pulmonary artery wedge pressure at peak exercise was 25 mm Hg, similar to that seen in exercising heart failure patients[151] and compared with only approximately 10 mm Hg in normal volunteers.[152] Left ventricular volumes were not measured in this study.

Frenneaux et al.[153] reported results of invasive (Swann-Ganz) exercise testing in 23 HCM patients several of whom had LVOTO. Subjects were relatively young (mean age, 34 years) and mildly symptomatic or asymptomatic as most (87%) were in New York Heart Association (NYHA) functional class I or II with only a moderate depression of

20. Hypertrophic Cardiomyopathy

maximal oxygen consumption during exercise. Cardiac index increased by 340%, and peak cardiac index correlated well with maximal oxygen consumption. However, pulmonary artery wedge pressure at rest or with exercise, a major determinant of LV end-diastolic stretch, was unrelated to maximal oxygen consumption. Patients did, however, demonstrate large changes in mean pulmonary artery wedge pressure; supine 15 ± 5 mm Hg, erect resting 5 ± 6 mm Hg, and erect peak exercise 24 ± 11 mm Hg. Resting and exercise LV volumes were not measured.

Lele et al.[146] expanded on this study to examine how increased cardiac output was related to heart rate and stoke volume responses. Their findings were that increases in stroke volume rather than heart rate were the major determinant of peak exercise capacity. The authors concluded that although capacity is not limited by symptoms resulting from elevated pulmonary venous pressures, it is dependent on increments in cardiac output resulting from augmentation of end-diastolic volume (preload reserve). However, an analysis of their data shows a poor relationship between exercise-induced augmentation of stroke volume and increases in pulmonary artery wedge pressure ($R^2 = 0.05$). Thus, although cardiac index in exercise is correlated strongly with exercise performance, and pulmonary artery wedge pressure increases to levels associated with pulmonary edema, there is no simple relationship between mean filling pressures and cardiac output. Similar findings are reported by Kitzman et al.[154] in a mixed group of patients with LV hypertrophy; there is a failure to augment stroke volume despite significant increases in preload — as measured by mean pulmonary artery wedge pressure.

The validity of mean pulmonary artery wedge pressure as an index for LV filling pressures is not certain; the correlation between mean pulmonary artery wedge pressure and LV end-diastolic pressure is particularly poor in patients with LV hypertrophy[85,155,156] Theoretically, at least, LV end-diastolic pressure or mean diastolic LV pressures are more appropriate measures of filling pressure, whereas mean pulmonary artery wedge pressure may better reflect the hydrostatic pressures resulting in dyspnea. Simultaneous LV PV measurements and those of LA function would more completely assess LV filling than any single pressure measurement. As yet, no studies compare PV characteristics with symptom status or functional parameters.

Echocardiographic Studies

Echocardiography can estimate chamber volumes and relaxation properties, and Doppler-derived measurements have recently been used to estimate LV filling pressures.[157-159]

Conventional Doppler

Echocardiographically derived diastolic abnormalities are consistently demonstrated in HCM, but an association of these to symptoms or exercise performance was not easy to demonstrate.[144-148,160,161] Using conventional *resting* transmitral Doppler measurements (E/A ratio), Maron et al.[160] detected abnormal diastolic indices in most HCM patients and noted that the severity of abnormality was increased in patients without LV obstruction. Nihoyannopoulos et al.[148] found similar patterns of abnormality in resting transmitral flow characteristics and showed a weak correlation with peak oxygen consumption during exercise testing. However, there were no differences in E/A Doppler ratios between symptomatic and asymptomatic patients, but pseudonormalized patterns were evident in the most symptomatic. In this study, and in a further study from the same group that employed radionuclide angiography,[145] evidence for left atrial systolic failure was also detected. In a study comparing exercise performance to transmitral Doppler measurements as well as pulmonary vein flow and left atrial fractional shortening, Briguori et al.[144] found no evidence for a relationship between resting transmitral flow indices and peak oxygen consumption but did find a reasonable correlation between left atrial fractional shortening and peak oxygen consumption.

Difficulties in demonstrating robust associations between symptoms and exercise performance are not surprising given the now well-described phenomena of pseudonormalization and load dependence of the E/A ratio. These parameters perform particularly poorly at estimating LV filling in HCM.[157,158]

Flow and Tissue Doppler Imaging

More recently studied echocardiographic measurements, including pulmonary vein Doppler imaging, mitral flow propagation velocity, tissue Doppler imaging, and a variety of derived ratios and intervals are more reliable at predicting LV filling pressures.[157,162,163] A brief description of these newer measurements may help in the interpretation of the HCM clinical studies that use them.

In HCM patients, Nagueh et al.[157] compared a variety of Doppler parameters (including E/A, the ratio of transmitral E to early mitral annular velocity [E/Ea]; early mitral propagation flow velocity; pulmonary vein inflow characteristics; and E and A acceleration/deceleration times) to a variety of LV diastolic pressure measurements (LV minimal pressure, pre-A LV end-diastolic pressure, and post-A LV end-diastolic pressure). The E/Ea and propagation velocity correlated well with pre-A LV end-diastolic pressure (r = 0.76 and r = 0.67, respectively). In a larger group of patients without HCM, they report that E/Ea and a different measure of LV filling pressure, the mean diastolic LV pressure, are strongly correlated.[159] However, the E/Ea ratios were in an indeterminate range in more than half of the patients for whom mean diastolic LV pressure could not be assigned as normal or elevated. Correlations between E/Ea and LV end-diastolic pressure have subsequently been shown by others but may be significantly better in patients with poor LV systolic function.[164] Data obtained from catheterized dogs suggest that E/Ea and LV end-diastolic pressure have an *inverse* correlation when preload is reduced.[164] In summary, although E/Ea may contribute to diastolic assessment, the available studies use quite different measures of LV filling pressure (pre-A LV end-diastolic pressure, mean diastolic LV pressure, LV end-diastolic pressure). The accuracy of filling pressures predicted by E/Ea may be altered by changes in preload and may be different in different patient populations.

In a study of 85 HCM patients, Matsumura et al.[147] found a reasonable correlation between resting E/Ea ratio and maximum oxygen consumption and that E/Ea values were highest in symptomatic patients. These findings have recently been validated in a group of patients with apical HCM.[161] However, although the r values were relatively modest (r = −0.42[147] and r = −0.47[161]), the studies' findings are all the more surprising when compared with the earlier studies in which filling pressures were measured invasively but no association was found with exercise performance.[146,153]

Atrial Function

To date, little has been written about the role of atrial function on preload reserve and exercise tolerance. Briguori et al.[144] reported an association between resting left atrial fractional shortening and exercise capacity. They suggest that left atrial fractional shortening reflects LV end-diastolic pressure and that elevated LV end-diastolic pressure determines exercise capacity. An alternative view is that left atrial systolic function contributes to LV end-diastolic pressure, preload reserve, and exercise capacity. Although Sachdev et al.[166] found that that left atrial size predicted exercise capacity in patients with nonobstructive HCM, they were unable to demonstrate that left atrial active emptying fraction, ejection force, and kinetic energy (all measurements obtained at rest) predicted exercise capacity.[167]

Left atrial PV studies and assessments of left atrial function during stress are largely lacking, although the few studies available for HCM suggest that decreased inotropic reserve and decreased atrial compliance accompany left atrial enlargement.[168–170] The role that primary abnormalities of atrial inotropic/reservoir function may have in abnormal LV filling remains largely theoretical. The potential for enhanced atrial function to compensate for abnormal LV relaxation/compliance and the characteristics of a secondary atrial myopathy that may develop in response to chronic and progressive LV disease deserve further evaluation.

Summary

There is ample evidence of diastolic abnormalities in HCM, but their role in determining functional status has been more difficult to demonstrate. More recent studies using tissue Doppler estimates of LV filling have demonstrated some relationship with exercise performance.

We have emphasized that HCM should not be regarded as a single disease, and that several abnormalities may be present concurrently. As such, it is not likely that a single pathophysiology leading to impaired LV filling will apply to all patients. An ability to parse abnormal filling into appropriate categories in terms of early relaxation, reduced LV passive chamber compliance, and abnormal atrial function requires the development of novel assessment strategies and will be essential for the design and testing of rational therapy.

Measurement Tools and Prospective Intervention Strategies

Therapeutic options for the symptomatic HCM patient without LVOTO are limited. Renin-angiotensin-aldosterone blockers, calcium antagonists, and statins have been suggested as potential treatments.[62,67,171–179] Each of these proposed therapies aims at a particular pathophysiologic abnormality, for example, at LV fibrosis/stiffness. The identification of appropriate patient groups and monitoring of therapy will require an ability to assess the components of LV filling. No readily available diagnostic techniques allow this, but echocardiographic approaches are likely to form the basis of any practical tool. The ideal tools will measure parameters that are load dependent in a linear or predictable way and will incorporate a mechanism to vary load. Noninvasive and easily obtained parameters or clinical surrogates would greatly assist in the monitoring of patients and treatments.

Novel Tools for Assessment and Monitoring

Doppler-derived indices may provide accurate estimates of LV filling abnormalities but will need to be validated against an acceptable gold standard in the appropriate patient group and clinical setting. This should involve prospective evaluation with comparisons with more than single LV filling pressure measurements under resting conditions.

A hybrid invasive–noninvasive tool using a combination of pulmonary artery catheterization and chamber volumes estimated by echocardiography has been used to demonstrate differences in LV compliance in sedentary versus athletic seniors.[137] A similar technique being developed for HCM incorporates load alteration by head-down and head-up tilting, measurement of chamber volumes and Doppler signals with echocardiography, and measurement of pressures with a pulmonary artery catheter (Figure 20.7). Preliminary results show significant alterations in LV filling pressures during tilt, allowing the construction of left atrial and LV PV curves.

Serum assays of collagen turnover and myocyte stretch may also prove useful for identifying target patient groups and for monitoring treatment but also should be validated. Collagen types I and III are generated from procollagens following the cleavage of small terminal peptides. The serum concentrations of procollagen type I C-terminal peptide (PIP) and procollagen type II N-terminal peptide (PIIINP) have been used as markers of LV fibrosis in patients with a variety of cardiac diseases. In patients with hypertensive heart disease,

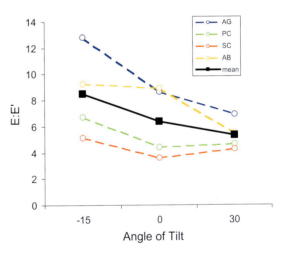

FIGURE 20.7. Echocardiographic tools for left ventricular filling assessment. Tilting will alter venous return and can provide a load stress for assessing left ventricular filling characteristics. This graph illustrates the changes in the value of E/Ea (see text) in four patients at three different angles of tilt: 15° head down, flat, and 15° head up. As E/Ea correlates with left ventricular filling pressure, the magnitude of change in E/Ea with tilt may reflect the magnitude of left ventricular diastolic pressure changes, providing a readily available noninvasive assessment parameter (unpublished data). Such parameters will need validation.

serum concentrations of both PIP and PIIINP are increased.[180–186] Concentrations of PIP correlate with the collagen volume fraction on endocardial biopsy, the magnitude of LV hypertrophy, the frequency of ventricular arrhythmias, and the echocardiographic measurements of diastolic abnormalities.[180–184,187]

Atrial natriuretic peptide and brain natriuretic peptide are circulating peptides synthesized and released by cardiac myocytes in response to wall stretch.[188] Plasma concentrations are elevated in patients with heart failure, HCM, and other valvular and myocardial diseases in which LV hypertrophy or chamber distention is prominent.[189–199] Patients with HCM have extremely elevated natriuretic peptide concentrations.[189,193–197,200] Concentrations at rest and changes following postural or exercise stress may parallel atrial distension and assist in the noninvasive assessment of diastolic function.

Potential Therapeutic Modalities

Although the expression of mutant sarcomeric protein function is fundamental for the development of myocardial disease in HCM, the mature disease phenotype incorporates consequences beyond the sarcomere as a result of unknown genetic and/or environmental interactions. Heterogeneity in the extent of these secondary effects must be responsible for some of the striking variability in disease expression and incomplete penetrance. The mechanisms underlying these secondary abnormalities are targets for intervention, the potential power of which is suggested by the spectrum of disease expression, which extends from a normal cardiac phenotype to severe hypertrophy, disabling symptoms and sudden death.

Although the various conditions causing LV hypertrophy concomitantly result in fibrosis, the development and regression of the two pathologic entities demonstrate temporal divergence and appear to be mechanistically dissimilar. In doses too small to cause regression of LV hypertrophy, the angiotensin-converting enzyme inhibitor lisinopril reduces fibrosis and normalizes myocardial stiffness in rats with spontaneous hypertension. Sub-antihypertensive doses of the aldosterone antagonist spironolactone prevent LV fibrosis but not LV hypertrophy in rats with hyperaldosteronism.[201,202] Similarly, in hypertensive patients, angiotensin receptor blockade with losartan reduces myocardial fibrosis and chamber stiffness. In contrast, reduction in both blood pressure and LV hypertrophy with the β-blocker labetalol is not accompanied by a reduction in collagen content or myocardial stiffness. These findings suggest that reverse remodeling of the collagen matrix may be possible by interventions aimed directly at the fibrotic process such as modulation of the renin-angiotensin-aldosterone system. Recently performed therapeutic studies with animals[171] and humans[62] with HCM provide strong initial evidence that renin-angiotensin-aldosterone inhibition also interrupts the fibrotic process in HCM. Clinical studies examining the efficacy in terms of prognosis and symptom status are currently lacking.

These and other potential therapies, including statin therapy,[203] calcium antagonists,[204–206] and even resynchronization pacing,[172] can be claimed, based on theoretical considerations, to improve LV filling in HCM; we need a better description of abnormal LV filling in HCM and better measurement tools to assess their plausibility and to evaluate their efficacy.

References

1. Elliott P, McKenna WJ. Hypertrophic cardiomyopathy. Lancet 2004;363(9424):1881–1891.
2. Maron BJ. Hypertrophic cardiomyopathy: a systematic review. JAMA 2002;287(10):1308–1320.
3. Cecchi F, et al. The Italian Registry for hypertrophic cardiomyopathy: a nationwide survey. Am Heart J 2005;150(5):947–954.
4. Maron BJ, et al. Epidemiology of hypertrophic cardiomyopathy-related death: revisited in a large non-referral-based patient population. Circulation 2000;102(8):858–864.
5. Kofflard MJ, et al. Hypertrophic cardiomyopathy in a large community-based population: clinical outcome and identification of risk factors for sudden cardiac death and clinical deterioration. J Am Coll Cardiol 2003;41(6):987–993.
6. Elliott PM, et al. Historical trends in reported survival rates in patients with hypertrophic cardiomyopathy. Heart 2006;92(6):785–791.
7. Maron BJ, et al. Clinical course of hypertrophic cardiomyopathy with survival to advanced age. J Am Coll Cardiol 2003;42(5):882–888.

8. Chikamori T, et al. Comparison of clinical features in patients greater than or equal to 60 years of age to those less than or equal to 40 years of age with hypertrophic cardiomyopathy. Am J Cardiol 1990; 66(10):875–878.

9. Lewis JF, Maron BJ. Elderly patients with hypertrophic cardiomyopathy: a subset with distinctive left ventricular morphology and progressive clinical course late in life. J Am Coll Cardiol 1989;13(1): 36–45.

10. Chen HH, et al. Diastolic heart failure in the community: clinical profile, natural history, therapy, and impact of proposed diagnostic criteria. J Card Fail 2002;8(5):279–287.

11. Redfield MM, et al. Burden of systolic and diastolic ventricular dysfunction in the community: appreciating the scope of the heart failure epidemic. JAMA 2003;289(2):194–202.

12. Redfield MM, et al. Age- and gender-related ventricular–vascular stiffening: a community-based study. Circulation 2005;112(15):2254–2262.

13. Senni M, et al. Congestive heart failure in the community: a study of all incident cases in Olmsted County, Minnesota, in 1991. Circulation 1998; 98(21):2282–2289.

14. Senni M, Redfield MM. Heart failure with preserved systolic function. A different natural history? J Am Coll Cardiol 2001;38(5):1277–1282.

15. Kitzman DW. Diastolic heart failure in the elderly. Heart Fail Rev 2002;7(1):17–27.

16. Maurer MS, et al. Left heart failure with a normal ejection fraction: identification of different pathophysiologic mechanisms. J Card Fail 2005;11(3):177–187.

17. Yang Z, et al. Danon disease as an underrecognized cause of hypertrophic cardiomyopathy in children. Circulation 2005;112(11):1612–1617.

18. Fananapazir L, et al. Missense mutations in the beta-myosin heavy-chain gene cause central core disease in hypertrophic cardiomyopathy. Proc Natl Acad Sci USA 1993;90(9):3993–3997.

19. Murphy RT, et al. Adenosine monophosphate-activated protein kinase disease mimics hypertrophic cardiomyopathy and Wolff-Parkinson-White syndrome: natural history. J Am Coll Cardiol 2005; 45(6):922–930.

20. Anastasakis A, et al. Subclinical skeletal muscle abnormalities in patients with hypertrophic cardiomyopathy and their relation to clinical characteristics. Int J Cardiol 2003;89(2–3):249–256.

21. Poetter K, et al. Mutations in either the essential or regulatory light chains of myosin are associated with a rare myopathy in human heart and skeletal muscle. Nat Genet 1996;13(1):63–69.

22. Wigle ED. Cardiomyopathy: the diagnosis of hypertrophic cardiomyopathy. Heart 2001;86(6): 709–714.

23. Fananapazir L, Epstein ND. Prevalence of hypertrophic cardiomyopathy and limitations of screening methods. Circulation 1995;92(4):700–704.

24. Maron BJ, et al. Prevalence of hypertrophic cardiomyopathy in a general population of young adults. Echocardiographic analysis of 4111 subjects in the CARDIA Study. Coronary Artery Risk Development in (Young) Adults. Circulation 1995; 92(4):785–789.

25. Marian AJ, Salek L, Lutucuta S. Molecular genetics and pathogenesis of hypertrophic cardiomyopathy. Minerva Med 2001;92(6):435–451.

26. Ahmad F, Seidman JG, Seidman CE. The genetic basis for cardiac remodeling. Annu Rev Genomics Hum Genet 2005;6:185–216.

27. Spirito P, Maron BJ. Absence of progression of left ventricular hypertrophy in adult patients with hypertrophic cardiomyopathy. J Am Coll Cardiol 1987;9(5):1013–1017.

28. Maron BJ, et al. Development and progression of left ventricular hypertrophy in children with hypertrophic cardiomyopathy. N Engl J Med 1986; 315(10):610–614.

29. Thaman R, et al. Progressive left ventricular remodeling in patients with hypertrophic cardiomyopathy and severe left ventricular hypertrophy. J Am Coll Cardiol 2004;44(2):398–405.

30. Koga Y, et al. Natural history of hypertrophic cardiomyopathy: Japanese experience. J Cardiol 2001; 37(Suppl 1):147–154.

31. Thaman R, et al. Prevalence and clinical significance of systolic impairment in hypertrophic cardiomyopathy. Heart 2005;91(7):920–925.

32. Biagini E, et al. Dilated-hypokinetic evolution of hypertrophic cardiomyopathy: prevalence, incidence, risk factors, and prognostic implications in pediatric and adult patients. J Am Coll Cardiol 2005;46(8):1543–1550.

33. Olivotto I, et al. Impact of atrial fibrillation on the clinical course of hypertrophic cardiomyopathy. Circulation 2001;104(21):2517–2524.

34. Doi Y, Kitaoka H. Hypertrophic cardiomyopathy in the elderly: significance of atrial fibrillation. J Cardiol 2001;37(Suppl 1):133–138.

35. Maron BJ, et al. Clinical profile of stroke in 900 patients with hypertrophic cardiomyopathy. J Am Coll Cardiol 2002;39(2):301–307.

36. Maron MS, et al. Effect of left ventricular outflow tract obstruction on clinical outcome in hypertrophic cardiomyopathy. N Engl J Med 2003;348(4): 295–303.

37. Wigle ED, et al. Hypertrophic cardiomyopathy. The importance of the site and the extent of hypertrophy. A review. Prog Cardiovasc Dis 1985;28(1):1–83.

38. Sherrid MV, et al. Systolic anterior motion begins at low left ventricular outflow tract velocity in obstructive hypertrophic cardiomyopathy. J Am Coll Cardiol 2000;36(4):1344–1354.

39. He S, et al. Importance of leaflet elongation in causing systolic anterior motion of the mitral valve. J Heart Valve Dis 1997;6(2):149–159.

40. Levine RA, et al. Papillary muscle displacement causes systolic anterior motion of the mitral valve. Experimental validation and insights into the mechanism of subaortic obstruction. Circulation 1995;91(4):1189–1195.

41. Yoganathan AP, et al. A three-dimensional computational investigation of intraventricular fluid dynamics: examination into the initiation of systolic anterior motion of the mitral valve leaflets. J Biomech Eng 1995;117(1):94–102.

42. Marin-Garcia J, Goldenthal MJ. Understanding the impact of mitochondrial defects in cardiovascular disease: a review. J Card Fail 2002;8(5):347–361.

43. Wilkins BJ, Molkentin JD. Calcium–calcineurin signaling in the regulation of cardiac hypertrophy. Biochem Biophys Res Commun 2004;322(4):1178–1191.

44. Chu G, Haghighi K, Kranias EG. From mouse to man: understanding heart failure through genetically altered mouse models. J Card Fail 2002;8(6 Suppl):S432–S449.

45. Richard P, et al. Hypertrophic cardiomyopathy: distribution of disease genes, spectrum of mutations, and implications for a molecular diagnosis strategy. Circulation 2003;107(17):2227–2232.

46. Mohiddin SA, et al. Utility of genetic screening in hypertrophic cardiomyopathy: prevalence and significance of novel and double (homozygous and heterozygous) beta-myosin mutations. Genet Test 2003;7(1):21–27.

47. Van Driest SL, et al. Myosin binding protein C mutations and compound heterozygosity in hypertrophic cardiomyopathy. J Am Coll Cardiol 2004;44(9):1903–1910.

48. Perkins MJ, et al. Gene-specific modifying effects of pro-LVH polymorphisms involving the renin-angiotensin-aldosterone system among 389 unrelated patients with hypertrophic cardiomyopathy. Eur Heart J 2005;26(22):2457–2462.

49. Marian AJ. Modifier genes for hypertrophic cardiomyopathy. Curr Opin Cardiol 2002;17(3):242–252.

50. Semsarian C, et al. A polymorphic modifier gene alters the hypertrophic response in a murine model of familial hypertrophic cardiomyopathy. J Mol Cell Cardiol 2001;33(11):2055–2060.

51. Tsoutsman T, Lam L, Semsarian C. Genes, calcium and modifying factors in hypertrophic cardiomyopathy. Clin Exp Pharmacol Physiol 2006;33(1–2):139–145.

52. Watkins H, et al. Characteristics and prognostic implications of myosin missense mutations in familial hypertrophic cardiomyopathy. N Engl J Med 1992;326(17):1108–1114.

53. Epstein ND, et al. Differences in clinical expression of hypertrophic cardiomyopathy associated with two distinct mutations in the beta-myosin heavy chain gene. A 908Leu–Val mutation and a 403Arg–Gln mutation. Circulation 1992;86(2):345–352.

54. Varnava AM, et al. Hypertrophic cardiomyopathy: histopathological features of sudden death in cardiac troponin T disease. Circulation 2001;104(12):1380–1384.

55. Karibe A, et al. Hypertrophic cardiomyopathy caused by a novel alpha-tropomyosin mutation (V95A) is associated with mild cardiac phenotype, abnormal calcium binding to troponin, abnormal myosin cycling, and poor prognosis. Circulation 2001;103(1):65–71.

56. Gruver EJ, et al. Familial hypertrophic cardiomyopathy and atrial fibrillation caused by Arg663His beta-cardiac myosin heavy chain mutation. Am J Cardiol 1999;83(12A):13H–18H.

57. Hughes SE, McKenna WJ. New insights into the pathology of inherited cardiomyopathy. Heart 2005;91(2):257–264.

58. Chung MW, Tsoutsman T, Semsarian C. Hypertrophic cardiomyopathy: from gene defect to clinical disease. Cell Res 2003;13(1):9–20.

59. Seidman JG, Seidman C. The genetic basis for cardiomyopathy: from mutation identification to mechanistic paradigms. Cell 2001;104(4):557–567.

60. Nagueh SF, et al. Evolution of expression of cardiac phenotypes over a 4-year period in the beta-myosin heavy chain-Q403 transgenic rabbit model of human hypertrophic cardiomyopathy. J Mol Cell Cardiol 2004;36(5):663–673.

61. Yamaji K, et al. Does the progression of myocardial fibrosis lead to atrial fibrillation in patients with hypertrophic cardiomyopathy? Cardiovasc Pathol 2001;10(6):297–303.

62. Araujo AQ, et al. Effect of Losartan on left ventricular diastolic function in patients with nonobstructive hypertrophic cardiomyopathy. Am J Cardiol 2005;96(11):1563–1567.

63. Lim DS, et al. Angiotensin II blockade reverses myocardial fibrosis in a transgenic mouse model of human hypertrophic cardiomyopathy. Circulation 2001;103(6):789–791.

64. Kawano H, et al. Valsartan decreases type I collagen synthesis in patients with hypertrophic cardiomyopathy. Circ J 2005;69(10):1244–1248.

65. Varnava AM, et al. Hypertrophic cardiomyopathy: the interrelation of disarray, fibrosis, and small vessel disease. Heart 2000;84(5):476–482.

66. Fassbach M, Schwartzkopff B. Elevated serum markers for collagen synthesis in patients with hypertrophic cardiomyopathy and diastolic dysfunction. Z Kardiol 2005;94(5):328–335.

67. Lombardi R, et al. Myocardial collagen turnover in hypertrophic cardiomyopathy. Circulation 2003;108(12):1455–1460.

68. Almquist AK, et al. Cardioverter-defibrillator implantation in high-risk patients with hypertrophic cardiomyopathy. Heart Rhythm 2005;2(8):814–819.

69. Begley DA, et al. Efficacy of implantable cardioverter defibrillator therapy for primary and secondary prevention of sudden cardiac death in hypertrophic cardiomyopathy. Pacing Clin Electrophysiol 2003;26(9):1887–1896.

70. Maron BJ, et al. Efficacy of implantable cardioverter-defibrillators for the prevention of sudden death in patients with hypertrophic cardiomyopathy. N Engl J Med 2000;342(6):365–373.

71. Elliott PM, et al. Sudden death in hypertrophic cardiomyopathy: identification of high risk patients. J Am Coll Cardiol 2000;36(7):2212–2218.

72. Knollmann BC, et al. Familial hypertrophic cardiomyopathy-linked mutant troponin T causes stress-induced ventricular tachycardia and Ca^{2+}-dependent action potential remodeling. Circ Res 2003;92(4):428–436.

73. Westfall MV, et al. Myofilament calcium sensitivity and cardiac disease: insights from troponin I isoforms and mutants. Circ Res 2002;91(6):525–531.

74. Varnava AM, et al. Relation between myocyte disarray and outcome in hypertrophic cardiomyopathy. Am J Cardiol 2001;88(3):275–279.

75. Cecchi F, et al. Coronary microvascular dysfunction and prognosis in hypertrophic cardiomyopathy. N Engl J Med 2003;349(11):1027–1035.

76. Frenneaux MP. Assessing the risk of sudden cardiac death in a patient with hypertrophic cardiomyopathy. Heart 2004;90(5):570–575.

77. Seggewiss H, Rigopoulos A. Management of hypertrophic cardiomyopathy in children. Paediatr Drugs 2003;5(10):663–672.

78. Hess OM, Sigwart U. New treatment strategies for hypertrophic obstructive cardiomyopathy: alcohol ablation of the septum: the new gold standard? J Am Coll Cardiol 2004;44(10):2054–2055.

79. Maron BJ, et al. The case for surgery in obstructive hypertrophic cardiomyopathy. J Am Coll Cardiol 2004;44(10):2044–2053.

80. Courtois M, Ludbrook PA, Kovacs SJ. Unsolved problems in diastole. Cardiol Clin 2000;18(3):653–667.

81. Zile MR, Brutsaert DL. New concepts in diastolic dysfunction and diastolic heart failure. Part II: causal mechanisms and treatment. Circulation 2002;105(12):1503–1508.

82. Kovacs SJ, Meisner JS, Yellin EL. Modeling of diastole. Cardiol Clin 2000;18(3):459–487.

83. Lemmon JD, Yoganathan AP. Computational modeling of left heart diastolic function: examination of ventricular dysfunction. J Biomech Eng 2000;122(4):297–303.

84. Kass DA. Assessment of diastolic dysfunction. Invasive modalities. Cardiol Clin 2000;18(3):571–586.

85. Braunwald E, Frahm C. Studies on Starling's law of the heart; IV. Observations on the hemodynamic functions of the left atrium in man. Circulation 1961;24:633–641.

86. Williams JF Jr, Sonnenblick EH, Braunwald E. Determinants of atrial contractile force in the intact heart. Am J Physiol 1965;209(6):1061–1058.

87. Hoit BD, et al. In vivo assessment of left atrial contractile performance in normal and pathological conditions using a time-varying elastance model. Circulation 1994;89(4):1829–1838.

88. Friedman HS, et al. Effects of cardiac glycosides on atrial contractile dysfunction after short-term atrial fibrillation. Chest 2000;118(4):1116–1126.

89. Lewis JF, Maron BJ. Cardiovascular consequences of the aging process. Cardiovasc Clin 1992;22(2):25–34.

90. Fleg JL. Alterations in cardiovascular structure and function with advancing age. Am J Cardiol 1986;57(5):33C–44C.

91. Galetta F, et al. Left ventricular diastolic function and carotid artery wall in elderly athletes and sedentary controls. Biomed Pharmacother 2004;58(8):437–442.

92. Cheitlin MD. Cardiovascular physiology-changes with aging. Am J Geriatr Cardiol 2003;12(1):9–13.

93. Gottdiener JS, et al. Left atrial volume, geometry, and function in systolic and diastolic heart failure of persons ±65 years of age (the cardiovascular health study). Am J Cardiol 2006;97(1):83–89.

94. Tabata T, et al. Influence of aging on left atrial appendage flow velocity patterns in normal subjects. J Am Soc Echocardiogr 1996;9(3):274–280.

95. Kistler PM, et al. Electrophysiologic and electroanatomic changes in the human atrium associated with age. J Am Coll Cardiol 2004;44(1):109–116.

96. Bers DM. Cardiac excitation-contraction coupling. Nature 2002;415(6868):198–205.

97. Cheng H, et al. Calcium sparks and $[Ca^{2+}]i$ waves in cardiac myocytes. Am J Physiol 1996;270(1 Pt 1):C148–C159.

98. Somura F, et al. Reduced myocardial sarcoplasmic reticulum Ca^{2+}-ATPase mRNA expression and biphasic force–frequency relations in patients with hypertrophic cardiomyopathy. Circulation 2001;104(6):658–663.

99. Semsarian C, et al. The L-type calcium channel inhibitor diltiazem prevents cardiomyopathy in a mouse model. J Clin Invest 2002;109(8):1013–1020.

100. Szczesna-Cordary D, et al. Familial hypertrophic cardiomyopathy-linked alterations in Ca^{2+} binding of human cardiac myosin regulatory light chain affect cardiac muscle contraction. J Biol Chem 2004;279(5):3535–3542.

101. Kirschner SE, et al. Hypertrophic cardiomyopathy-related beta-myosin mutations cause highly variable calcium sensitivity with functional imbalances among individual muscle cells. Am J Physiol Heart Circ Physiol 2005;288(3):H1242–H1251.

102. Kohler J, et al. Mutation of the myosin converter domain alters cross-bridge elasticity. Proc Natl Acad Sci USA 2002;99(6):3557–3562.

103. Keller DI, et al. Human homozygous R403W mutant cardiac myosin presents disproportionate enhancement of mechanical and enzymatic properties. J Mol Cell Cardiol 2004;36(3):355–362.

104. Crilley JG, et al. Hypertrophic cardiomyopathy due to sarcomeric gene mutations is characterized by impaired energy metabolism irrespective of the degree of hypertrophy. J Am Coll Cardiol 2003; 41(10):1776–1782.

105. Gomes AV, Venkatraman G, Potter JD. The miscommunicative cardiac cell: when good proteins go bad. Ann NY Acad Sci 2005;1047:30–37.

106. Oliveira SM, et al. Mutation analysis of AMP-activated protein kinase subunits in inherited cardiomyopathies: implications for kinase function and disease pathogenesis. J Mol Cell Cardiol 2003; 35(10):1251–1255.

107. Hughes SE. The pathology of hypertrophic cardiomyopathy. Histopathology 2004;44(5):412–427.

108. Breisch EA, White FC, Bloor CM. Myocardial characteristics of pressure overload hypertrophy. A structural and functional study. Lab Invest 1984;51(3):333–342.

109. Saetersdal TS, et al. Ultrastructural studies on the growth of filaments and sarcomeres in mechanically overloaded human hearts. Virchows Arch B Cell Pathol 1976;21(2):91–112.

110. Mundhenke M, et al. Myocardial collagen type I and impaired left ventricular function under exercise in hypertrophic cardiomyopathy. Thorac Cardiovasc Surg 2002;50(4):216–222.

111. Sugihara N, et al. Quantitation of myocardial fibrosis and its relation to function in essential hypertension and hypertrophic cardiomyopathy. Clin Cardiol 1988;11(11):771–778.

112. Tanaka M, et al. Quantitative analysis of myocardial fibrosis in normals, hypertensive hearts, and hypertrophic cardiomyopathy. Br Heart J 1986; 55(6):575–581.

113. Factor SM, et al. Pathologic fibrosis and matrix connective tissue in the subaortic myocardium of patients with hypertrophic cardiomyopathy. J Am Coll Cardiol 1991;17(6):1343–1351.

114. Anderson KR, Sutton MG, Lie JT. Histopathological types of cardiac fibrosis in myocardial disease. J Pathol 1979;128(2):79–85.

115. Moon JC, et al. The histologic basis of late gadolinium enhancement cardiovascular magnetic resonance in hypertrophic cardiomyopathy. J Am Coll Cardiol 2004;43(12):2260–2264.

116. Debl K, et al. Delayed hyperenhancement: frequent finding in magnetic resonance imaging of left ventricular hypertrophy due to aortic stenosis and hypertrophic cardiomyopathy. Heart 2006;92: 1447–1451.

117. Boerrigter G, et al. Immunohistochemical video-microdensitometry of myocardial collagen type I and type III. Histochem J 1998;30(11):783–791.

118. Jugdutt BI. Remodeling of the myocardium and potential targets in the collagen degradation and synthesis pathways. Curr Drug Targets Cardiovasc Haematol Disord 2003;3(1):1–30.

119. Diez J, et al. Mechanisms of disease: pathologic structural remodeling is more than adaptive hypertrophy in hypertensive heart disease. Nat Clin Pract Cardiovasc Med 2005;2(4):209–216.

120. Iida K, et al. Comparison of percentage area of myocardial fibrosis and disarray in patients with classical form and dilated phase of hypertrophic cardiomyopathy. J Cardiol 1998 32(3):173–180.

121. Spirito P, Watson RM, Maron BJ. Relation between extent of left ventricular hypertrophy and occurrence of ventricular tachycardia in hypertrophic cardiomyopathy. Am J Cardiol 1987;60(14):1137–1142.

122. Spirito P, et al. Diastolic abnormalities in patients with hypertrophic cardiomyopathy: relation to magnitude of left ventricular hypertrophy. Circulation 1985;72(2):310–316.

123. De Marchi SF, Allemann Y, Seiler C. Relaxation in hypertrophic cardiomyopathy and hypertensive heart disease: relations between hypertrophy and diastolic function. Heart 2000;83(6):678–684.

124. Wachtell K, et al. Left ventricular filling patterns in patients with systemic hypertension and left ventricular hypertrophy (the LIFE study). Losartan Intervention For Endpoint. Am J Cardiol 2000;85(4):466–472.

125. Redaelli A, et al. Haemodynamics and mechanics following partial left ventriculectomy: a computer modeling analysis. Med Eng Phys 2004;26(1):31–42.

126. Tsang TS, et al. Left atrial volume as a morphophysiologic expression of left ventricular diastolic dysfunction and relation to cardiovascular risk burden. Am J Cardiol 2002;90(12):1284–1289.

127. Simek CL, et al. Relationship between left ventricular wall thickness and left atrial size: comparison with other measures of diastolic function. J Am Soc Echocardiogr 1995;8(1):37–47.

128. Bouchard RJ, Gault JH, Ross J Jr. Evaluation of pulmonary arterial end-diastolic pressure as an estimate of left ventricular end-diastolic pressure in patients with normal and abnormal left ventricular performance. Circulation 1971;44(6):1072–1079.

129. Rahimtoola SH, et al. Left atrial transport function in myocardial infarction. Importance of its booster pump function. Am J Med 1975;59(5):686–694.

130. Dardas PS. et al. Noninvasive indexes of left atrial diastolic function in hypertrophic cardiomyopathy. J Am Soc Echocardiogr 2000;13(9):809–817.

131. Oki T, et al. Transesophageal pulsed Doppler echocardiographic evaluation of left atrial systolic performance in hypertrophic cardiomyopathy: combined analysis of transmitral and pulmonary venous flow velocities. Clin Cardiol 1997;20(1):47–54.

132. Reiser PJ, et al. Human cardiac myosin heavy chain isoforms in fetal and failing adult atria and ventricles. Am J Physiol Heart Circ Physiol 2001;280(4):H1814–H1820.

133. Schiaffino S, et al. Myosin changes in hypertrophied human atrial and ventricular myocardium. A correlated immunofluorescence and quantitative immunochemical study on serial cryosections. Eur Heart J 1984;5(Suppl F):95–102.

134. Pak PH, et al. Marked discordance between dynamic and passive diastolic pressure–volume relations in idiopathic hypertrophic cardiomyopathy. Circulation 1996;94(1):52–60.

135. Pak PH, et al. Mechanism of acute mechanical benefit from VDD pacing in hypertrophied heart: similarity of responses in hypertrophic cardiomyopathy and hypertensive heart disease. Circulation 1998;98(3):242–248.

136. Kass DA, et al. Use of a conductance (volume) catheter and transient inferior vena caval occlusion for rapid determination of pressure–volume relationships in man. Cathet Cardiovasc Diagn 1988;15(3):192–202.

137. Arbab-Zadeh A, et al. Effect of aging and physical activity on left ventricular compliance. Circulation 2004;110(13):1799–805.

138. Maron BJ, et al. Hypertrophic cardiomyopathy. Interrelations of clinical manifestations, pathophysiology, and therapy (1). N Engl J Med 1987;316(13):780–789.

139. Maron BJ, et al. Hypertrophic cardiomyopathy. Interrelations of clinical manifestations, pathophysiology, and therapy (2). N Engl J Med 1987;316(14):844–852.

140. Bonow RO, et al. Atrial systole and left ventricular filling in hypertrophic cardiomyopathy: effect of verapamil. Am J Cardiol 1983;51(8):1386–1391.

141. Alvares RF, Goodwin JF. Non-invasive assessment of diastolic function in hypertrophic cardiomyopathy on and off beta adrenergic blocking drugs. Br Heart J 1982;48(3):204–212.

142. Betocchi S, et al. Isovolumic relaxation period in hypertrophic cardiomyopathy: assessment by radionuclide angiography. J Am Coll Cardiol 1986;7(1):74–81.

143. Chen YT, et al. Left ventricular diastolic function in hypertrophic cardiomyopathy: assessment by radionuclide angiography. Int J Cardiol 1987;15(2):185–193.

144. Briguori C, et al. Exercise capacity in hypertrophic cardiomyopathy depends on left ventricular diastolic function. Am J Cardiol 1999;84(3):309–315.

145. Chikamori T, et al. Mechanisms of exercise limitation in hypertrophic cardiomyopathy. J Am Coll Cardiol 1992;19(3):507–512.

146. Lele SS, et al. Exercise capacity in hypertrophic cardiomyopathy. Role of stroke volume limitation, heart rate, and diastolic filling characteristics. Circulation 1995;92(10):2886–2894.

147. Matsumura Y, et al. Left ventricular diastolic function assessed using Doppler tissue imaging in patients with hypertrophic cardiomyopathy: relation to symptoms and exercise capacity. Heart 2002;87(3):247–251.

148. Nihoyannopoulos P, et al. Diastolic function in hypertrophic cardiomyopathy: relation to exercise capacity. J Am Coll Cardiol 1992;19(3):536–540.

149. Yetman AT, et al. Exercise capacity in children with hypertrophic cardiomyopathy and its relation to diastolic left ventricular function. Am J Cardiol 2001;87(4):491–493, A8.

150. Chan WL, et al. Effect of preload change on resting and exercise cardiac performance in hypertrophic cardiomyopathy. Am J Cardiol 1990;66(7):746–751.

151. Janicki JS, et al. The pressure–flow response of the pulmonary circulation in patients with heart failure and pulmonary vascular disease. Circulation 1985;72(6):1270–1278.

152. Higginbotham MB, et al. Regulation of stroke volume during submaximal and maximal upright exercise in normal man. Circ Res 1986;58(2):281–291.

153. Frenneaux MP, et al. Determinants of exercise capacity in hypertrophic cardiomyopathy. J Am Coll Cardiol 1989;13(7):1521–1526.

154. Kitzman DW, et al. Exercise intolerance in patients with heart failure and preserved left ventricular systolic function: failure of the Frank-Starling mechanism. J Am Coll Cardiol 1991;17(5):1065–1072.

155. Falicov RE, Resnekov L. Relationship of the pulmonary artery end-diastolic pressure to the left ventricular end-diastolic and mean filling pressures in patients with and without left ventricular dysfunction. Circulation 1970;42(1):65–73.

156. Gomez CM, Palazzo MG. Pulmonary artery catheterization in anaesthesia and intensive care. Br J Anaesth 1998;81(6):945–956.

157. Nagueh SF, et al. Doppler estimation of left ventricular filling pressures in patients with hypertrophic cardiomyopathy. Circulation 1999;99(2):254–261.

158. Nishimura RA, et al. Noninvasive Doppler echocardiographic evaluation of left ventricular filling pressures in patients with cardiomyopathies: a simultaneous Doppler echocardiographic and cardiac catheterization study. J Am Coll Cardiol 1996;28(5):1226–1233.

159. Ommen SR, et al. Clinical utility of Doppler echocardiography and tissue Doppler imaging in the estimation of left ventricular filling pressures: a comparative simultaneous Doppler-catheterization study. Circulation 2000;102(15):1788–1794.

160. Maron BJ, et al. Noninvasive assessment of left ventricular diastolic function by pulsed Doppler echocardiography in patients with hypertrophic cardiomyopathy. J Am Coll Cardiol 1987;10(4):733–742.

161. Ha JW, et al. Tissue Doppler–derived indices predict exercise capacity in patients with apical hypertrophic cardiomyopathy. Chest 2005;128(5):3428–3433.

162. Naqvi TZ, Diastolic function assessment incorporating new techniques in Doppler echocardiography. Rev Cardiovasc Med 2003;4(2):81–99.

163. Gibson DG, Francis DP. Clinical assessment of left ventricular diastolic function. Heart 2003;89(2):231–238.

164. Kidawa M, et al. Comparative value of tissue Doppler imaging and M-mode color Doppler mitral flow propagation velocity for the evaluation of left ventricular filling pressure. Chest 2005;128(4):2544–2550.

165. Jacques DC, et al. Influence of alterations in loading on mitral annular velocity by tissue Doppler echocardiography and its associated ability to predict filling pressures. Chest 2004;126(6):1910–1918.

166. Sachdev V, et al. Left atrial volumetric remodeling predicts functional capacity in hypertrophic cardiomyopathy. J Am Coll Cardiol 2003;41.

167. Shizukuda Y, et al. Is functional capacity related to left atrial contractile function in nonobstructive hypertrophic cardiomyopathy? Congest Heart Fail 2005;11(5):234–240.

168. Sanada H, et al. Increased left atrial chamber stiffness in hypertrophic cardiomyopathy. Br Heart J 1993;69(1):31–35.

169. Sanada H, et al. Left atrial afterload mismatch in hypertrophic cardiomyopathy. Am J Cardiol 1991;68(10):1049–1054.

170. Sanada H, et al. [Left atrial booster pump function in patients with hypertrophic cardiomyopathy and essential hypertension: evaluations based on left atrial pressure–volume relationship.] J Cardiol 1992;22(1):99–106.

171. Tsybouleva N, et al. Aldosterone, through novel signaling proteins, is a fundamental molecular bridge between the genetic defect and the cardiac phenotype of hypertrophic cardiomyopathy. Circulation 2004;109(10):1284–1291.

172. Waggoner AD, et al. Cardiac resynchronization therapy acutely improves diastolic function. J Am Soc Echocardiogr 2005;18(3):216–220.

173. Izawa H, et al. Effect of nicorandil on left ventricular end-diastolic pressure during exercise in patients with hypertrophic cardiomyopathy. Eur Heart J 2003;24(14):1340–1348.

174. Mottram PM, et al. Effect of aldosterone antagonism on myocardial dysfunction in hypertensive

175. Westermann D, et al. Diltiazem treatment prevents diastolic heart failure in mice with familial hypertrophic cardiomyopathy. Eur J Heart Fail 2006;8:115–121.

176. Hess OM, Grimm J, Krayenbuehl HP. Diastolic function in hypertrophic cardiomyopathy: effects of propranolol and verapamil on diastolic stiffness. Eur Heart J 1983;4(Suppl F):47–56.

177. Bakris GL, et al. Advanced glycation end-product cross-link breakers. A novel approach to cardiovascular pathologies related to the aging process. Am J Hypertens 2004;17(12 Pt 2):23S–30S.

178. Fedak PW, et al. Cardiac remodeling and failure: from molecules to man (part I). Cardiovasc Pathol 2005;14(1):1–11.

179. Muller-Ehmsen J, Schwinger RH. TNF and congestive heart failure: therapeutic possibilities. Expert Opin Ther Targets 2004;8(3):203–209.

180. Diez J, et al. Increased serum concentrations of procollagen peptides in essential hypertension. Relation to cardiac alterations. Circulation 1995;91(5):1450–1456.

181. Maceira AM, et al. Ultrasonic backscatter and serum marker of cardiac fibrosis in hypertensives. Hypertension 2002;39(4):923–928.

182. Maceira AM, et al. Ultrasonic backscatter and diastolic function in hypertensive patients. Hypertension 2002;40(3):239–243.

183. Lopez B, et al. Usefulness of serum carboxy-terminal propeptide of procollagen type I in assessment of the cardioreparative ability of antihypertensive treatment in hypertensive patients. Circulation 2001;104(3):286–291.

184. Diez J, et al. Clinical aspects of hypertensive myocardial fibrosis. Curr Opin Cardiol 2001 16(6):328–335.

185. Lindsay MM, Maxwell P, Dunn FG. TIMP-1: a marker of left ventricular diastolic dysfunction and fibrosis in hypertension. Hypertension 2002;40(2):136–141.

186. Sato A, Hayashi M, Saruta T. Relative long-term effects of spironolactone in conjunction with an angiotensin-converting enzyme inhibitor on left ventricular mass and diastolic function in patients with essential hypertension. Hypertens Res 2002;25(6):837–842.

187. Querejeta R, et al. Serum carboxy-terminal propeptide of procollagen type I is a marker of myocardial fibrosis in hypertensive heart disease. Circulation 2000;101(14):1729–1735.

188. Ruskoaho H, et al. Mechanisms of mechanical load-induced atrial natriuretic peptide secretion: role of endothelin, nitric oxide, and angiotensin II. J Mol Med 1997;75(11–12):876–885.

189. Murakami Y, et al. New insights into the mechanism of the elevation of plasma brain natriuretic polypeptide levels in patients with left ventricular hypertrophy. Can J Cardiol 2002;18(12):1294–1300.

190. Hasegawa K, et al. Light and electron microscopic localization of brain natriuretic peptide in relation to atrial natriuretic peptide in porcine atrium. Immunohistocytochemical study using specific monoclonal antibodies. Circulation 1991;84(3):1203–1209.

191. Pucci A, et al. Localization of brain and atrial natriuretic peptide in human and porcine heart. Int J Cardiol 1992;34(3):237–247.

192. Chen HH, Burnett JC. Natriuretic peptides in the pathophysiology of congestive heart failure. Curr Cardiol Rep 2000;2(3):198–205.

193. Fahy GJ, et al. Plasma atrial natriuretic peptide is elevated in patients with hypertrophic cardiomyopathy. Int J Cardiol 1996;55(2):149–155.

194. Nishigaki K, et al. Marked expression of plasma brain natriuretic peptide is a special feature of hypertrophic obstructive cardiomyopathy. J Am Coll Cardiol 1996;28(5):1234–1242.

195. Nakamura T, et al. Increased plasma brain natriuretic peptide level as a guide for silent myocardial ischemia in patients with non-obstructive hypertrophic cardiomyopathy. J Am Coll Cardiol 2002;39(10):1657–1663.

196. Sakamoto T, et al. B-type natriuretic peptide after percutaneous transluminal septal myocardial ablation. Int J Cardiol 2002;83(2):151–158.

197. Yoshibayashi M, et al. Increased plasma levels of brain natriuretic peptide in hypertrophic cardiomyopathy. N Engl J Med 1993;329(6):433–434.

198. Freitag MH, et al. Plasma brain natriuretic peptide levels and blood pressure tracking in the Framingham Heart Study. Hypertension 2003;41(4):978–983.

199. Gerber IL, et al. Increased plasma natriuretic peptide levels reflect symptom onset in aortic stenosis. Circulation 2003;107(14):1884–1890.

200. Begley D, et al. Brain natriuretic peptide in hypertrophic cardiomyopathy caused by sarcomeric gene mutations: a marker for poor outcome? J Am Coll Cardiol 2000;35(2 Suppl):191A.

201. Brilla CG, Maisch B. Regulation of the structural remodelling of the myocardium: from hypertrophy to heart failure. Eur Heart J 1994;15(Suppl D):45–52.

202. Brilla CG, Janicki JS, Weber KT. Cardioreparative effects of lisinopril in rats with genetic hyperten-

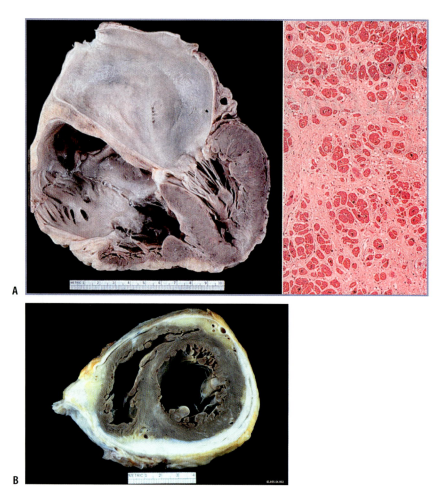

FIGURE 21.1. (A) Pathologic specimen of restrictive cardiomyopathy characterized by slightly thickened ventricular walls and biatrial enlargement due to limitation of ventricular filling. Microscopically, there was significant fibrosis in the ventricular myocardium. (B) Pathologic specimen of typical constrictive pericarditis. The pericardium was thickened circumferentially. Because of the abnormal pericardial encasement of both ventricles, the ventricular filling was limited with hemodynamic presentation similar to that of restrictive cardiomyopathy. (Courtesy of William Edwards, MD.)

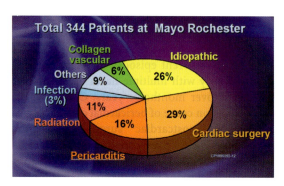

FIGURE 21.2. Diagram demonstrating etiologies of constrictive pericarditis at the Mayo Clinic, Rochester, Minnesota, in 344 patients who underwent pericardiectomy from 1998 to 2002. The most common causes of constriction were previous cardiac surgery, followed by previous pericarditis and radiation therapy. An idiopathic constrictive pericarditis represents a patient group with no known cause but is most likely related to a previous viral pericarditis.

constriction. Furthermore, the inflamed visceral and parietal pericardial layers become adherent and can cause constrictive physiology, which may be transient or progress to chronic irreversible constriction with a thickened and fibrotic pericardium.

Other etiologies of constriction include previous radiation therapy, collagen vascular diseases, rheumatoid arthritis, infection, and cardiac trauma. Tuberculosis may be an important cause of constriction in some parts of the world but is uncommon in modern societies. In a substantial number of cases, a definite etiology cannot be identified. Patients with idiopathic constrictive pericarditis usually have a longer duration of symptoms and increased incidence of calcified pericardium.[5] The constrictive process is usually gradual, and often the final presentation of constrictive pericardial syndrome can be remote from the inciting event.[6]

Pathophysiology

Constriction impacts diastolic filling of left and right cardiac chambers, which results in elevated left and right ventricular diastolic filling pressures as well as left and right atrial filling pressures. The reduced intracardiac volume results in reduced cardiac output, low blood pressure, and poor renal perfusion. Poor renal perfusion activates the renin-angiotensin-aldosterone system and compensatory salt and water retention, worsening volume load in the systemic venous system.[7] Tachycardia partially compensates for the low cardiac output because stroke volume remains fixed. In advanced or prolonged cases of pericardial constriction, left ventricular (LV) systolic function may also be depressed because of myocardial fibrosis or cellular atrophy.[8] During early diastole the atria and ventricles are in equilibration, and pressure changes in the right chambers are transmitted to the jugular veins. In fact, the atrial and jugular venous wave shows a prominent diastolic "Y" descent and a slightly less pronounced "X" single descent shortly after commencement of ventricular systole. During inspiration, failure of transmission of the negative intrathoracic pressure to the intrapericardial chambers translates into failure of the vena cava and right atrial pressures to decline. In fact, there may be an inspiratory increase in the right atrial and caval pressures recognized as Kussmaul's sign.[9] The thickened pericardium seals intracardiac hemodynamic changes from the intrathoracic pressure changes. With inspiration, the pressure gradient from the lungs via the pulmonary veins to the left cardiac chambers decreases, resulting in lower transmitral blood flow and decreased diastolic pulmonary venous flows. The reduced filling to the left ventricle allows an intraventricular septal shift to the left and an incremental flow across the tricuspid valve into the right ventricle. This results in increased diastolic hepatic vein forward flow and increased transtricuspid valve flow. With expiration, the opposite changes occur with enhanced pulmonary venous and transmitral flow; concomitantly there is reduced right heart flow and diastolic flow reversals in the hepatic veins (Figure 21.3).[10]

The disease is usually in the chronic phase when the diagnosis is made, and the clinical presentation is that of volume overload as manifested by peripheral edema, pleural effusions, and ascites

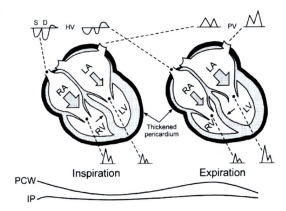

FIGURE 21.3. A diagram of a heart with a thickened pericardium to illustrate the respiratory variation in ventricular filling and the corresponding Doppler features of the mitral valve, tricuspid valve, pulmonary vein (PV), and hepatic vein (HV). These changes are related to discordant pressure changes in the thorax and to the intracardiac pressures. Pulmonary capillary wedge pressure (PCW) represents the pressure in the thorax, and intrapericardium (IP) represents the intracardiac pressures. The pressure difference between PCW and IP represents a driving pressure gradient to the left side of the heart that decreases with inspiration and increases with expiration. LA, left atrium; LV, left ventricle; RA, right atrium; RV, right ventricle. (Reprinted with permission from Oh JK, et al. The Second Echo Manual. Philadelphia: Lippincott Williams & Wilkins; 1999).

with exertional dyspnea. Not infrequently, patients with constrictive pericarditis are misdiagnosed as a primary gastrointestinal or hepatic disease and undergo unnecessary diagnostic procedures such as gastric endoscopy, liver biopsy, or even abdominal exploration.[4] However, cardiovascular examination is always abnormal with elevated jugular venous pressure, a prominent third heart sound, or pericardial knock. The electrocardiogram may show low voltages, because the thickened pericardium poorly transmits the electrical voltages of the myocardium. Mild electrolyte abnormalities of hyponatremia, hypokalemia, hypomagnesemia, and contraction metabolic alkalosis may be present either because of activation of the rennin-angiotensin-aldosterone system or because of aggressive and protracted diuretic use.

Diagnosis

The most important step for identifying constrictive pericarditis in patients with heart failure is to consider this entity especially when the ejection fraction is normal and one of the predisposing factors is present. If a chest x-ray demonstrates calcified pericardium in a patient with heart failure, the diagnosis of constrictive pericarditis is almost certain (Figure 21.4). However, calcified pericardium is detected in less than 25% of patients with constriction.[5] Although a thickened pericardium of 4 mm or more is helpful in diagnosing pericardial constriction, a normal pericardial thickness does not exclude the diagnosis. Inspection and measurement of surgically excised pericardia from patients with constriction failed to showed increased pericardial thickness in 18%.[11] Transthoracic echocardiography is not a good technique for detecting increased pericardial thickness, and transesophageal echocardiography is superior in assessing pericardial thickness.[12] However, computed tomography and magnetic resonance imaging are the best imaging techniques for measuring pericardial thickness (Figure 21.5).

The most available diagnostic modality that can reliably identify patients with constrictive pericarditis and differentiate it from restrictive cardiomyopathy or other myocardial diseases is comprehensive echocardiography.[10,13] By paying attention to structural, functional, and hemodynamic details of echocardiographic findings, we should be able to secure the diagnosis of constriction or restriction in almost all cases encountered in our clinical practice.

Ventricular septal motion is characteristically abnormal in patients with constrictive pericarditis because of the differential ventricular filling with respiration and increased interventricular dependence. Atria are enlarged more so in restrictive cardiomyopathy and constriction, but atrial enlargement cannot be used to differentiate one condition from the other. Inferior vena cava, hepatic vein, and pulmonary veins are dilated in both restrictive cardiomyopathy and constrictive pericarditis unless well treated with a diuretic agent. In constriction, the atrial ventricular groove may be indented with their characteristic waist appearance. In almost all patients, if not all, with restrictive cardiomyopathy, longitudinal systolic and diastolic motion of the heart is reduced.[14,15] This can be best assessed by tissue Doppler imaging but may be obvious on visual inspection of the mitral annulus from the parasternal long axis or apical four-chamber view. The longitudinal motion is relatively normal or even increased in constrictive pericarditis. Therefore two-dimensional echocardiography can provide several features of restriction or constriction if carefully observed; however, a definitive diagnosis requires documentation of unique hemodynamic features of constriction or restriction. Because atrial and diastolic filling pressures are elevated in symptomatic patients with both conditions, restrictive mitral and tricuspid inflow velocity is expected in constriction and restriction; the E/A ratio usually

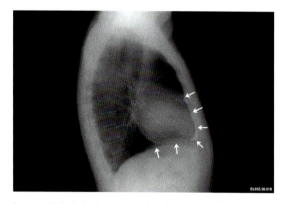

FIGURE 21.4. Lateral view of the chest x-ray demonstrating marked calcification of the pericardium (arrows). Anterior and diaphragmatic surfaces of the heart were covered by the calcified pericardium.

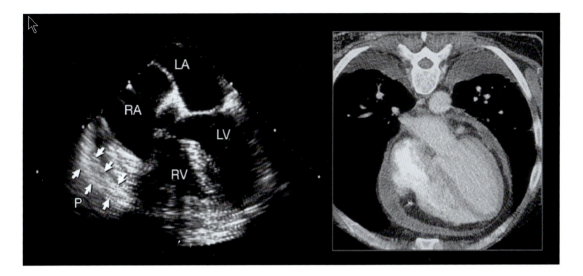

FIGURE 21.5. Transesophageal echocardiographic imaging of thickened pericardium (arrows; P) **(left)** and electron beam computed tomography scan **(right)** of the pericardium from the same patient showing thickened pericardium. LA, left atrium, LV, left ventricle; RA, right atrium; RV, right ventricle. (Reprinted with permission from Oh JK, et al. The Second Echo Manual. Philadelphia: Lippincott Williams & Wilkins; 1999).

of >1.5, and the E velocity deceleration time is <160 ms.

Additionally, however, in constrictive pericarditis there is usually, but not always, a characteristic variation in mitral early diastolic velocity E due to the following mechanism.[10,13] A thickened or inflamed pericardium prevents full transmission of the intrathoracic pressure changes that occur with respiration to the pericardial and intrathoracic cavities, creating respiratory variations in the left-side filling pressure gradient (the pressure difference between the pulmonary vein and the left atrium). With inspiration intrathoracic pressure falls 3–5 mm Hg normally, and the pressure in other intrathoracic structures such as pulmonary vein and pulmonary capillaries falls to a similar degree. This inspiratory pressure change is not fully transmitted to the intracardiac cavities in constrictive pericarditis (Figure 21.6). As a result, the driving pressure gradient for LV filling decreases immediately after inspiration and increases with expiration. This characteristic hemodynamic pattern is best illustrated by simultaneous pressure recordings from the LV and the pulmonary capillary wedge pressure together with the mitral inflow velocities. Therefore, the peak E velocity is reduced with inspiration.

Initially Hatle et al.[10] proposed 25% or greater variation of mitral inflow E velocity as diagnostic for constrictive pericarditis based on their observation of seven patients with constriction. However, further clinical experience with a larger number of patients suggested that a substantial portion of the patients with constriction may have less than 25% variation or even no respiratory variation because of additional myocardial disease or markedly elevated filling pressure.[16,17] Unlike myocardial disease, a deceleration time of mitral E velocity shortens in constrictive pericarditis further with a reduced E velocity with inspiration (Figure 21.7). There is a corresponding respiratory variation in pulmonary venous diastolic forward flow velocities in constrictive pericarditis. Respiratory variation in tricuspid inflow velocity is completely opposite to that of mitral inflow velocity. Hepatic vein flow velocity has more predominant diastolic forward flow velocity in both restrictive cardiomyopathy and constriction, but hepatic vein flow reversals occur during opposite respiratory cycles in these conditions (Figure 21.8A). In restrictive cardiomyopathy, hepatic vein diastolic flow reversal is mostly during inspiration when systemic venous return is increased and exceeds the filling capacity of the diseased myocardium (Figure 21.8B). Therefore, both forward and reverse flow in the hepatic vein increases with the inspiration and decreases with expiration in restrictive cardiomyopathy.

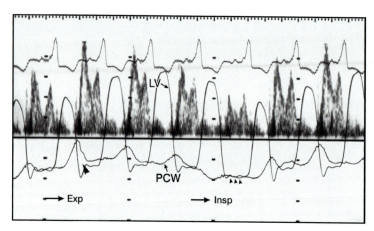

FIGURE 21.6. Simultaneous recordings from the left ventricle (LV) and the pulmonary capillary wedge pressure (PCW) together with mitral inflow Doppler velocities. The onset of the respiratory phase is indicated at the bottom. Exp, expiration; Insp, inspiration. With the onset of expiration, PCW increases much more than the LV diastolic pressures, creating a large increase in pressure gradient (large arrowhead). With inspiration, however, PCW decreases much more than the LV diastolic pressure, with a decreased driving pressure gradient (three small arrowheads). This respiratory change in the LV filling gradient is well reflected by the changes in the mitral inflow velocities recorded on Doppler echocardiography. (Reprinted with permission from Oh JK, et al. The Second Echo Manual. Philadelphia: Lippincott Williams & Wilkins; 1999).

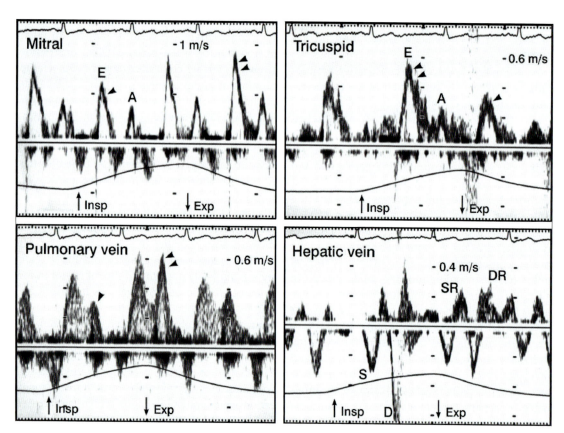

FIGURE 21.7. Pulsed-wave Doppler recording of the mitral inflow, tricuspid inflow, pulmonary vein, and hepatic vein velocities of constrictive pericarditis with a simultaneous recording of respiration. Exp, expiration; Insp, inspiration; SR, systolic reversal; DR, diastolic reversal. (Reprinted with permission from Oh JK, et al. The Second Echo Manual. Philadelphia: Lippincott Williams & Wilkins; 1999).

21. Pericarditis and Cardiomyopathy

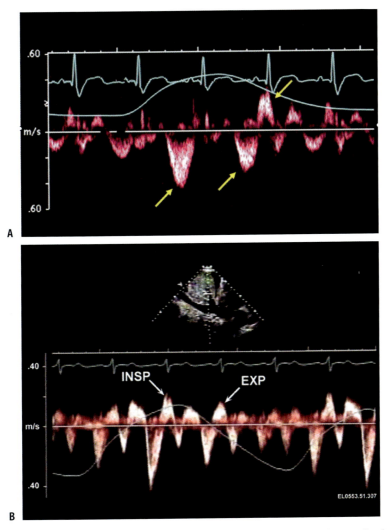

FIGURE 21.8. **(A)** Hepatic vein pulsed-wave Doppler recording of constrictive pericarditis along with simultaneous respirometry recording. With inspiration, forward velocity increases (first upward arrow), but with expiration forward flow velocity decreases (second upward arrow) and diastolic flow reversal increases markedly (downward arrow). These findings are typical of constrictive pericarditis. **(B)** Hepatic vein Doppler recording from a patient with a myopathy. With inspiration (INSP), both forward flow and reverse flow increase. With expiration (EXP), both forward and reversed flow decrease opposite to the hepatic vein of constrictive pericarditis shown in A. On top, a dilated hepatic vein is shown with a sample volume for Doppler examination.

However, in constriction, right ventricular cavity size becomes larger during inspiration because of the decreased LV filling and the ventricular septal shift to the left (Figure 21.9). With expiration, the right ventricle becomes smaller with the ventricular septal shift to the right, and there is increased diastolic flow reversal as well as a decreased forward flow velocity. This is completely paradoxical to respiratory phasic changes of hepatic venous flow seen in restrictive cardiomyopathy. This characteristic hepatic venous flow velocity pattern in constriction has been observed even in the concomitant presence of atrial fibrillation or with severe tricuspid valve regurgitation. The sensitivity of two-dimensional and Doppler echocardiography using the above criteria for detecting constriction is greater than 85% but has been enhanced by additional tissue Doppler imaging which increased the specificity of Doppler echocardiography for diagnosing constrictive

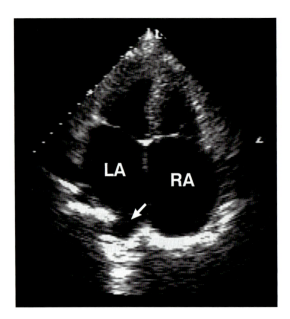

FIGURE 21.12. Typical apical four-chamber view of primary restrictive cardiomyopathy. Ventricular dimensions are normal, but both atria are markedly enlarged, as well as the pulmonary vein (arrow). LA, left atrium; RA, right atrium.

graphic equipment. Extracardiac manifestations of the underlying disease or other two-dimensional features such as apical thrombus with peripheral eosinophilia help make the diagnosis of hypereosinophilic syndrome (Figure 21.13). In Doppler studies, there is no ventricular interdependence. Hepatic vein Doppler imaging demonstrates diastolic flow reversal with inspiration in symptomatic patients with restrictive cardiomyopathy (see Figure 21.8B).

The other differentiating features on echocardiography in restrictive cardiomyopathy are the absence of respiratory variation in cardiac hemodynamics across the left and right atrioventricular valves and the reduced Ea velocity of the mitral annulus (Figure 21.14). Color M-mode echocardiography demonstrated a reduced propagation velocity of mitral inflow in restrictive cardiomyopathy, whereas it is relatively normal in constriction.[14–16] If LV cavity size is small, it is, however,

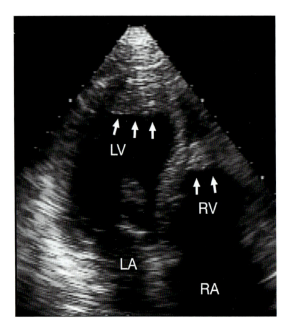

FIGURE 21.13. Apical four-chamber view of hypereosinophilic syndrome involving the heart. Both apices are filled with eosinophilic thrombus (arrows). LA, left atrium; LV, left ventricle; RA, right atrium; RV, right ventricle.

21. Pericarditis and Cardiomyopathy

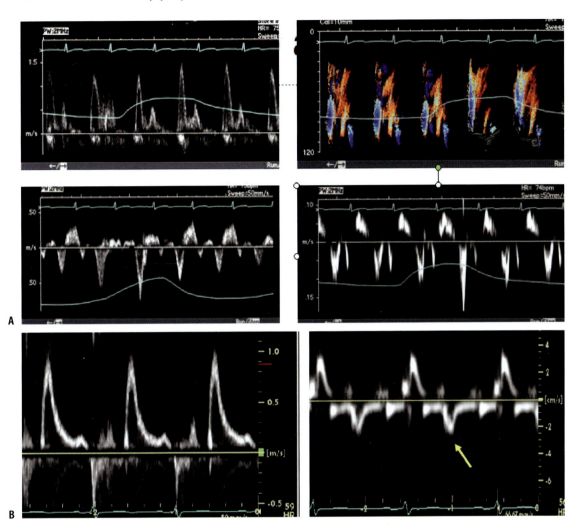

FIGURE 21.14. (A) Characteristic Doppler findings in constrictive pericarditis: mitral inflow velocity (upper left), color M-mode image of mitral inflow with normal propagation velocity and respiratory variation of E velocity (upper right), hepatic vein velocity with diastolic flow reversal with expiration (lower left), and tissue Doppler velocity of the mitral annulus showing increased early diastolic velocity with respiratory variation (lower right). (B) Mitral inflow velocity (left) and tissue Doppler recording (right) of restrictive cardiomyopathy. Mitral inflow velocity has characteristic restrictive inflow with increased E velocity and a short deceleration time. Early diastolic mitral annulus velocity (arrow, 2 cm/s) is markedly reduced.

possible to have falsely normal mitral inflow propagation velocity. Because color propagation velocity as determined by color M-mode and tissue Doppler imaging of the mitral annulus provide similar information, color-M mode does not appear to have increased diagnostic value.

Cardiac amyloid is the most common of the secondary restrictive cardiomyopathies. It is recognized by the presence of extra cardiac amyloid (renal, carpal tunnel syndrome, etc.). Cardiac involvement in amyloidosis portends a poor prognosis.[40,41] Regardless of the type of amyloid (primary, secondary to myeloma, senile, or due to chronic inflammatory conditions), the cardiac findings are essentially the same. Cardiac amyloid is characterized by increased left and right ventricular wall thickness, although normal wall thickness cannot exclude the diagnosis of small pericardial effusion and multivalvular mild regurgitation due to amyloid infiltration of the valve. There may be LV outflow obstruction with systolic anterior motion of the mitral valve.[42]

Restrictive diastolic function is noted when advanced in the presentation. Idiopathic hypereosinophilic syndrome is defined as an elevated eosinophil count exceeding 1,500/μL for at least 6 months and absence of an underlying cause for the eosinophilia.[43]

Cardiac involvement has three stages: asymptomatic necrotic stage, intracavitary thrombi stage, and the final fibrotic stage with endomyocardial fibrosis and damage to the atrioventricular valve. Echocardiographic findings usually demonstrate apical obliteration by thrombus, atrial enlargement, diastolic dysfunction, and relatively preserved systolic function.[44] Atrioventricular valve involvement is common. Computed tomography and magnetic resonance imaging in restrictive cardiomyopathy have a limited role, as wall thickness and the morphology of the atria and ventricles can be assessed by echocardiography.

Treatment

The prognosis for restrictive cardiomyopathy is heterogeneous and depends on the underlying etiology. However, even in the same etiologic category, prognosis differs and depends on extracardiac involvement in part or on the extent of myocardial involvement in a particular patient. The pattern of diastolic dysfunction also has a prognostic implication within the same disease class.[40] Treatment essentially is directed at symptomatic relief, which lowers systemic venous overload and pulmonary venous congestion. Diuretics should be used with the cognition that excess may worsen cardiac output and precipitate fatigue and hypotension. Digoxin should not be used in amyloid heart disease or in a restrictive cardiomyopathy that exhibits relative bradycardia or elements of heart block. The most curative therapy is cardiac transplantation.

New Invasive Hemodynamic Features to Differentiate Constriction From Restriction

Despite the different pathophysiologic mechanisms of constrictive pericarditis and restrictive cardiomyopathy, they share many similar invasive hemodynamic findings. Both have increased atrial pressures and equalization of end-diastolic pressures, although the equalization is more common in constrictive pericarditis. The dip and plateau pattern seen in ventricular diastolic pressure tracings have classically been associated with constriction. This finding reflects rapid early diastolic filling of the ventricles, followed by an abrupt cessation of filling in mid and late diastole. This pattern is also found in restrictive cardiomyopathy and is the result of the noncompliant myocardium limiting mid and late diastolic filling.

As in noninvasive evaluation, one must use respiratory variation in ventricular filling to differentiate between constriction and restriction during cardiac catheterization. The dissociation between intrathoracic and intracardiac pressures in constriction causes a respiratory variation in pressure difference between pulmonary capillary wedge pressure and LV diastolic pressure (see Figure 21.6) Therefore, there is less filling of the LV and the LV systolic pressure decreases with inspiration, while filling increases in the right ventricle resulting in an increase in right ventricular systolic pressure. With expiration, LV filling increases, which raises LV systolic pressure, and right ventricular filling decreases, resulting in a lower right ventricular systolic pressure. This reciprocal diastolic filling in the left and right ventricles causes a discordant systolic pressure change between them in constriction.[39] Because this respiratory differential filling originates from the left side of the heart, the LV pressure will decrease at an early phase of inspiration and the right ventricular systolic pressure increases toward the end of inspiration (Figure 21.15). In restrictive cardiomyopathy, however, hemodynamic changes are the result of the stiff ventricular myocardium. The intrathoracic pressures are transmitted to the myocardium, and the pressure gradient between the pulmonary capillary wedge pressure and the LV diastolic pressure remains constant throughout the respiratory cycle. Simultaneous pressure measurement of the left and right ventricles will be concordant throughout the respiratory cycle so that with inspiration the decrease in intrathoracic pressure causes a decrease in LV and right ventricular systolic pressures equally. Therefore, the unique hemodynamic features of constriction, interventricular interaction, variation in ventricu-

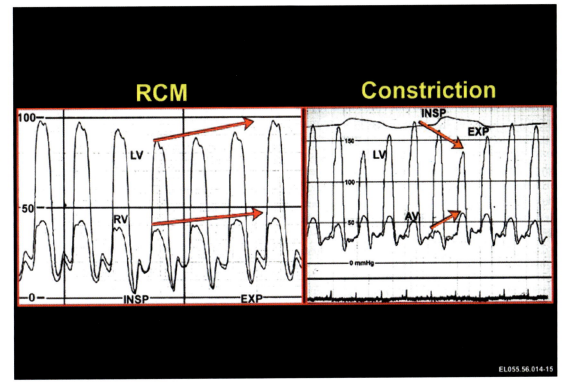

FIGURE 21.15. Simultaneous left ventricular (LV) and right ventricular (RV) pressure tracings from restrictive cardiomyopathy and constrictive pericarditis. In both conditions, there is equalization of ventricular end-diastolic pressures and "square root" sign (or "dip and plateau"). However, in restrictive cardiomyopathy there was a concordant change in the LV and RV systolic pressures with respiration, whereas there was a discordant pressure change in the LV and RV systolic pressures with respiration in constrictive pericarditis. EXP, expiration; INSP, inspiration.

lar filling with respiration, and discordant systolic pressure change in the right and left ventricles need to be demonstrated to diagnose constrictive pericarditis.

Endomyocardial Biopsy

An endomyocardial biopsy procedure may be performed for patients expected to have restrictive cardiomyopathy. The biopsy is usually done to exclude a specific heart muscle disease such as amyloid or sarcoidosis. Biopsy tissue may show idiopathic restrictive cardiomyopathy that demonstrates nonspecific fibrosis with increased collagen deposition and myocellular hypertrophy without necrosis or disarray. The diagnostic yield is low and rarely useful in distinguishing restrictive cardiomyopathy from constrictive pericarditis.

Conclusion

The differentiation of pericardial constriction from restrictive cardiomyopathy remains a diagnostic challenge for clinicians. For patients presenting with symptoms of congestive heart failure and a normal ejection fraction for whom a diagnosis of pericardial constriction or restrictive cardiomyopathy is under consideration, the distinction is of paramount importance because management and prognosis hinge on an accurate diagnosis. Noninvasive testing is increasingly beneficial with detailed echocardiographic examinations including a complete Doppler study with function are not well known because of limited access to invasive measures in healthy individuals. The effect on LV relaxation has been investigated in only one small human study, and it failed to show an effect of normal aging on global LV relaxation.[14] A number of animal studies, however, suggest that aging is associated with slowing of LV relaxation, possibly because of decreased Ca^{2+} uptake by the sarcoplasmic reticulum. Furthermore, LV diastolic compliance may be reduced in the elderly, an effect that may be secondary to deconditioning.[15]

Diastolic function in the elderly should be assessed using the same methods as for younger individuals. In the elderly, however, normal values are different, and filling patterns that are considered abnormal in young people may be quite normal in the elderly. This implies that age should be taken into account when the Doppler techniques are used to measure diastolic function. There is a need for more studies that define normality for transmitral velocities and tissue Doppler variables in the elderly.

How to Diagnose Diastolic Heart Failure

The diagnosis of heart failure is based on history, clinical examination, and objective measures of cardiac dysfunction. Symptoms and signs include dyspnea, tachypnea, cough, and abnormal auscultatory findings over heart and lungs. There may also be secondary right-sided heart failure with distended neck veins and other signs of elevated central venous pressure. The hemodynamic hallmarks of diastolic dysfunction are impaired LV relaxation and increased diastolic stiffness, which lead to compensatory elevation of LV filling pressure.

Consistent with the recent consensus report from the European Study Group on Diastolic Heart Failure,[3] we recommend that the diagnosis of DHF be restricted to patients for whom there is objective evidence that supports the diagnosis. Because invasive studies are rarely available, the objective diagnostic evidence is most often limited to noninvasive data. The most important diagnostic information comes from Doppler echo-

cardiographic examinations and includes cardiac functional as well as structural data. Atrial natriuretic peptides provide additional diagnostic information, but have a limited role.

Invasive Methods

Measurement of Left Ventricular Filling Pressure

The term *left ventricular filling pressure* is used for both left atrial mean pressure and LV end-diastolic pressure. There is often a slight difference between the two pressures, but this is rarely of clinical significance as long as there is no mitral stenosis. Left atrial pressure is a more direct determinant of pulmonary capillary pressure, whereas LV end-diastolic pressure is the best measure of preload when studying LV mechanical function. In rare cases, left atrial pressure and LV end-diastolic pressure do not reflect preload, as in cardiac tamponade and during mechanical ventilation with positive end-expiratory pressure, when LV end-diastolic pressure is elevated because of increased pressure external to the ventricle. In these cases, LV transmural pressure provides a measure of true preload as discussed in Chapter 3. In general, however, both left atrial pressure and LV end-diastolic pressure are excellent measures of LV preload, and for clinical purposes they can be used interchangeably.

In patients undergoing left heart catheterization, LV filling pressure can be measured directly as LV end-diastolic pressure, and during right heart catheterization LV filling pressure can be estimated using balloon-tipped, flow-directed pulmonary artery catheters. The latter approach provides pulmonary capillary wedge pressure, which is an indirect and in most cases an accurate measure of mean left atrial pressure. Alternatively, one may use pulmonary artery diastolic pressure as an estimate of mean left atrial pressure, provided there is normal pulmonary circulation and no significant mitral regurgitation.

Measurement of Left Ventricular Relaxation

Global LV relaxation can be quantified by measuring how rapidly LV pressure falls during iso-

22. Summary

volumic relaxation. This is measured as the time constant of LV isovolumic pressure fall (*tau*). When *tau* is prolonged, it indicates slowing of global LV relaxation. Measurement of *tau* requires high sensitivity catheters and cannot be done with the fluid-filled catheters that are used during routine left heart catheterization. Special catheters with a micropressure sensor mounted at the tip of the catheter are needed to obtain satisfactory data quality. These micromanometer-tipped catheters, however, are too expensive to be used in routine catheterizations. Furthermore, the added diagnostic value of measuring tau has not been fully explored. Therefore, invasive assessment of LV relaxation is rarely justified in clinical practice.

Assessment of Left Ventricular Stiffness

Evaluation of LV passive elastic properties is done almost exclusively as part of research protocols, but understanding the underlying concepts is important for interpretation of noninvasive measures of diastolic function. The evaluation of passive elastic properties requires combined measurement of LV pressures and dimension and preferably LV pressure–volume curves, as explained in Chapter 9. In this regard, it is important to understand the distinction between LV chamber properties and myocardial properties. Left ventricular myocardial passive elastic properties are difficult to measure in patients, even with the most sophisticated invasive methodology. What can be measured in patients are LV chamber properties, which are calculated from simultaneous measurements of LV intracavitary pressure and volume, giving rise to the LV diastolic pressure–volume relationship. The slope and the position of the LV diastolic pressure–volume curve define LV passive elastic properties. Both a reduction in slope, which implies a reduction in chamber compliance, and a parallel upward shift in the diastolic pressure–volume so that a higher pressure is needed to obtain a similar LV volume indicate a stiffer ventricle. In principle, LV chamber stiffness can change because of a change in LV myocardial properties but also because of interactions with the right ventricle, the pericardium, and with the lungs. In Chapter 3 it is explained how elevated right ventricular dia-

stolic pressure, as during pulmonary embolism, can shift the interventricular septum toward the left ventricle and reduce LV diastolic volume. The chapter also explains how changes in pericardial pressure can modify the LV diastolic pressure–volume relationship. The most well-known example of the latter is cardiac tamponade, which leads to an increase in LV chamber stiffness but no change in myocardial stiffness. Interactions with the lungs are clinically important during mechanical ventilation with positive end-expiratory pressure. Because of elevated pleural pressure during positive end-expiratory pressure, the LV becomes compressed, leading to a shift in the LV diastolic pressure–volume curve, consistent with a less compliant left ventricle. Importantly, in all these examples of changes in extraventricular pressure there is no change in the passive elastic properties of the LV myocardium. As outlined in Chapter 3, in experimental studies it is possible to differentiate between changes in LV chamber properties and changes in LV myocardial properties ("true myocardial compliance") by measuring simultaneous LV and pericardial pressures, thereby obtaining the LV transmural pressure–volume curve.

Noninvasive Methods

Evaluation of Left Ventricular Filling Patterns

Pulmonary venous, transmitral, and intraventricular filling patterns reflect changes in LV diastolic function, and a myriad of indices have been proposed for evaluation of diastolic function. In daily routine, however, measurements can be restricted to transmitral flow velocities and mitral annular velocities. Based on these variables, three different patterns of transmitral filling have been defined and serve as a means to grade diastolic dysfunction (see Chapters 6 and 10).

In the early stages of diastolic dysfunction there is typically slowing of LV relaxation, which causes a decrease in peak E velocity and a compensatory increase in peak A velocity. This shift in filling from early to late diastole, measured as a decrease in the E/A ratio, is described as a pattern of *impaired relaxation* (see Chapter 10). As heart failure progresses and left atrial pressure becomes elevated, there is an increase in the early diastolic transmitral pressure gradient, which increases peak E velocity, and the E/A ratio may become normal. This is described as a *pseudonormalized* filling pattern. When heart failure progresses further, left atrial pressure may become markedly elevated, and the early diastolic transmitral pressure gradient increases, leading to supernormal peak E velocity. Because elevation in LV diastolic pressure causes the ventricle to operate on a steeper portion of its pressure–volume curve, indicating reduced chamber compliance, there is little further increase in LV volume during atrial contraction. This is measured as a small and abbreviated transmitral A velocity. Furthermore, because of reduced LV chamber compliance, the early transmitral filling velocity decelerates rapidly. This filling pattern with increased E/A ratio and short E deceleration time is described as *restrictive physiology*. An additional feature of this filling pattern is abbreviated isovolumic relaxation time due to premature opening of the mitral valve caused by the elevated left atrial pressure.

Because assessment of mitral flow velocities alone does not differentiate between pseudonormal and true normal filling, there is need for an additional technique. The best and easiest additional method is measurement of peak early diastolic mitral annulus velocity (E′), which is reduced in patients with pseudonormalized filling. In patients with impaired relaxation and restrictive physiology there is also reduced E′ (Figure 22.1).

In simple terms, E′ can be considered an index of early diastolic filling volume, and transmitral E

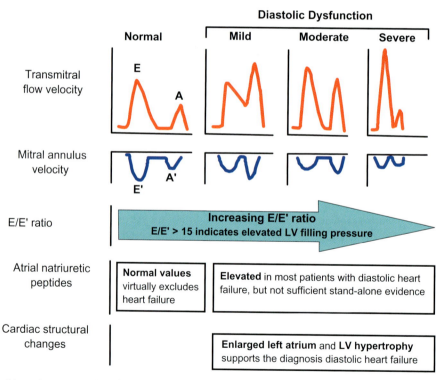

FIGURE 22.1. Schematic representation of noninvasive methods to diagnose diastolic heart failure. Diastolic dysfunction is supported by demonstration of abnormal transmitral and mitral ring velocities. Progression from mild to severe diastolic dysfunction is associated with an increasing E/E′ velocity ratio and reflects an increasing left ventricular (LV) filling pressure; an E/E′ >15 supports filling pressures >15 mm Hg, and an E/E′ ratio <8 supports a normal filling pressure. For an E/E′ ratio of 8–15, other indices should be used to estimate filling pressure. Atrial natriuretic peptide levels are used mainly to exclude heart failure and have limited positive predictive value. An enlarged left atrium and left ventricular hypertrophy support the diagnosis of diastolic heart failure.

22. Summary

reflects the transmitral pressure gradient. If transmitral E is tall and E′ is low, it means that a high transmitral driving pressure results in only a small filling volume and is consistent with a stiff ventricle and thus with diastolic dysfunction.

Estimation of Left Ventricular Filling Pressure

Over the past two decades a number of Doppler echocardiographic indices have been proposed as clinical semiquantitative measures of LV filling pressure. Most of these indices, however, have only a weak or variable relationship to LV filling pressure and are not suited for clinical decision making. One approach, however, the ratio between peak early diastolic mitral flow velocity and mitral annular velocity (E/E′), has proven clinically useful and is currently the best noninvasive method for estimating LV filling pressure.

There are two factors that explain why an increased E/E′ is associated with elevated left atrial pressure. First, peak transmitral flow velocity (E) is determined by the transmitral pressure difference, and therefore a tall transmitral E means a high transmitral pressure gradient. Second, a reduced E′ implies slow LV relaxation and therefore minimum diastolic pressure is elevated. The combination of an elevated transmitral pressure difference (tall E) and an elevated minimum LV diastolic pressure (reduced E′) means that left atrial pressure is elevated. One advantage of considering the E/E′ ratio is that effects of normal aging appear to be eliminated, and the ratio becomes an index of filling pressure.

When the E/E′ exceeds 15 it is associated with an LV filling pressure >15 mm Hg, and an E/E′ <8 suggests normal filling pressure. In the E/E′ range of 8–15, other information must be applied to estimate LV end-diastolic pressure. These methods are described in Chapter 13. In patients with a well-defined pulmonary venous flow reversal, it is possible to measure peak velocity and duration of retrograde flow during atrial contraction, and these measures can be used to estimate level of LV filling pressure. It is important to be aware that the values for E/E′ ratios are based on E′ recorded by pulsed tissue Doppler imaging, which gives peak velocities. This is in contrast to measuring E′

by two-dimensional color mode, which provides mean velocities and are approximately 20%–30% lower than peak velocities.

Another method is based on estimation of systolic pulmonary artery pressure from the systolic tricuspid gradient by continuous wave Doppler. If pulmonary artery pressure is elevated, it most likely is due to elevated LV filling pressure. Important limitations to this approach are lung disease and severe mitral regurgitation, but both of these conditions can usually be sorted out. Systolic pulmonary artery pressure is estimated as the sum of right atrial pressure and the systolic tricuspid pressure gradient.

Estimation of Right Atrial Pressure

In contrast to the left side of the heart, the venous system on the right side can be inspected clinically, and its pressure level can be assessed with reasonable accuracy. The jugular veins can be evaluated in most patients and are well suited for estimating central venous pressure. In particular, the internal jugular veins are suited, as there is only a trivial pressure gradient between the veins and the right atrium because there are no valves in this segment of the veins. Therefore, the internal jugular vein represents a "manometer" of right atrial pressure. Importantly, the vein column is not visible as a vessel, but the pulsations of the veins can be seen, and the highest level of venous pulsations indicates the venous pressure level. The patient is placed at an angle that allows the upper level of the venous column to be identified. The vertical distance from the sternal angle to the upper level of the pulsations is measured. Because the sternal angle is approximately 4–5 cm above the right atrium regardless of the patient's position, central venous pressure is calculated at the sum of vertical height plus 4–5 cm. There is also an echocardiographic method to estimate right atrial pressure based on vena cava diameter reduction during inspiration.

Magnetic Resonance Imaging, Nuclear Methods, and Computed Tomography

Magnetic resonance imaging, radionuclide-based methods, and computed tomography have no role in the routine evaluation of patients with suspected DHF. There are exceptions, such as constrictive pericarditis, that require more comprehensive imaging.

Structural Changes

Increased left atrial volume may also be used as objective evidence of diastolic function. Furthermore, LV hypertrophy is consistent with impaired diastolic function and supports the diagnosis.

Blood Markers

Elevated brain natriuretic peptide and N-terminal prohormone brain natriuretic peptide may be used to support the diagnosis DHF, but their presence is not considered sufficient stand-alone evidence for diastolic dysfunction. Natriuretic peptide measurements are recommended mainly for the exclusion of the diagnosis, which is justified by its high negative predictive value for heart failure.

Differential Diagnosis

Because symptoms and signs of DHF are relatively nonspecific, it is important to exclude noncardiac etiologies, in particular, lung disease. It is also important to exclude other cardiac disorders, such as valvular heart disease and coronary artery disease. Valvular heart disease is a well-known cause of heart failure and is easily identified by echocardiography. Symptoms of coronary artery stenosis can mimic those of heart failure, in particular, in diabetic patients. Therefore, a stress test or coronary angiography should be considered.

A diagnostic work-up for patients with suspected DHF can be done at low cost in almost every cardiology practice. When invasive data are not available, echocardiography is the preferred method to determine if there is LV diastolic dysfunction. In general practice, blood markers such as brain natriuretic peptide may be used as the initial method, and when brain natriuretic peptide level is normal, it is very unlikely that the patient has any form of heart failure. Importantly, this does not mean that the patient has no heart disease, and a search for valve disease, coronary artery disease, or other cardiac disorders may

be needed. When blood markers are elevated, however, heart failure is likely, and the patient should be referred for echocardiography to define underlying pathology and to confirm the diagnosis.

Why Assess Diastolic Function in Systolic Heart Failure?

Evaluation of LV diastolic function is useful not only for patients with DHF but also for patients with SHF by providing an estimate of LV filling pressure. Therefore, assessment of diastolic function is of interest for virtually every heart failure patient provided that the examination has a clear objective.

Prognosis and Treatment

Patients with heart failure and a preserved EF represent about 50 % of all patients with heart failure. Their prognosis is almost as severe as that for patients with heart failure with reduced EF.

An effective treatment of DHF has yet not been established, but ongoing clinical trials may provide some answers. Because of the limited documentation available, it is difficult to give firm recommendations. At present, it seems reasonable to treat symptoms with drugs similar to those used for heart failure with reduced systolic function.

Currently, six drug classes are used in patients with heart failure due to diastolic dysfunction: beta-adrenergic receptors blockers, calcium channel blockers, angiotensin converting enzyme inhibitors, angiotensin receptor blockers, diuretics and aldosterone antagonists. The rationale for their administration includes elimination of ischaemia, slowing heart rate, regression of myocardial hypertrophy and fibrosis, and also their proven effect in patients with systolic dysfunction. Other treatments likely to favorably affect diastolic function, are being developed.

The most solid data on treatment that are in our possession now include:

1. Treatment of the underlying condition, with a special focus on adequate control of

blood pressure in patients with arterial hypertension.

2. Use of diuretics in patients with signs and symptoms of congestion.

3. Avoidance of heart rate acceleration.

In practice, all approaches for which there is evidence of efficacy and safety in patients with systolic heart failure, need to be also used in patients with diastolic heart failure, as long as the necessary evidence specific to diastolic heart failure is accumulated.

References

1. Gandhi SK, Powers JC, Nomeir AM, Fowle K, Kitzman DW, Rankin KM, Little WC. The pathogenesis of acute pulmonary edema associated with hypertension. N Engl J Med 2001;344(1):17–22.

2. Yu C-H, Lin H, Yang H, Kong S-L, Zhang Q, Lee SW-A. Progression of systolic abnormalities in patients with "isolated" diastolic heart failure and diastolic dysfunction. Circulation 2002;105:1195–1201.

3. Paulus WJ, et al. How to diagnose diastolic heart failure. A consensus statement on the diagnosis of heart failure with normal left ventricular ejection fraction. By the Heart Failure and Echocardiography Associations of the European Society of Cardiology. Eur Heart J. Advance Access published on April 11, 2007.

4. Vasan RS, Levy D. Defining diastolic heart failure. A call for standardized diagnostic criteria. Circulation 2000;101:2118–2121.

5. Bursi F, Weston SA, Redfield MM, Jacobsen SJ, Pakhomov S, Nkomo VT, Meverden RA, Roger VL. Systolic and diastolic heart failure in the community. JAMA 2006;296(18):2209–2216.

6. Gheorghiade M, Abraham WT, Albert NM, Greenberg BH, O'Connor CM, She L, Stough WG, Yancy CW, Young JB, Fonarow GC, OPTIMIZE-HF Investigators and Coordinators. Systolic blood pressure at admission, clinical characteristics, and outcomes in patients hospitalized with acute heart failure. JAMA 2006;296(18):2217–2226.

7. Kawaguchi M, Hay I, Fetics B, Kass DA. Combined ventricular systolic and arterial stiffening in patients with heart failure and preserved ejection fraction: implications for systolic and diastolic reserve limitations. Circulation 2003;107(5):714–720.

8. Kitzman DW, Higginbotham MB, Cobb FR, Sheikh KH, Sullivan MJ. Exercise intolerance in patients with heart failure and preserved left ventricular systolic function: failure of the Frank-Starling mechanism. J Am Coll Cardiol 1991;17(5):1065–1072.

9. Lakatta EG. Age-associated cardiovascular changes in health: impact on cardiovascular disease in older persons. Heart Fail Rev 2002;7:29–49.

10. Chen CH, Nakayama M, Nevo E, Fetics BJ, Maughan WL, Kass DA. Coupled systolic-ventricular and vascular stiffening with age: implications for pressure regulation and cardiac reserve in the elderly. J Am Coll Cardiol 1998;32(5):1221–1227.

11. Redfield MM, Jacobsen SJ, Borlaug BA, Rodeheffer RJ, Kass DA. Age- and gender-related ventricular-vascular stiffening: a community-based study. Circulation 2005;112(15):2254–2262.

12. Mottram PM, Haluska BA, Leano R, Carlier S, Case C, Marwick TH. Relation of arterial stiffness to diastolic dysfunction in hypertensive heart disease. Heart 2005;91(12):1551–1556.

13. Wandt B, Bojo L, Hatle L, Wranne B. Left ventricular contraction pattern changes with age in normal adults. J Am Soc Echocardiogr 1998;11(9):857–863.

14. Yamakado T, Takagi E, Okubo S, Imanaka-Yoshida K, Tarumi T, Nakamura M, et al. Effects of aging on left ventricular relaxation in humans. Analysis of left ventricular isovolumic pressure decay. Circulation 1997;95:917–923.

15. Arbab-Zadeh A, Dijk E, Prasad A, Fu Q, Torres P, Zhang R, Thomas JD, Palmer D, Levine BD. Effect of aging and physical activity on left ventricular compliance. Circulation 2004;110(13):1799–1805.

Index

A

AC. *See* Aortic closure
ACE. *See* Angiotensin-converting enzyme
ACE-I. *See* Angiotensin-converting enzyme inhibitors
Acidosis, 257
Actin, 30, 31, 62
α-actin, 31, 62
Acute myocardial ischemia, 93
Acute pulmonary edema, 235
  hypertension and, 77
  venous system and, 77
Acute pulmonary hypertension, 45–47
  EDP and, 45
Adenosine diphosphate, 244
Adenosine triphosphate, 30, 257, 293
β-adrenergic receptor blockers, 227–229, 231, 233
β-adrenergic receptors, 192
β-adrenergic response, 58
β-adrenergic stimulation, 7
AFFIRM trial, 64–65
Afterload, 8
  aortic stenosis and, 59
  dilated cardiomyopathy and, 59
  neurohormones and, 71
  RV and, 45
  ventricular stiffness and, 59
Aging, 14, 34, 266
  DHF and, 206–207, 331–332
  LVEF and, 214
  mortality and, 217–218
  systolic blood pressure and, 77, 263–264

Alagebrium chloride (ALT-711), 234
Aldosterone, 72–74
  diabetes mellitus and, 279
  myocardial fibrosis and, 73–74
  myocardial hypertrophy and, 73–74
Aldosterone antagonists, 71, 229–230
  for HCM, 302
Aldosterone Antagonist Therapy in Adults with Preserved Ejection Fraction Congestive Heart Failure (TOPCAT), 224, 230
ALT-711. *See* Alagebrium chloride
Amiodarone, 233
Amyloidosis, 231, 233
  digoxin and, 324
Anemia, 25
  DHF and, 210
  SHF and, 71
Angina pectoris, 24
Angioplasty, 42
Angiotensin-converting enzyme (ACE), angiotensin II and, 71–72
Angiotensin-converting enzyme inhibitors (ACE-I), 71–73, 231, 236, 289
  for diabetes mellitus, 279
  for HF, 223–227
Angiotensin I (AT$_1$), 72, 75–76
Angiotensin II, 32–33
  ACE and, 71–72
  cardiomyocytes and, 73
  LA and, 54
  myocardial hypertrophy and, 32

receptors of, 21
vasoconstriction by, 71
Angiotensin receptor blockers (ARB), 74, 224–227, 232
  mortality and, 225
  for myocardial fibrosis, 225
  for myocardial hypertrophy, 225
ANP. *See* Atrial natriuretic peptide
Aorta, coarctation of, 263
Aortic closure (AC), 30, 101
Aortic opening (AO), 101
Aortic regurgitation, 196
Aortic stenosis, 26, 29, 231, 259
  afterload and, 59
Apical hypertrophy, 286
Apical suction, intraventricular pressure gradients and, 92
Apoptosis, norepinephrine and, 76
ARB. *See* Angiotensin receptor blockers
Arrhythmias, 71
  norepinephrine and, 76
Arrhythmic sudden death, HCM and, 290–291
Arterial elastance (Ea), 35–36
Arterial stiffness, filling pressures and, 35
Arterial system, 77
Asymmetric septal hypertrophy, 286
Asymptote pressure, 140
Asynchrony
  isoproterenol-induced, 30
  of local diastolic function, 109–110
  pacing-induced, 30
AT$_1$. *See* Angiotensin I
Atenolol, 227
Atherosclerosis, 34, 265

339

Index

Atrial compliance, 64
Atrial contraction phase, 4
Atrial fibrillation, 61, 158, 231, 235
calcium overload and, 64
CHARM and, 210
DHF and, 207, 209–210
diastolic dysfunction and, 158, 265
E waves and, 158
filling pressures in, 197–198
LA and, 64–65
LVEF and, 182
A waves and, 150
Atrial-induced filling, 89–90
Atrial-induced reversed velocity (Ar), 82–85, 121, 190
atrial fibrillation and, 196–199
Atrial natriuretic peptide (ANP), 53–54
cardiomyocytes and, 175–176
Atrial remodeling, 58, 60–65, 85
Atrial septal defect, 47
Atrial stiffness, 57, 60–61
basement membrane proteins and, 63
collagen and, 63
ECM and, 63
elastin and, 63
Atrial strain, 61–62
Atrial suction, 83
Atrial systole, 58
Atrial volumes, 167
Atrioventricular coupling, 286
A waves, 89, 91
atrial fibrillation and, 150

B

Bainbridge reflex, 54
Balloon coronary occlusion ischemia, 245–250, 253–254
LV and, 246
perfusion and, 246
tissue build up in, 257–258
Basement membrane proteins, 7–8, 31
atrial stiffness and, 63
Benzoensulfonic acid (MCC-135), 234
Bernoulli equation, 86
Bivariate Cox model, 63
β-blockers, 76, 232
Blood flow. See Cardiac output
Blood urea nitrogen, mortality and, 218

BNP. See Brain natriuretic peptide
Body mass index, 14. See also Obesity
BNP and, 179
NT-pro-BNP and, 178
Bone marrow cell transfer, 233
Bone Marrow Transfer to Enhance ST Elevation Infarct Regeneration study, 233
Bradykinin, 258
Brain natriuretic peptide (BNP), 4, 53–54, 208, 336. See also N-terminal prohormone BNP
algorithm for, 176
body mass index and, 179
CAD and, 176
cardiomyocytes and, 175
CHF and, 76
combined DHF/SHF and, 181–182
determinants of, 177
diabetes mellitus and, 278
diastolic dysfunction and, 179
echocardiography and, 110
guidelines for, 182–183
hypertension and, 267
LVEF and, 179
measurement of, 175
obesity and, 177
renal dysfunction and, 177
systolic blood pressure and, 179
treatment and, 182
Breathing Not Properly study, 181
Bucindolol, 76
Burned out hypertrophy, 286

C

CABG. See Coronary artery bypass graft
CAD, DHF and, 210
Calcification, 34
CT and, 167
of pericardium, 314
Calcium channel blockers, 229, 232
Calcium homeostasis, 5–6
Calcium overload, 62–63
atrial fibrillation and, 64
CALM II study, 278
Candesartan in Heart Failure-Assessment of Reduction in Mortality and Morbidity (CHARM), 75, 214, 216–217, 218, 224, 225–227
atrial fibrillation and, 210
DHF and, 73

diabetes and, 278
mortality and, 226
Canrenone, 229–230
Cardiac amyloidosis, 169
Cardiac autonomic neuropathy, 277
Cardiac cycle, 23–27
diastole and, 24–27
LA in, 54–58
Cardiac endothelium. See Endothelium
Cardiac hypertrophy, norepinephrine and, 76
Cardiac nociceptors, 258
Cardiac output, 9. See also Pulmonary venous flow
with DHF, 126
LA and, 53–54
with SHF, 126
Cardiomyocytes, 5, 62
angiotensin II and, 73
ANP and, 175–176
BNP and, 175
calcium homeostasis and, 5–6
cross-bridge detachments and, 6–7
cytoskeletal abnormalities in, 7
excitation-contraction in, 29
HCM and, 290
inactivation-relaxation in, 29
myocardial stiffness and, 30–31
PKA and, 32
Cardiovascular congestion, 21–23
in DHF, 22–23
filling pressures and, 22
in overload, 21–22
in SHF, 22
Cardiovascular Health Study, 210, 215, 285
Cardiovascular magnetic resonance (CMR)
atrial volume and, 167
vs. echocardiography, 163
as echocardiography complement, 166–167
MF and, 167
perfusion and, 170
pericardium and, 167
problems with, 170
septum and, 167–170
for tissue characterization, 170
tricuspid inflow velocity and, 167

Index 341

Carvedilol, 227–228
Catecholamines, 73–74
Catheterization, 207
  in constrictive pericarditis, 319
Cavity size, 25–26
Chamber compliance, 89
CHARM. *See* Candesartan in Heart
  Failure-Assessment of
  Reduction in Mortality and
  Morbidity
CHF. *See* Congestive heart failure
Chronic heart failure
  DHF and, 11–15
  phenotypes of, 13–15
  progression of, 11–13
  treatment of, 223–234
Chronic obstructive pulmonary
  disease (COPD), 210–211
Chronic pulmonary hypertension,
  47
  septum and, 47
  TSG and, 47
Chymase pathway, 72
CMR. *See* Cardiovascular magnetic
  resonance
CNP. *See* C-type natriuretic
  peptide
Coarctation, of aorta, 263
Collagen, 7–8, 31
  atrial stiffness and, 63
  renin-angiotensin-aldosterone
    system and, 63
Column motion, 94
Combined diastolic and systolic
  heart failure, 181–182
Compliance
  atrial, 64
  diastolic, 41
  filling velocities and, 81
  loss of, 34
  LV chamber, 89
  ventricular, 5–9
Computed tomography (CT),
  335–336
  calcification and, 167
Concentric hypertrophy, 122
  sarcomeres and, 122
Congestive heart failure (CHF), 45,
  47–49, 110, 137
  BNP and, 76
  exercise and, 76
  MF and, 189
  pacing-induced, 128
  rapid-pacing model of, 48

REACH, 215
  stroke work and, 47
  TOPCAT, 224, 230
  transmitral flow velocities and,
    90
CONSENSUS trial, 224
Constrictive pericarditis, 169,
  311–320
  catheterization in, 319
  diagnosis of, 314–319
  echocardiography for, 314–319
  effusive, 319–320
  MF with, 315
  transient, 320
  treatment for, 319–320
Constrictive physiology, 167
Contraction-relaxation cycle, 3
Convective term, in Bernoulli
  equation, 86
COPD. *See* Chronic obstructive
  pulmonary disease
Coronary artery bypass graft
  (CABG), 21–22, 259
Coronary artery disease (CAD),
  231, 243–260
  BNP and, 176
  DHF and, 210
  diabetes mellitus and, 272
Coronary Artery Surgery Study,
  217
Coronary revascularization, 233
Coronary sinus washout, 250–251
Coronary vascular turgor, 254–257
Corticosteroids, 233
Coupling, 34–36, 286
Cox model, 63
C-peptide, 279
Creatine phosphate, 257
Cross-bridge detachments, 6–7
Cross-linking, 31, 278, 279
  diastole and, 292
CT. *See* Computed tomography
C-type natriuretic peptide (CNP),
  53, 177
Cyclophosphamide, 233
Cytokines, 11, 192
Cytoskeleton. *See* Cardiomyocytes
Cytosolic calcium, 62–63

D
D. *See* Diastole
Decompensated diastolic heart
  failure, 181
Dementia, DHF and, 210

DENSE. *See* Displacement encoding
  with stimulated echoes
Desferrioxamine, 233
Desmin, 7, 31, 62
DHF. *See* Diastolic heart failure
Diabetes, 14, 15, 34, 109, 208, 231
  CHARM and, 278
  DHF and, 207, 210, 336
  LVEF and, 182
Diabetes mellitus
  ACE-I for, 279
  aldosterone and, 279
  BNP and, 278
  CAD and, 272
  diastolic dysfunction and,
    271–279
  EF and, 272
  filling pressures and, 279
  free fatty acids and, 275
  glucose and, 275
  HF with, 278
  hypertension and, 271
  myocardial dysfunction and,
    272–274
  myocardial fibrosis and,
    276–277, 279
  obesity and, 277
  protein glycation with, 275
  pseudonormalized filling and,
    271
  SERCA2 and, 275
  systolic dysfunction and, 272
Diabetic lung disease, 277
Diabetic vascular disease, 277
Diastasis, 4, 55
Diastole (D), 4
  cardiac function in, 24–27
  components of, 292
  cross-linking and, 292
  IVRT in, 86
  LA and, 55
  LV and, 23, 24
  PLA in, 86
  PLV in, 86
  relaxation and, 9
  strain and, 103
  transmural pressure and, 41
Diastolic calcium sparks, 6
Diastolic compliance, 41
Diastolic deformation indexes,
  111–112
Diastolic dysfunction. *See also*
  Pseudonormalized filling
  atrial fibrillation and, 158, 265

Heart transplantation, 233
Helsinki Aging Study, 215
Hemochromatosis, 231
Hemodynamic pump, 9–10
    failure of, 11–12
Hepatic disease, 313
Hepatic vein velocities, 153–156
HF. *See* Heart failure
HFNEF. *See* Heart failure with
    normal ejection fraction
HFPEF. *See* Heart failure with
    preserved ejection fraction
HFREF. *See* Heart failure with
    reduced ejection fraction
Hong-Kong Diastolic Heart Failure
    study, 227
Hospital admissions, 218–219
Hydroxychloroquine, 233
Hyperaldosteronism, 263, 302
Hyperemia, 254–257
Hyperhomocysteinemia, 266
Hyperlipidemia, 266
    DHF and, 210
Hyperplasia, 293
Hypertension, 15, 29, 34, 109, 208,
    231, 263–267
    acute pulmonary edema and, 77
    BNP and, 267
    DHF and, 180–181, 207, 209
    diabetes mellitus and, 271
    dyspnea and, 193
    flash pulmonary edema and, 36
    left ventricular hypertrophy and,
    77
    LVEF and, 182
    neurohormones and, 267
    NT-pro-BNP and, 267
    pulmonary, 45–47
Hypertensive pulmonary edema,
    23
Hypertrophic cardiomyopathy
    (HCM), 231, 285–302
    aldosterone antagonists for, 302
    ARB for, 233
    asymptomatic, 291
    cardiomyocytes and, 290
    diastolic abnormalities in, 293
    dilated cardiomyopathy and,
    286–288, 294
    echocardiography of, 299–302
    ECM and, 293
    exercise and, 298–299
    histological abnormalities in,
    293–294

ICDs and, 290
left ventricular filling pressure
    with, 188
LV filling and, 291–292
molecular variants in, 288–290
morphologic variants of,
    286–288
mutations and, 288–290
myocardial fibrosis and, 294
myocellular abnormalities in,
    293
preload reserve and, 291–292
prognostic therapy for, 289
PV and, 296–298
renin-angiotensin-aldosterone
    system and, 302
spironolactone for, 302
symptomatic, 291
verapamil for, 229
wedge pressure and, 298–299
Hypertrophy. *See also* Left
    ventricular hypertrophy;
    Myocardial hypertrophy
    concentric, 122
    eccentric, 122–123
    maron-type obstructive, 286
    midcavity, 286
    norepinephrine and, 76
    reversed asymmetric septal,
    286
    ventricular, 7
Hypoxemia, 249–250
    tissue build up in, 257–258
Hypoxia, 243, 244

I

Idiopathic dilated cardiomyopathy.
    See Dilated cardiomyopathy
Implantable cardioverter
    defibrillators (ICDs), 233
    HCM and, 290
    MRI and, 166
Inactivation-relaxation, in
    cardiomyocytes, 29
IN-CHF Registry, 210
Inertial term, in Bernoulli
    equation, 86
Inferior vena cava, 168
Inferior vena occlusion, 43
Insulin resistance, 278–279
Interactions
    biventricular, 259
    direct, 44–45
    heart-lung, 44

during mechanical ventilation,
    49–50
ventricular, 41–50
Intermediate filaments. *See*
    Desmin
Interstitial fibrosis, 192, 276
Interstitial myocardial fibrosis, 7
Intracoronary bone marrow cell
    transfer, 233
Intraventricular filling, 91–93
Intraventricular pressure
    gradients, apical suction
    and, 92
I-PRESERVE. *See* Irbesartan in
    Heart Failure with Preserved
    Systolic Function
Irbesartan in Heart Failure with
    Preserved Systolic Function
    (I-PRESERVE), 224, 227
Ischemia, 231–232, 235, 243, 244.
    See also Balloon coronary
    occlusion ischemia; Pacing-
    induced ischemia
    acute, 93
    exercise-induced, 253
    myocardial stretch during,
    254–257
    norepinephrine and, 76
    perfusion and, 170
    unequal intensity of, 258–259
    vascular turgor during,
    254–257
ISD. *See* Isosorbide dinitrate
Isoproterenol-induced asynchrony,
    30
Isosorbide dinitrate (ISD), 59
Isovolumic relaxation time
    (IVRT), 86, 91, 189, 191, 198,
    199, 259
    in diastole, 86
IVRT. *See* Isovolumic relaxation
    time

K

Kaplan-Meier survival curves, 130
    SCD and, 230

L

LA. *See* Left atrium
Labetalol, 235
Lactate, 250–251
Laminin, 8, 31
Left atrial pressure (PLA), 82
    in diastole, 86

Index

vs. operative atrial stiffness, 57
pulmonary venous flow and, 82, 84
Left atrium (LA), 53–66
  angiotensin II and, 54
  atrial fibrillation and, 64–65
  in cardiac cycle, 54–58
  cardiac output and, 53–54
  as conduit, 57–58
  as control center, 53–54
  diastole and, 55
  elasticity of, 60–61
  ET-1 and, 54
  filling of, 82
  mitral regurgitation and, 65
  operative stiffness in, 57
  pressure in, 57
  as pump, 58
  remodeling of, 62–63
  as reservoir, 56–57
  stiffness of, 60–61, 63
  as transit chamber, 53
  ventricular filling and, 54–58
Left ventricle (LV), 4
  balloon coronary occlusion ischemia and, 246
  diastole and, 23, 24
  distensibility of, 25, 140–142
  EDP in, 45
  EF and, 119
  filling of, 82, 127, 291–292, 333–335
  filling velocities of, 81–95
  function of, 123–126
  glycemic control and, 275–276
  pacing-induced ischemia and, 246
  pressure fall in, 27
  PV in, 43, 140, 296–298
  stiffness of, 142
  structure of, 122–123
  suction of, 87, 158
  torsion of, 168
  transmural pressure in, 42
Left ventricular diastolic performance, 119–121
Left ventricular ejection fraction (LVEF), 11, 13, 187, 329
  aging and, 214
  atrial fibrillation and, 182
  BNP and, 179
  DHF and, 205–211, 213–219
  diabetes and, 182
  HF and, 182

hypertension and, 182
left ventricular filling pressures and, 196–197
SHF and, 71
Left ventricular end-diastolic pressure, 191
Left ventricular end-diastolic volume (LVEDV), 43, 46, 138
  LVSW and, 48
Left ventricular filling pressures, 332
  estimation of, 335
  left ventricular relaxation and, 191
  LVEF and, 196–197
  MF and, 188–189
  mitral valve disease and, 198–199
  pulmonary venous flow and, 190
Left ventricular hypertrophy, 72, 122–123, 158
  hypertension and, 77
Left ventricular internal diameter (LVID), 23
Left ventricular intracavity filling, in HF, 94–95
Left ventricular outflow tract, 189
Left ventricular outflow tract obstruction (LVOTO), 285, 288, 291
Left ventricular pressure (LVP), 28, 35, 82
  decay of, 139
  in diastole, 86
Left ventricular relaxation, 81, 137–140, 191–192, 332–333
  left ventricular filling pressures and, 191
Left ventricular stiffness, 333
Left ventricular stroke work (LVSW), 46
  LVEDP and, 48
Left ventricular systolic performance, 119
LIFE trial, 278
Little old ladies' heart, 263
Load. *See also* Afterload; Preload
  myocardial relaxation and, 27–28
Longitudinal myocardial fibers, 9
LOS. *See* Losartan
Losartan (LOS), 21, 74, 278
Loss of compliance, 34

L-type channels, 58, 293
LV. *See* Left ventricle
LVEDV. *See* Left ventricular end-diastolic volume
LVEF. *See* Left ventricular ejection fraction
LVID. *See* Left ventricular internal diameter
LVOTO. *See* Left ventricular outflow tract obstruction
LVP. *See* Left ventricular pressure
LVSW. *See* Left ventricular stroke work
L waves, 89

M

Magnesium adenosine triphosphate, 244
Magnetic resonance imaging (MRI), 99, 104–106, 163–171, 335–336
  ICDs and, 166
  pacemakers and, 166
  techniques of, 163–166
Maron-type obstructive hypertrophy, 286
MC. *See* Mitral closure
MCC-135. *See* Benzoensulfonic acid
Mechanical ventilation, ventricular interaction during, 49–50
Methotrexate, 233
Metoprolol, 76, 227
MF. *See* Mitral flow
Microfilaments. *See* Actin
Microtubules, 31, 62
Midcavity hypertrophy, 286
Mid-diastolic filling, 87–88
Mitral annular motion, 151–152
  MF and, 158–159
Mitral annulus, peak velocities of, 108
Mitral annulus velocity, 266
  echocardiography and, 191–194
Mitral closure (MC), 102
Mitral flow (MF), 100, 196, 198, 266
  CHF and, 189
  CMR and, 166, 167
  with constrictive pericarditis, 315
  Doppler echocardiography and, 151, 153
  dyspnea and, 193, 194

Mitral flow (MF) (*cont.*)
  left ventricular end-diastolic pressure and, 191
  left ventricular filling pressures and, 188–189
  mitral annular motion and, 158–159
  pseudonormalized filling and, 59, 99, 189–190
  wedge pressure and, 197
Mitral inflow. *See* Mitral flow
Mitral opening (MO), 30, 102
Mitral regurgitation, 25, 196
  LA and, 65
  overload and, 65
Mitral valve disease, left ventricular filling pressures and, 198–199
Mitral valve repair, 233
M-mode, 63, 94, 105, 120–121, 191
MO. *See* Mitral opening
MONICA study, 179, 208
Morphine, 235
Mortality
  aging, 217–218 and
  ARB and, 225
  blood urea nitrogen and, 218
  CHARM and, 226
  with DHF, 213–214
  predictors of, 217–218
  renal dysfunction and, 218
  serum creatinine and, 218
M protein, 31, 62
MRI. *See* Magnetic resonance imaging
Muscle stiffness, 143–145
Muscular pump, 4
Mutations, HCM and, 288–290
Myocardial backscatter, 276
Myocardial deformation, 111–112. *See also* Strain
Myocardial dysfunction, diabetes mellitus and, 272–274
Myocardial fibrosis, 12, 72
  aldosterone and, 73–74
  ARB for, 225
  diabetes mellitus and, 276–277, 279
  HCM and, 294
Myocardial hibernation, 243
Myocardial hypertrophy, 11, 15, 72
  aldosterone and, 73–74
  angiotensin II and, 32

ARB for, 225
ET-1 and, 32
Myocardial inactivation, determinants of, 29
Myocardial infarction, 208, 209
Myocardial ischemia, 243
Myocardial necrosis, 12
Myocardial relaxation, 21–36, 24
  determinants of, 27–30
  load and, 27
  time course of, 27–30
Myocardial stiffness, 34, 143–145
  cardiomyocytes and, 30–31
Myocardial stretch, 254–257
Myocardial tagging, 166
Myocardial velocities, 99–112
  assessment of, 99–100
  diastolic deformation indexes, 111–112
  diastolic dysfunction and, 107–108
  interpretation of, 106–107
  parameters of, 100–106
Myocarditis, 166
Myocytes. *See* Cardiomyocytes
Myomesin, 31, 62
Myosin, 54
β-myosin heavy chain mutations, 288

N
N2B, 7
N2BA, 7
National Heart Failure Project (NHF), 209
Natriuretic peptides, 71, 76–77, 207. *See also* Brain natriuretic peptide; N-terminal prohormone BNP
  clinical use of, 178
  DHF and, 175–183
  structure and mechanisms of, 175–178
Nebivolol, 227–229
Nebulin, 62
Necrosis, norepinephrine and, 76
Nesiritide, 76
Neurohormonal hypothesis, 123
Neurohormones, 5, 9, 71–77
  afterload and, 71
  DHF and, 71–77
  distensibility and, 27
  hypertension and, 267
  vasoconstriction and, 71

New York Heart Association (NYHA) classifications, 12, 13, 112, 180, 214, 224
NHF. *See* National Heart Failure Project
Nitrales, 232
Nitric oxide, 8, 32
Nitroglycerin, 47, 235
Nitroprusside, 42, 235
  for SHF, 22
N-Methylethanolamine, 234
Nociceptors, 258
Nonuniformity, relaxation and, 30
Norepinephrine
  apoptosis and, 76
  arrhythmias and, 76
  cardiac hypertrophy and, 76
  ischemia and, 76
  necrosis and, 76
N-terminal prohormone BNP (NT-pro-BNP), 4, 336
  body mass index and, 178
  cardiomyocytes and, 176
  determinants of, 177
  hypertension and, 267
  measurement of, 175
  renal dysfunction and, 177
NT-pro-BNP. *See* N-terminal prohormone BNP
NYHA. *See* New York Heart Association classifications

O
Obesity, 15, 108, 208, 231
  BNP and, 177
  DHF and, 206–207
  diabetes mellitus and, 277
Obstructive airway disease, 194
Operative atrial stiffness, *vs.* left atrial pressure, 57
Overload
  cardiovascular congestion in, 21–22
  mitral regurgitation and, 65

P
Pacemakers, 233
  MRI and, 166
Pacing-induced asynchrony, 30
Pacing-induced CHF, 128
Pacing-induced ischemia, 245–249, 253
  LV and, 246
  tissue build up in, 257–258

Index

Paracrine substances, 5, 8, 258
Parietal fibrosis, 63
Pathologic parietal fibrosis, 63
PCWP. *See* Pulmonary capillary wedge pressure
Peak velocities, 86, 93, 104, 150, 154, 167, 196–197, 335
  early diastolic, 106
  E wave, 158
  of mitral annulus, 108
PEP-CHF. *See* Perindopril in Elderly People with Chronic Heart Failure study
Perfusion, 252
  balloon coronary occlusion ischemia and, 246
  CMR and, 170
  ischemia and, 170
Pericarditis. *See* Constrictive pericarditis
Pericardium
  calcification of, 314
  CMR and, 167
  PV and, 42
  transmural pressure and, 41–44
  ventricular interaction via, 41–50
Perindopril, 224
Perindopril in Elderly People with Chronic Heart Failure study (PEP-CHF), 217, 223, 224, 225
Peripheral vasculature, 71–77
Phenotypes, 108
  of chronic heart failure, 13–15
Phenotypical trajectories, 13
Pheochromocytoma, 235, 263
Phlebotomy, 47
pH measurements, 250–251
Phonocardiography, 191
Phosphate isomerase, 244
Phospholamban, 6, 29, 62–63
Phosphorylation
  of PKA, 31
  titin and, 31
PKA. *See* Protein kinase A
PLA. *See* Left atrial pressure
Plasma renin activity (PRA), 74
PLVF. *See* Preserved left ventricular function
Potassium, 73–74, 250–251
PRA. *See* Plasma renin activity; Right atrial pressure
Pre-A, 188
Preload, 8

Preload reserve, 291–293
Preserved left ventricular function (PLVF), 208, 223
Pressure-volume relation (PV), 22, 25, 292. *See also* Diastolic pressure-volume
  atrial diastolic, 85
  HCM and, 296–298
  in LV, 43, 140, 296–298
  pericardium and, 42
  ventricular remodeling and, 15
Propagation velocity (V_p), 191, 196
  EF and, 191
Protein glycation, with diabetes mellitus, 275
Protein kinase A (PKA), 32
  cardiomyocytes and, 32
  hyperphosphorylation of, 6
  phosphorylation of, 31
Proteoglycans, 7
Pseudonormalized filling, 61, 91, 100, 104, 107–108, 120–121, 153–158, 265–266, 271–272, 299
  diabetes mellitus and, 271
  echocardiography and, 195
  mitral flow and, 59, 99, 189–190
  relaxation and, 178, 180
Pulmonary capillary wedge pressure (PCWP), 42, 316
  stroke volume and, 49
Pulmonary edema, 36, 77, 235
  hypertensive, 23
Pulmonary hypertension, 45–47
  acute, 45–47
  chronic, 47
Pulmonary regurgitation, 195
Pulmonary venous flow, 55, 56, 167, 189, 266
  deceleration of, 84–85
  early, 83
  late-diastolic, 83
  left ventricular end-diastolic pressure and, 191
  left ventricular filling pressures and, 190
  mid-diastolic, 83
  PLA and, 82, 84
  velocity of, 150–151
Pulmonary venous flow velocities, 81–85
PV. *See* Pressure-volume relation

Q
QRS complex, 55

R
Race, 218
Radiation therapy, 313
Rapid early diastolic filling, 86–87
REACH. *See* Resource Utilization Among Congestive Heart Failure
Receiver operating characteristic (ROC), 178–179, 193
Relaxation. *See also* Isovolumic relaxation time; Myocardial relaxation
  contraction-relaxation cycle, 3
  diastole and, 9
  diastolic, 29
  in HF, 88
  nonuniformity and, 30
  pseudonormalized filling and, 178, 180
  S and, 9
  ventricular, 5–9
Remodeling, 228, 289, 331. *See also* Atrial remodeling; Ventricular remodeling
RENAAL trial, 278
Renal artery stenosis, 263
Renal dysfunction, 76
  BNP and, 177
  DHF and, 210–211
  mortality and, 218
  NT-pro-BNP and, 177
Renal parenchymal disease, 263
Renin-angiotensin-aldosterone system, 8, 31, 71–74
  CNP and, 53
  collagen and, 63
  HCM and, 302
  sympathetic nervous system and, 76
Resource Utilization Among Congestive Heart Failure (REACH), 215
Restrictive cardiomyopathy, 311–326
  diagnosis of, 321–324
  diuretics for, 324
  ECG for, 321
  echocardiography for, 321–324
  pathophysiology of, 321
  treatment for, 324

Restrictive physiology, 91, 108, 154, 158, 167, 334
Revascularization, 233
Reversed asymmetric septal hypertrophy, 286
Reverse epidemiology, 14
Rheumatoid arthritis, 313
Right atrial pressure (PRA), 42
  estimation of, 335
Right ventricle (RV), 27
  afterload and, 45
  diastolic function of, 153–156
  EDP in, 45
  hepatic vein velocities, 153–156
  superior vena cava velocities, 156
  tricuspid inflow velocity, 153
ROC. *See* Receiver operating characteristic
RV. *See* Right ventricle
Ryanodine receptors (RyRs), 6, 293
RyRs. *See* Ryanodine receptors

S
S. *See* Systole
Sarcoidosis, 231, 233
Sarcomeres, 7, 31, 49, 255–256, 288, 302
  concentric hypertrophy and, 122
  eccentric hypertrophy and, 122
Sarcoplasmic reticulum (SR), 5, 28
  re-uptake of, 65
Sarcoplasmic reticulum Ca^{2+} (SERCA2), 5–6, 15, 293
  diabetes mellitus and, 275
Sarcoplasmic reticulum Ca^{2+} ATPase (SERCA2a), 28–29
SCD. *See* Serum digitalis concentration
SENIORS. *See* Study of the Effects of Nebivolol Intervention on Outcomes and Rehospitalizations
Septal ablation, 233
Septum, 319
  chronic pulmonary hypertension and, 47
  CMR and, 167–170
  ventricular interaction via, 41–50
Septum-to-left ventricular free wall diameter (SLVFW), 44
Septum-to-right ventricular free wall diameter (SRVFW), 44

SERCA2. *See* Sarcoplasmic reticulum Ca^{2+}
SERCA2a. *See* Sarcoplasmic reticulum Ca^{2+} ATPase
Series interaction, 44–45
Serum creatinine, mortality and, 218
Serum digitalis concentration (SCD), 230
Serum potassium, 73–74
SHF. *See* Systolic heart failure
Simplus balloon catheters (USCI), 246
Sinus node, 54
Sinus rhythm, 61
Sinus tachycardia, filling pressures in, 197
Sinus washout, 250–251
Smoking, 266
  DHF and, 210
Sodium-calcium exchanger, 6, 28
Sodium nitroprusside, 42, 235
Speckle tracking echocardiography, 103
Sphygmomanometer cuff, 194
Spironolactone, 74, 230, 232
  for HCM, 302
Spontaneous coronary spasm, 253
SR. *See* Sarcoplasmic reticulum
SRVFW. *See* Septum-to-right ventricular free wall diameter
Statins, 232, 233–234
Stiffness. *See also* Atrial stiffness; Myocardial stiffness; Ventricular stiffness
  with DHF, 77
  diastolic myocardial, 143–145
  end-diastolic, 21–36
  of LA, 60–61, 63
  of LV, 142
  muscle, 143–145
Strain, 100, 170
  atrial, 61–62
  D and, 103
  imaging and, 102
  systolic, 112, 229
Strain rate, 61–62, 100, 103, 111–112, 229
  diastolic, 112
  imaging and, 102
Stress-induced tachycardia, 54
Stress-strain relation, 143–145
Stroke volume (SV), 9, 34, 64, 166
  with DHF, 126

PCWP and, 49
  with SHF, 126
Stroke work, 9–10
  CHF and, 47
  LVSW, 46
  transmural pressure and, 45
Study of the Effects of Nebivolol Intervention on Outcomes and Rehospitalizations (SENIORS), 224, 228–229
Suction, 99, 168
  apical, 92
  atrial, 83
  diastolic, 24, 82, 87
  of LV, 87, 158
Sudden death, HCM and, 290–291
Superior vena cava velocities, 156
SV. *See* Stroke volume
S waves, 83
Swedish Evaluation of Diastolic Dysfunction Treated with Carvedilol study, 228
Sympathetic nervous system, 71
  renin-angiotensin-aldosterone system and, 76
Systole (S), 3, 4
  asynchrony of, 109
  atrial, 58
  relaxation and, 9
Systolic activation, 11
Systolic blood pressure, 72–73
  aging and, 77, 263–264
  BNP and, 179
  exercise and, 75
Systolic dysfunction, 11
  diabetes mellitus and, 272
Systolic heart failure (SHF), 9, 14, 22
  aldosterone antagonists for, 229–230
  anemia and, 71
  β-blockers for, 76
  cardiac output with, 126
  cardiovascular congestion in, 22
  definition of, 121
  vs. DHF, 119–131
  DHF with, 181–182
  diastolic dysfunction and, 123
  diastolic pressure-volume and, 26
  eccentric hypertrophy and, 123
  elastic recoil and, 123
  LV and, 121–126

Index

LVEF and, 71
nitroprusside for, 22
stroke volume with, 126
symptoms of, 129

T
Tachycardia, 4, 197
  stress-induced, 54
Task Force on Acute Heart Failure
    of the European Society of
    Cardiology, 235
TDE. *See* Echocardiography
Time velocity integral (TVI), 190
Tissue Doppler echocardiography
    (TDE). *See* Echocardiography
Titin, 7, 31, 62
  phosphorylation and, 31
TOPCAT. *See* Aldosterone
    Antagonist Therapy in Adults
    with Preserved Ejection
    Fraction Congestive Heart
    Failure
Torsion, 88, 99, 103, 168, 170
  of LV, 168
  twist, 104
  ventricular, 104
Transient constrictive pericarditis,
    320
Transmitral flow velocities, 86–91,
    194
  CHF and, 90
  Doppler echocardiography and,
    150
  IVRT, 86
  rapid early diastolic filling,
    86–87
Transmitral pressure gradient,
    192
Transmural LV end-diastolic
    pressure (TransLVEDP), 48
Transmural pressure
  diastole and, 41
  in LV, 42

pericardium and, 41–44
  stroke work and, 45
Transplantation, 233
Transseptal pressure gradient
    (TSG), 44
  chronic pulmonary hypertension
      and, 47
Tricuspid inflow velocity, 153, 168
  CMR and, 166, 167
Tricuspid regurgitation, 195, 196
Triphasic mitral inflow pattern,
    158
Troponin C, 30
Troponin I phosphorylation, 28
TSG. *See* Transseptal pressure
    gradient
Tubulin, 7, 31
Turgor, 254–257
TVI. *See* Time velocity integral

U
UK-HEART. *See* United Kingdom
    Heart Failure Evaluation and
    Assessment of Risk Trial
United Kingdom Heart Failure
    Evaluation and Assessment of
    Risk Trial (UK-HEART), 215
USCI. *See* Simplus balloon
    catheters

V
Valsalva maneuver, 157, 189, 277
Valvular heart disease, 187
  DHF and, 336
Vascular clips, 166
Vascular system, 77
Vascular turgor, 254–257
Vasoconstriction
  by angiotensin II, 71
  by ET-1, 75
  neurohormones and, 71
Vasodilator in Heart Failure Trials,
    224

Velocity Vector Imaging, 103
Venous flow velocities, 81–85
Venous system, 77
  acute pulmonary edema and, 77
Venous vasoconstriction, 21
Ventricular artery coupling, 34–36
Ventricular compliance, 5–9
Ventricular filling, LA and, 54–60
Ventricular hypertrophy, 7, 14
Ventricular interaction, 44–45
  during mechanical ventilation,
      49–50
  via pericardium, 41–50
  via septum, 41–50
Ventricular muscular pump, 3–4,
    10
Ventricular relaxation, 5–9
Ventricular remodeling, 10, 12,
    14, 71, 108, 125, 129, 181,
    294
  concentric, 130–131, 211
  eccentric, 123
  PV and, 15
Ventricular septum (VS). *See*
    Septum
Ventricular stiffness
  afterload and, 59
  in LV, 333
Verapamil, 229
Veterans Administration
    Cooperative Study, 213
V_p. *See* Propagation velocity
VS. *See* Septum

W
Washout, 250–251
Wedge pressure, 192. *See also*
    Pulmonary capillary wedge
    pressure
  HCM and, 298–299
  MF and, 197
Wiggers cycle, 23
Women, DHF and, 209